Clinical and Diagnostic Virology

'This comprehensive text will provide an excellent guide to all the many healthcare professionals, including those in training, who deal with patients who have, or may have, a virus infection. The rigorous structure to each chapter, with clear tables and concise factual exposition makes it easy to look up specific queries, or to learn about a specific infection in depth. This is a timely and very welcome addition to the canon of medical textbooks, given the increasing importance and relevance of clinical virology to general medicine.'

Will Irving, Professor and Honorary Consultant in Virology, University of Nottingham and Nottingham University Hospitals NHS Trust

'This concise guide proves invaluable for those working within clinical virology and studying for CICE/FRCPath Part 1. As it is organised by individual viruses and clinical syndromes, it serves as both a quick reference guide and an effective teaching tool. Personally, I have found the first edition of this book to be very useful throughout my career so far, so an updated second edition is most welcome!'

Dr Hayley Colton, Specialty Registrar in Medical Virology/Infectious Diseases, Sheffield Teaching Hospitals NHS Foundation Trust

Clinical and Diagnostic Virology

Second Edition

Tim Wreghitt
Addenbrooke's Hospital

Goura Kudesia
Sheffield Teaching Hospitals

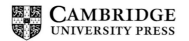
CAMBRIDGE
UNIVERSITY PRESS

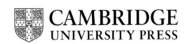

Shaftesbury Road, Cambridge CB2 8EA, United Kingdom

One Liberty Plaza, 20th Floor, New York, NY 10006, USA

477 Williamstown Road, Port Melbourne, VIC 3207, Australia

314–321, 3rd Floor, Plot 3, Splendor Forum, Jasola District Centre, New Delhi – 110025, India

103 Penang Road, #05-06/07, Visioncrest Commercial, Singapore 238467

Cambridge University Press is part of Cambridge University Press & Assessment, a department of the University of Cambridge.

We share the University's mission to contribute to society through the pursuit of education, learning and research at the highest international levels of excellence.

www.cambridge.org
Information on this title: www.cambridge.org/9781009334419

DOI: 10.1017/9781009334389

First edition © G. Kudesia and T. Wreghitt 2009
Second edition © Tim Wreghitt and Goura Kudesia 2024

First published 2009
Second edition 2024

A catalogue record for this publication is available from the British Library

A Cataloging-in-Publication data record for this book is available from the Library of Congress

ISBN 978-1-009-33441-9 Paperback

....

Contents

Section 4 – Laboratory Diagnosis

Section 5 – Patient Management

Preface

This book is a comprehensive overview of clinical and diagnostic virology for those healthcare professionals who are caring for people who have or may have viral infections. There are embedded links to relevant websites, where detailed, up-to-date advice on clinical management can be found.

The book is intended for use by infection speciality trainees as well as primary care practitioners, trainee doctors, healthcare scientists, infection control nurses and other healthcare professionals (doctors, nurses and healthcare staff) working in non-infection specialities who deal with patients with suspected virus infections.

The aim of the book is for it to be a quick reference guide to differential diagnosis, giving information on which specimens and tests are best for laboratory diagnosis and how to interpret results, which treatments to use and what the implications are for control of infection.

The book has easily accessible information, with tables, figures and algorithms to aid easy reference for the busy clinician. After a chapter on basic virology, the book is divided into four main sections:

- An alphabetically arranged series of chapters on individual viruses. We have used a standard chapter format throughout, to enable the reader to access important information (e.g. epidemiology, route of spread, prevalence, clinical presentation, laboratory diagnosis and interpretation of results and treatment) quickly and easily.
- A set of clinical syndromes (e.g. hepatitis and skin rashes) where different viruses and their clinical syndromes are presented.
- A laboratory diagnosis section.
- A patient management section, giving information on the use of antiviral drugs, viral vaccines, occupational health, and public health and pandemic preparedness.

We are aware that most virologists in the UK deal with some non-viral pathogens (e.g. chlamydia, toxoplasma, atypical pneumonia organisms), so chapters on these pathogens are also included.

In revising this book for the second edition, we have updated all the chapters in the previous edition and added chapters on SARS-CoV-2, viral zoonotic infections, quality control and laboratory accreditation, and public health and pandemic preparedness.

We hope you enjoy reading this book and find it a useful source of information. We hope it will help you manage patients and resources better or learn more about viruses and their impact on human health.

Acknowledgements

Figures 7.2, 7.3 and 11.1 were prepared by Philip M. Ball MA FMAA.

We acknowledge the help and advice of Dr Jim Gray, Mr Gordon Sutehall, Dr Anna Smielewska and Dr Martin Curran in reviewing chapters.

We are grateful to Centers for Disease Control and Prevention, the UK Health Security Agency and Sheffield Virology Laboratory for allowing us to reproduce the images in the book.

Abbreviations

AIDS	acquired immunodeficiency syndrome
ALT	alanine transaminase
ART	antiretroviral therapy
ATL	adult T-cell leukaemia/lymphoma
BAL	bronchoalveolar lavage
BASL	British Association for Study of Liver Disease
BBV	blood-borne virus
BHIVA	British HIV Association
BMT	bone marrow transplant
CDC	Centers for Disease Control and Prevention
CJD	Creutzfeldt-Jakob disease
CMV	cytomegalovirus
CNS	central nervous system
CSF	cerebrospinal fluid
DAA	direct-acting antiviral
DNA	deoxyribonucleic acid
DS	double stranded
EASL	European Association for Study of Liver Disease
EBV	Epstein–Barr virus
EDTA	ethylenediaminetetraacetic acid
EI	erythema infectiosum
EIA	enzyme immunoassay
ELISA	enzyme-linked immunosorbent assay
EM	electron microscopy
FVU	first-void urine
HIV	human immunodeficiency virus
HAV	hepatitis A virus
HBV	hepatitis B virus
HCV	hepatitis C virus
HCW	healthcare worker
HDV	hepatitis D virus
HEV	hepatitis E virus
HHV	human herpes virus
hMPV	human metapneumovirus
HNIG	human immunoglobulin
HPV	human papillomavirus
HSV	herpes simplex virus
HTLV	human T-cell lymphotropic virus
ICU	intensive care unit
IF or IFT	immunofluorescence test
I/V	intravenous
LRTI	lower respiratory tract infection
MERS	Middle East respiratory syndrome
MMR	measles, mumps and rubella
mRNA	messenger RNA
MSM	men who have sex with men
NAAT	nucleic acid amplification techniques/test
NHS	National Health Service
NK	natural killer
PCR	polymerase chain reaction
PEP	post-exposure prophylaxis

PIV	parainfluenza virus
POC	point of care
POCT	point of care testing
PrEP	pre-exposure prophylaxis
PTLD	post-transplant lymphoproliferative disease
PWIDs	persons who inject drugs
RNA	ribonucleic acid
RSV	respiratory syncytial virus
RT-PCR	reverse transcription polymerase chain reaction
SARS	severe acute respiratory syndrome
SARS-CoV-2	SARS coronavirus 2
SIV	simian immunodeficiency virus
SS	single stranded
STI	sexually transmitted infection
STLV	simian T-lymphotropic virus
TBE	tick-borne encephalitis
TCR	T-cell receptor
TSE	transmissible spongiform encephalopathy
UKHSA	UK Health Security Agency
VCA	viral capsid antigen
vCJD	variant Creutzfeldt-Jakob disease
VLP	virus-like particle
VZIG	varicella-zoster immune globulin
VZV	varicella-zoster virus
WHO	World Health Organization
YFV	yellow fever virus
ZV	Zika virus

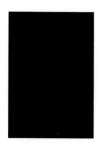

Introduction
Basic Virology

History of Viruses

The existence of viruses was first suspected in the nineteenth century when it was shown that filtered extract of infective material, when passed through filters small enough to stop all known bacteria, could still be infectious, and hence the word 'virus' (Latin for poisonous liquid) was first introduced. However, viral diseases such as smallpox and poliomyelitis had been known to affect mankind for many centuries before that.

Subsequent to the discovery of the existence of viruses, the next major step in elucidating their role in human disease was the invention of electron microscopy, followed by cell culture and now molecular techniques to detect the presence of viruses in infected material. Many new viruses have been discovered in the past two to three decades, but it was the discovery of human immunodeficiency virus (HIV) in 1983, the etiological agent of the AIDS epidemic, that brought clinical virology to the forefront as a significant speciality. There was a concerted effort by the scientific community to identify the causative agent of AIDS and then by the pharmaceutical industry for drug development. This was followed a few years later by the discovery of hepatitis C and hepatitis E viruses. Since then, molecular technology (e.g. cloning and sequencing) has been applied to rapidly identify new viral threats, such as severe acute respiratory syndrome (SARS), Middle East respiratory syndrome (MERS) and SARS coronavirus 2 (SARS-CoV-2).

The availability of rapid and sensitive molecular diagnostic techniques and effective antiviral drug therapy means that patients can now be treated in real time. Almost all physicians and healthcare workers have to deal with the consequences of viral infections. The aim of this book is to demystify virology, provide sufficient information to enable the reader to deal with day-to day virus-related problems and achieve the most rapid diagnosis and beneficial treatment.

To do this we must first understand some basic principles of virology.

Viral Taxonomy

Unlike all other organisms, viruses have either DNA or RNA genomes (never both). Viruses are classified in *families* on the basis of their genome (RNA or DNA) and whether it is single or double stranded (SS or DS). SS RNA viruses are further split on the basis of whether they carry a negative (−RNA) or a positive (+RNA) strand as this affects their replication strategy. As a rule of thumb *all DNA viruses except those belonging to Parvoviridae are DS and all RNA viruses except those belonging to Reoviridae are SS.*

Other features of viruses to take into account are their size and shape, and the presence or absence of a lipid envelope, which some viruses acquire as they bud out of cells. RNA viruses generally tend to be enveloped and have outer proteins (required for attachment to the cell surface) projecting out of this lipid envelope.

The viral genome is packaged within a nucleoprotein (capsid), which consists of a repetition of structurally similar amino acid subunits. The viral genome and the capsid are together referred to as the nucleocapsid. The viral nucleoprotein or capsid gives the virus its shape (helical or icosahedral).

Virus Replication

Viruses are obligate intracellular pathogens and require cellular enzymes to help them to replicate. Unlike bacteria, which replicate by binary fission, viruses have to 'disassemble' their structure before they can replicate. The steps of viral replication can be broadly divided into:

- attachment
- cell entry
- virus disassembly or uncoating
- transcription and translation of viral genome
- viral assembly and release.

The structure of the viral genome dictates the steps in its replication cycle.

Attachment

The first step in the replication cycle is the attachment of the virus particle to the cell surface. To do this, different viruses use specific cellular receptors on the cell surface, which are therefore very specific in the cell type that they can infect – this gives them their 'cell tropism' and is important in disease pathogenesis (i.e. why some viruses only affect certain organs). Influenza viruses use the haemagglutinin protein to attach to the sialic acid–containing oligosaccharides on the cell surface. Viruses may use more than one cell receptor, for example HIV uses the CD4 receptor to attach to the CD4-T-helper cells, but it also uses a chemokine receptor CCR5 as a co-receptor. It is now believed that most viruses use more than one receptor on the cell surface in a sequential binding process.

Cell Entry

Viruses may enter the cell directly by endocytosis or, for enveloped viruses, by fusion of their lipid envelope with the cell membrane.

Virus Disassembly or Uncoating

Before the virus can replicate, the viral genome has to be exposed by removal of the associated viral proteins. This is usually mediated by the endocytosed viral particle merging with cellular lysosomes; the resulting drop in pH dissociates the viral genome from its binding protein.

Transcription and Translation of the Viral Genome

How the virus replicates is dictated by the structure of its viral genome.

- Viruses containing SS +RNA use their +RNA as messenger RNA (mRNA) and utilize the cell's ribosomes and enzymes to translate the information contained in this

+RNA to produce viral proteins. One of the first proteins to be produced is RNA-dependent RNA polymerase, which then transcribes viral RNA into further RNA genomes. These viruses, because they can subvert the cellular system for their own replication, do not need to carry the information for the initial replication enzymes within their genome.

- Viruses containing SS −RNA need to convert it first to +RNA strand, which is then used as an mRNA template for translation or direct transcription to the genomic −RNA. They therefore need to carry a viral-specific RNA-dependent RNA polymerase.
- DS RNA viruses have to first convert the −RNA strand of the DS RNA into a complementary +RNA to be used as mRNA. The +RNA strand of the DS RNA acts as a template for viral genome replication. These viruses also need to carry the RNA-dependent RNA polymerase to initiate the first steps of viral replication.
- Retroviruses are unique SS +RNA viruses. Instead of using the SS +RNA as an mRNA template, the RNA is first transcribed into complementary DNA by an RNA-dependent DNA polymerase in a process called reverse transcription (hence the name – retro = reverse). The normal transcription is always from DNA to RNA. Further transcription then occurs as for other SS DNA viruses.
- DNA virus mRNA is transcribed from the DS DNA viruses in a similar fashion to cellular DNA replication. These viruses can therefore completely depend upon cellular processes to replicate. The genome of these viruses (e.g. cytomegalovirus (CMV), Epstein–Barr virus (EBV)) needs to carry information to code for the virus-specific proteins only. Regulatory proteins and those required for viral DNA synthesis are coded early on and the later proteins are generally structural proteins.
- SS DNA viruses are first converted into double stranded, and then mRNA is transcribed as for DS DNA viruses.

Viral Assembly and Release

Before the virus particle can be released, its proteins and genome have to be assembled within the cell as a 'viral package'. This process may require the cell to alter viral proteins by glycosylation, etc. Viral release may occur either through cell death or through viral budding from cell membrane. Enveloped viruses use the latter mechanism and acquire their lipid envelope at this stage. Viral enzymes may be required for the viruses released via budding (e.g. the neuraminidase of influenza viruses acts on the sialic-acid bond on the cell surface to release the infectious virus particle).

Immune Response to Viruses

Immune response can be divided into two types of responses:

- Innate immunity: innate immune response is the first immediate response to an insult/injury including viral infections. It can be defined as a system of rapid immune responses that are present from birth and not specific to a particular microorganism.
- Adaptive immunity: immunity that develops when the immune system responds to a foreign substance or microorganism for the first time. Unlike the innate immune response, which is immediate, the adaptive immune response may take days or weeks to develop. It is specific for the microorganism and results in immune memory so the

host is able to prevent disease in the future by mounting a quick immune response when exposed to the same pathogen. Adaptive immunity lasts for a long time or may be lifelong.

Innate and adaptive immunity are not mutually exclusive but are complementary defence mechanisms, with defects in either system affecting the host mechanism.

Innate Immune Response

These host defence mechanisms are evolutionarily found in all multicellular organisms, and expressed in humans as conserved elements. There is a vast array of physical, cellular and chemical defence involved in this response. The first line of defence is physical barriers like skin, mucous membrane and mucus, and cilia, which may trap microorganisms. The cellular component is comprised of phagocytic cells (e.g. neutrophils, monocytes and macrophages), which engulf the microorganism and destroy it. In addition, natural killer (NK) cells, a type of T-cell, plays a role in both innate and adaptive immunity. They play a major role in the destruction of cells infected by viruses. Infected cells are destroyed by the release of perforins and granzymes (proteins that cause lysis of target cells) from NK cells, which induce apoptosis (programmed cell death). Chemical defence involves chemokines, cytokines and interferon, which are secreted by the cells of the innate immune system and help regulate the immune response as they do for adaptive immunity.

Adaptive Immunity

The adaptive immune response is aided by the actions of the innate immune response. The adaptive immune response acts by recognition of specific 'non-self' antigens. It is composed of a cell-mediated response effected through T-cells, and antibody-mediated response, mediated through B-cells, which differentiate into plasma cells to produce antibodies.

Cell-mediated response: T-cells are derived from hematopoietic stem cells in bone marrow. T-cells are activated when they encounter a foreign antigen, which is recognised by the unique antigen-binding receptors on their membrane, known as the T-cell receptor (TCR). This process requires the antigen presenting cells (APCs; usually dendritic cells, but also macrophages, B-cells, fibroblasts and epithelial cells). APCs express proteins called major histocompatibility complex (MHC) on their surface, which are classified into MHC class I (present on the surface of almost all nucleated cells) and class II (found on the cell surface of cells of the immune system). The foreign antigen complexed with the appropriate MHC on the APCs is presented to the TCR for activation of T-cells. This stimulates the T-cells to differentiate, primarily into either cytotoxic T-cells (CD8+ cells) or T-helper (Th) cells (CD4+ cells). CD8+ cytotoxic T-cells are primarily involved in the destruction of viral-infected cells. Clonal expansion of cytotoxic T-cells produces effector cells which release substances that induce apoptosis of target cells. Most effector cells die after clearance of infection, but a few of these cells remain as memory cells.

CD4+ Th cells have no cytotoxic or phagocytic activity but they 'mediate' the immune response by directing other cells to perform these tasks and regulate the type of immune response that develops by releasing cytokines that influence the activity of many cell types, including the APCs that activate them.

Antibody-mediated response: This is effected via B-cells which also arise from the hematopoietic stem cells in the bone marrow. Like T-cells, they also carry unique antigen-binding receptors on their cell surface, but unlike T-cells, which require APCs, the B-cell antigen binding receptor can directly bind to foreign antigens that it recognises. Once activated, the B-cells undergo proliferation and differentiate into antibody-secreting plasma cells or memory B-cells which are long lived and can be called upon to eliminate an antigen quickly on re-exposure, by producing the appropriate antibodies. Five major types of antibodies are produced: IgA, IgD, IgE, IgG and IgM. These antibody classes can be further subdivided according to their functionality (e.g. to fix complement, opsonisation (coating of antigen) for destruction, neutralisation of viruses, etc.).

Both the cell-mediated and antibody-mediated responses are interdependent on each other and act in unison to clear infections. T-helper cells secrete cytokines that help the B-cell multiply and direct the type of antibody that will be produced subsequently. Some cytokines, such as IL-6, help B-cells to mature into antibody-secreting plasma cells. The secreted antibodies bind to antigens, flagging them for destruction through complement activation or promotion of phagocytosis by the cells of the immune system, etc.

Viral Pathogenesis

Viral pathogenesis can be described as the process by which the virus interacts with its host to produce disease. As this is a process which involves virus–host interaction, both viral and host factors have a bearing on the pathogenesis of viral disease.

Viral Tropism

The disease manifestation depends upon the organs infected, which in turn depends upon viral tropism. The ability of viruses to infect only certain cell types due to the presence of specific viral receptors on the cell surface has already been discussed. Other factors that affect this tropism are the route of viral entry (e.g. viruses that infect through the respiratory or genital route generally tend to be limited to infections of those systems).

Viral Spread

The mechanism of viral spread is important in pathogenesis. Up to a million potentially infectious particles can be produced as a result of sneezing. The smaller the particle size the more likely it is to escape the mechanical trapping barriers within the respiratory system. The lipid envelope of the enveloped viruses can be easily stripped by detergents or 70% alcohol; such viruses can be easily destroyed in the environment. Only those viruses that can resist the acidity of the stomach can cause gastrointestinal infections. Enteric viruses that spread by the faecal-oral route need to be acid resistant to escape destruction by gastric juices, which may have a pH as low as 2.

Many viruses cause only localised infection as they are unable to spread. Viruses that spread further afield from the infecting site may use virus-encoded proteins to direct their transport within the cell in a way that enhances their spread via blood or along nerves (e.g. polio and rabies viruses). Other viruses, such as CMV, EBV and HIV, are carried by infected blood cells to distant parts.

Measles virus, varicella-zoster virus (chickenpox) and rubella virus all spread via the respiratory route but cause systemic infections. These viruses have a transient 'primary viraemia' just after infection to lodge in the reticuloendothelial system. The virus replicates there for a period of time (incubation period) without causing disease symptoms. This is followed by a second longer phase of viraemia (secondary viraemia) when the infection is spread to the target organs to manifest the disease symptoms.

Viral Persistence

Many viruses cause persistent infection, which can be latent, as in herpes virus infection, or chronic, as in hepatitis B virus infection. Many persistent/chronic viral infections can induce malignancies and this is discussed further in Chapter 46.

In latency, the virus lies dormant. The mechanisms of latency are not understood very well, but the virus reactivates from time to time to cause localised infection, as in the case of herpes simplex virus causing cold sores, or may spread along the nerves, as in the case of varicella-zoster virus (shingles). In chronic infection the virus replicates and continues to cause damage. Viruses are able to persist to cause chronic infection: (1) by escaping the immune system by constantly mutating, e.g. HIV; (2) by downregulating the host immune system, e.g. CMV, which codes for proteins that reduce the expression of major MHC class 1 receptors on the cell surface; and (3) by integrating in the viral genome and replicating with the cells, e.g. HIV and hepatitis B virus.

Viral Virulence Factors

Viral virulence is defined as the amount of virus required to produce disease or death in 50% of a cohort of experimentally infected animals. This virulence depends on virus and host factors. Viral virulence determinants are often viral surface proteins. Viruses can also induce apoptosis (genetically programmed cell death) or block apoptosis, depending upon the best strategy for its continued replication and spread.

Host Factors

Disease manifestations may be the direct result of infection or may be immune-mediated as a result of the host immune response to infection. The aplastic anaemia in parvovirus B19 infection is due to destruction of the red blood cells by the virus, whereas the rash is immune-mediated. Hepatocellular damage in hepatitis B infection is a result of destruction of infected hepatocytes by the cytotoxic T-cells. In influenza and Covid-19, most of the symptoms are mediated by the interferon and interleukin pathways as a result of the host response to the virus. Human immunodeficiency virus induces immunodeficiency by destroying the helper T-cells (CD4 cells) of the cell-mediated immune system.

Conclusion

The study of viruses is providing insight into many cellular mechanisms. Understanding of the steps in the viral replication cycle has enabled many 'designer' antiviral drugs (such as the influenza A virus neuraminidase inhibitor drug, oseltamivir) to be manufactured. It is hoped that this brief introduction to basic virology will enable the reader to understand some of the underlying mechanisms that are relevant to the subsequent chapters in this book, and help the reader to make the most of the information contained within.

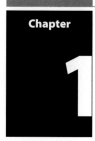

Adenoviruses

The Viruses

Adenoviruses are double-stranded DNA viruses and belong to the family Adenoviridae.

Epidemiology

Route of Spread

There are more than 50 different serotypes (each designated by a number) of adenoviruses and several disease syndromes associated with different serotypes. Respiratory adenoviruses are spread by the respiratory route. Enteric adenoviruses (adenovirus 40 and 41) are spread via the faecal-oral route, and adenoviruses causing conjunctivitis are very infectious and spread by direct contamination of the eye. Adenovirus infections in humans are generally caused by adenoviruses types B, C, E and F.

Prevalence

Adenovirus infections affect all ages. Respiratory adenovirus infections occur every year in the community, causing outbreaks in persons of all ages, often in children in schools and other institutions throughout the year. Severe disease is rare in people who are otherwise healthy. Adenovirus infection accounts for up to 10% of respiratory infections in children. Most cases are mild.

Enteric adenoviruses are a cause of sporadic diarrhoea and vomiting, mainly in young children, throughout the year. Although they cause small outbreaks, usually in community settings, they are not associated significantly with large outbreaks of diarrhoea and vomiting in hospitals and cruise ships.

Adenoviruses associated with conjunctivitis occur sporadically, often associated with clusters of cases. They happen throughout the year, and outbreaks can occur particularly in winter and spring, when they may spread more quickly in closed populations such as in hospitals, nurseries, long-term care facilities, schools and swimming pools.

A total of 75% of viral conjunctivitis cases are due to adenovirus infection.

Incubation Period

2–14 days.

Infectious Period

Patients are infectious while they are symptomatic. Spread occurs mainly when an infected person is in close contact with another person. This may occur by the faecal-oral route, airborne transmission or small droplets containing the virus. Less commonly, the virus may spread via contaminated surfaces.

At-Risk Groups

Immunocompromised persons, who often have prolonged carriage of the virus, especially in enteric infections.

Clinical

Symptoms

- Respiratory adenoviruses cause a range of respiratory symptoms from mild coryza to pneumonia. Clinical symptoms include fever, cough and sore throat due to pharyngitis and tonsillitis. Some infections are asymptomatic. It is difficult to differentiate adenovirus infection from other respiratory virus infections symptomatically, although adenoviruses, unlike influenza viruses, do not usually produce myalgia. Some adenoviruses can also cause a maculopapular rash. Rarely, death occurs due to disseminated adenovirus infection.
- Enteric adenoviruses cause diarrhoea, vomiting and fever, particularly in children less than 2 years of age. The diarrhoea lasts for an average of 8 days (range 3–11 days), longer than diarrhoea caused by rotaviruses.
- Ocular adenoviruses cause conjunctivitis with red, sore injected conjunctiva. It is a very infectious condition and scrupulous infection control procedures are necessary to prevent spread, particularly by the direct contact route. Large outbreaks have been reported. One famous outbreak called 'shipyard eye' occurred in a shipyard in the north of England, when metal workers were treated for metal slivers in their eyes. Contaminated eye instruments were blamed for transmitting the virus.
- In the spring of 2022, the UK Health Security Agency identified a growing cluster of acute hepatitis cases in children under the age of 10 years with no association with travel and hepatitis viruses A–E. Of the children, 66% had adenoviruses (adenovirus 41) detected, and a case control study confirmed this association. Some children had severe infection, necessitating liver transplantation. Adenovirus-associated viruses were also found in the majority of cases. Several different factors are thought to be associated with this outbreak, which was not a point source outbreak, with several adenovirus 41 lineages detected.

Immunocompromised Patients

Organ transplant recipients, especially children, infected with respiratory adenoviruses can have measles-like symptoms (e.g. measles-like rash and conjunctivitis but no Koplik's spots). Bone marrow transplant recipients can experience severe or fatal infection. Enteric adenoviruses can cause prolonged symptoms and viral excretion in transplant recipients, especially children. Many paediatric centres therefore follow their high-risk bone marrow transplant recipients with regular laboratory screens for adenovirus infection.

Table 1.1 Laboratory diagnosis of adenoviruses

Clinical indication	Specimens	Test	Interpretation of positive result
Respiratory symptoms	Nose and throat swab in virus transport medium. Bronchoalveolar lavage fluid. Nasopharyngeal aspirate.	NAAT	Indicates adenovirus infection. Type-specific primers can be used to distinguish between different types of adenoviruses.
Conjunctivitis	Conjunctival swab in virus transport medium.	NAAT	Indicates adenovirus infection. Type-specific primers can be used to distinguish between different types of adenoviruses.
Diarrhoea and vomiting	Faeces.	NAAT	Indicates adenovirus infection. Type-specific primers can be used to distinguish between different types of adenoviruses.
		Rapid test devices	Indicates adenovirus infection.

Adenoviruses may cause myocarditis, meningoencephalitis or hepatitis in immunocompromised people.

Laboratory Diagnosis

Several laboratory methods and clinical specimens can be used to diagnose adenovirus infection (Table 1.1). Nucleic acid amplification techniques (NAAT), like polymerase chain reaction (PCR), are the method of choice (although virus culture, immunofluorescence and electron microscopy can be used if available).

Figure 1.1 shows an electron micrograph of a group of adenoviruses.

Management

Treatment

Aerosolised ribavirin can be given to children with bronchiolitis and intravenous ribavirin can be given (under expert advice) to immunocompromised children. Bone marrow transplant recipients can experience severe and fatal infections and can be treated with cidofivir (see Chapter 54).

Prophylaxis

There is no prophylaxis available. Currently, there is no adenovirus vaccine available to the general public, but a vaccine is available for the United States military for Types 4 and 7. US military personnel are the recipients of this vaccine because they may be at a higher risk of infection because of closer prolonged contact.

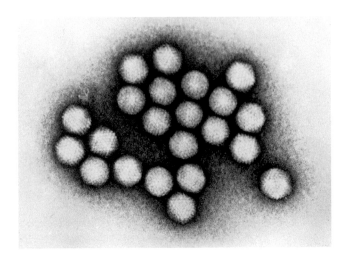

Figure 1.1 A group of negatively stained adenoviruses (courtesy of CDC)

Infection Control

All adenovirus infections are infectious and patients should be isolated whenever possible, especially when in the same ward as immunocompromised patients.

Chapter

2 Arboviruses

The Viruses

There are >500 recognised arbovirus species that cause infections in humans, animals and birds. They are divided into six main families:

- Flaviviridae
- Togaviridae
- Bunyaviridae
- Rhabdoviridae
- Reoviridae
- Orthomyxoviridae.

The majority of mosquito-borne viruses affecting humans are found in the first three families of viruses, and some of the important ones are described in this chapter. Table 2.1 details important arboviruses associated with human illness.

Epidemiology

Arboviruses are infections that are transmitted to humans by arthropod vectors (mosquitoes, ticks or biting flies). Some of these (e.g. dengue fever) can produce haemorrhagic symptoms. There are several different viruses with different geographical distributions, animal vectors and associated symptoms.

Prevalence

The origin of most, if not all, of the arboviral infections can be traced back to the African subcontinent, and they are most prevalent there and in the tropics, but the distribution is worldwide including the Americas, Australasia and Asia.

Details of some of the more important ones that cause human infections are shown next.

Family Flaviviridae (Genus *Flavivirus*)

Several important human pathogens belong to the genus *Flavivirus*.

• Dengue Fever Virus

Dengue fever virus (DENV) is the most common arbovirus infection in the UK, with infection being acquired abroad in tropical and subtropical regions of the world where malaria is also prevalent. These include South East Asia, Central and South America, the

Table 2.1 Important arboviruses associated with human illness

Virus		Endemic countries	Host	Illness	Arthropod vector	Diagnosis/management
Family Flavividae (genus *Favivirus*)	Dengue virus 1–4	Worldwide in tropics	Humans	Fever, headache, muscle/joint pain, petechial rash and haemorrhagic fever	Mosquitoes – *Aedes aegypti* and *Aedes albopictus*	Blood for PCR and specific IgM. Supportive treatment.
	West Nile virus	Africa, Asia, Europe, Americas	Humans/ birds	Fever, encephalitis	Mosquito – *Culex*	Blood and CSF for PCR. Supportive treatment.
	Japanese encephalitis	Asia, Pacific Islands	Humans/ wading birds/pigs	Fever, meningoencephalitis	Mosquito – *Culex*	Blood and CSF for PCR. Supportive treatment. Prevention is the mainstay. Effective vaccine is available and vaccination of at-risk population and travellers to endemic areas is recommended.
	Tick-borne encephalitis	Endemic in many countries in Europe and Asia.	Humans/ rodents/ domestic animals	Fever, headache, encephalitis	The virus is transmitted by ixodid ticks.	PCR on blood and CSF. Effective vaccine is available for prevention.
	Zika virus	Africa, Asia, Americas	Humans	Fever, headache, rash, Guillain–Barré syndrome. congenital Zika syndrome – microcephaly, hearing loss, etc.	Mosquito – *Aedes aegypti*. Also sexual and vertical transmission in humans.	PCR on blood. Public health message for avoidance of sexual and vertical transmission. Supportive treatment.

Family Togaviridae (genus *Alphavirus*)	Chikingunya	Africa, Asia	Humans/primates	Fever, arthralgia, rarely encephalitis	Mosquito – *Aedes*	PCR blood, specific IgM. Supportive treatment.
	Eastern equine virus	Americas	Humans/equine/birds	Fever, encephalitis	Mosquito – *Culex*	PCR on blood and CSF. Supportive treatment.
	Western equine virus	Americas	Humans/equine/birds	Fever, encephalitis	Mosquito – *Culex*	PCR blood and CSF. Supportive treatment.
Family Bunyaviridae (genus *Phlebovirus*)	Rift Valley fever	Africa and the Arabian peninsula	Humans/cattle/sheep	Haemorrhagic fever, hepatitis, encephalitis	Mosquito – *Culex* and *Aedes*. Contact with blood and organs of infected animals.	PCR on blood. Supportive treatment.

Caribbean and the Northern Territory of Australia. DENV is transmitted to humans by *Aedes aegypti* and *Aedes albopictus* mosquitoes. There are four different serotypes of dengue fever virus (DENV1–4) which are not cross-protective, so inhabitants of areas of the world where these viruses are endemic may experience infection with more than one serotype in their lifetime. The incubation period is 2–5 days. Symptoms usually begin with the sudden onset of fever, headache, muscle and joint pain and bright red petechial rash, which usually presents first on the chest and lower limbs but may become widespread over the body. The bone and muscle pain can be very severe, which is why the disease is known as 'break bone fever'. Milder forms of the disease may be confused with other diseases such as influenza or malaria. The mortality rate is low (unless the haemorrhagic form develops). Symptoms usually last for 5–7 days. Severe cases can develop into dengue haemorrhagic fever (DHF; see Chapter 38 on haemorrhagic fevers). It is estimated that 50–100 million cases of DENV infection and 250,000–500,000 cases of DHF occur every year worldwide. Large outbreaks of dengue occur every 5–6 years, but the disease is endemic in many countries with outbreaks every year. Recently, small outbreaks have occurred in Europe (e.g. Majorca).

There is no antiviral treatment; good supportive care is required. Infection cannot be transmitted from one human to another unless via a mosquito vector. It can be transmitted via blood donation.

• Yellow Fever

Yellow fever is a disease of the tropical regions of sub-Saharan Africa and South America and has caused several outbreaks there in the last decade. Yellow fever virus (YFV) is a flavivirus transmitted by *Aedes* mosquitoes. It has three types of transmission cycles:

- sylvatic or jungle – in which monkeys are the primary reservoir of infection
- mixed – in which mosquitoes transmit to both monkeys and humans
- urban – in which large outbreaks occur once the virus is introduced into areas with dense human and mosquito population leading to human-to-human transmission via mosquito bites.

Yellow fever has an incubation period of 3–6 days. Symptoms of the acute illness range from asymptomatic to non-specific symptoms such as fever, myalgia, malaise, headache, and nausea and vomiting. A small number of patients develop high fever and jaundice (hence the name yellow fever) in a second phase after a short asymptomatic period. Bleeding can occur from several sites with death occurring within 7–10 days of development of the severe illness. Mortality rates can be up to 30%. Treatment is supportive. There is an effective vaccine available, a single dose of which provides lifelong immunity; travellers to countries where the disease is endemic are strongly advised to be vaccinated. There is also concentrated effort for mass vaccination of populations in the endemic countries to break the cycle of transmission and to avoid future outbreaks by achieving high vaccination rates.

• West Nile Fever

West Nile fever is caused by a flavivirus which is transmitted to humans by mosquitoes. The infection has an incubation period of 1–6 days. West Nile fever has a wide geographical distribution: outbreaks occur in Africa, the Middle East, Asia, the USA and Europe. The virus emerged in the USA in New York in 1999, and outbreaks now occur throughout North America each year. The mosquitoes become infected when they bite birds; horses can be infected as incidental hosts too, like humans. Most infected people have no symptoms or mild illness with fever, headache and myalgia lasting 3–6 days. A maculopapular rash appears in about 50% of symptomatic patients. In a few people, especially the elderly, West Nile fever causes severe symptoms; it can cause permanent neurological damage. Severe headache, high fever and a stiff neck can herald the onset of encephalitis and coma. The death rate in hospitalised patients is 3–15%, but overall it is less than 1%. There is no specific treatment.

• Japanese Encephalitis Virus

Several countries in the South-East Asia and Western Pacific regions have endemic Japanese encephalitis virus (JEV) transmission with an estimated 60,000–70,000 clinical cases each year with approximately 15,000–20,000 deaths.

Transmission is via bites from infected *Culex* mosquitoes. The virus exists in an enzootic transmission cycle between mosquitoes and pigs/waterbirds. The disease occurs predominantly in rural areas, and large epidemics can occur especially during the rainy season.

Most JEV infections are mild with fever and headache, but 1 in 250 infections can result in severe disease which is characterised by rapid onset of high fever, headache, neck stiffness, coma, seizures and death with a fatality rate as high as 30%. Of the survivors, 20–30% may have neurological sequelae. JEV primarily affects children and is the most common cause of encephalitis in Asia.

There is no effective treatment, but effective vaccines are available for prevention, and the World Health Organization (WHO) recommends JE vaccination for control in endemic areas and also for travellers to those areas.

• Tick-Borne Encephalitis Virus

The tick-borne encephalitis virus includes three subtypes: European, Far Eastern and Siberian. The vector of transmission is *Ixodes* ticks, and tick-borne encephalitis (TBE) has become a challenge in Europe, including the UK, where recently indigenous cases have been found, with case numbers increasing dramatically over the last 30 years.

The majority of cases are asymptomatic, with clinical cases having a biphasic illness. The first phase lasts for 2–10 days and is associated with non-specific symptoms. This is followed by an asymptomatic phase lasting a few days to weeks, with subsequent presentation with meningoencephalitis or myelitis.

The European subtype is milder with 20–30% experiencing a second phase with a mortality rate of 0.5–2%. The Far Eastern subtype is associated with more severe monophasic illness with a mortality rate of up to 35%. The Siberian subtype is again associated with less severe disease.

There is an effective vaccine against TBE, and it is recommended for use in endemic areas and for travellers to those areas.

• Zika Virus

Zika virus (ZV) was first identified in Uganda in 1947, and subsequently sporadic human infections and outbreaks have been detected in Africa, Asia and the Americas. Most ZV infections are asymptomatic, but symptoms can include rash, fever, conjunctivitis, muscle/joint pain and headache and usually last for 2–7 days. Guillain–Barré syndrome, myelitis and neuropathy may occur as complications of infection.

During a large outbreak of ZV infection in 2015 in Brazil, an association was first made with vertical transmission of ZV infection from infected mothers to babies leading to congenital Zika syndrome. Birth defects include microcephaly, with other defects such as limb contracture, high muscle tone, eye abnormalities and hearing loss being also described. Infection during pregnancy may also cause fetal loss, still and pre-term birth. It is estimated that the risk of fetal infection varies between 5% and 15%.

Transmission is via mosquito vector *Aedes aegypti*, but sexual transmission from symptomatic or asymptomatic men to women and also from men to men and from women to men has been shown. Sexual transmission can occur before symptom onset, during acute illness and even after resolution of symptoms. ZV has been detected in semen (where it is known to survive for a long time), vaginal secretions, blood and saliva.

To avoid complications of ZV infection in pregnancy, the WHO recommends protected sex for 3 months for men and 2 months for women after infection or after return from an endemic area. In endemic areas sexually active men and women should be counselled regarding risk of infection in pregnancy, and pregnant women should refrain from unprotected sex.

Family Togaviridae (Genus *Alphavirus*)

• Chikungunya

Chikungunya virus is an alphavirus which is transmitted to humans by *Aedes aegypti* mosquitoes. The incubation period is 2–10 days. Symptoms usually start with a sudden onset of malaise, fever and joint pains. Myalgia and joint pains can be very severe. A maculopapular rash may appear with the onset of symptoms or several days later. Large outbreaks occur in Asia and sub-Saharan Africa, but there have been outbreaks in islands in the Indian Ocean and, more recently, in Italy. The fatality rate is low. In Africa, the virus also infects monkeys.

• Eastern Equine Encephalitis

Eastern equine encephalitis (EEE) is an alphavirus which is transmitted to humans by mosquitoes. Severe and sometimes lethal infection occurs in humans, horses and pheasants. After an incubation period of 3–10 days, the most severe cases have a dramatic onset of neurological symptoms, leading to coma and death in 30% of cases. Other symptoms include fever, myalgia, headache, photophobia and vomiting. Outbreaks occur, usually in the summer, from Ontario and Quebec to Wisconsin, Texas and the Caribbean. It also causes outbreaks in South America as far south as Argentina.

• Western Equine Encephalitis

Western equine encephalitis (WEE) is caused by an alphavirus which is transmitted by several mosquito species. Outbreaks occur in western USA, Canada, Mexico, Guyana, Brazil, Argentina and Venezuela. The incubation period is 2–10 days, and symptoms usually begin with a sudden onset of headache, dizziness, fever, chills, myalgia and malaise. The continuing headache, dizziness and drowsiness often prompt medical intervention. The overall mortality rate is 4%. The infection also occurs in birds and horses.

• Other Alphaviruses

Some other alphaviruses of note causing human infections are the O'nyong-nyong virus (Africa), Semliki Forest virus (Africa), Sindbis virus (Europe, Africa, Asia, Australia), Ross River virus (Australia, Pacific Islands) and Venezuelan equine encephalitis (this belongs to the same group of viruses as the EEE and WEE viruses). Mosquito vectors involved are *Aedes/Culex/Anopheles* depending on local epidemiology.

Family Bunyaviridae (Genus *Phlebovirus*)

• Rift Valley Fever Virus

Rift Valley fever virus (RVFV) was first described from the Rift Valley of Kenya, but several outbreaks have been reported from sub-Saharan and North Africa with cases also being reported from Saudi Arabia and Yemen. It primarily affects animals but can affect humans. It is transmitted by mosquitoes and by blood-feeding flies, but most human infections occur as a result of contact with blood and/or the organs of infected animals.

The disease ranges from mild flu-like illness to haemorrhagic fever in a small percentage.

Diagnosis

Since most of the arboviral infections present with non-specific symptoms, especially in the early stages, clinical diagnosis is difficult and depends on a good epidemiological and travel history. Specific diagnosis should be attempted, and the specimens of choice are EDTA blood for specific viral PCR and clotted blood for specific IgM antibody detection. All diagnostic tests should be done in category 4, high-security facilities.

Useful Websites

For more detailed and up-to-date information visit:

www.who.int/ith/en
www.ukhsa.gov.uk
www.cdc.gov/travel
www.traveldoctor.co.uk

Cytomegalovirus

The Virus

Cytomegalovirus (CMV) is a double-stranded DNA virus and member of the Herpesviridae family of viruses.

Epidemiology

Route of Spread

CMV is transmitted via saliva and sexual contact, from infected donated blood and organs or by intrauterine transmission.

Prevalence

CMV infection occurs worldwide and the prevalence of infection varies considerably. In the UK a rule of thumb is that the percentage of the community with CMV infection is equivalent to the age (e.g. approximately 20% of 20-year-olds will have had CMV infection). Prevalence tends to be higher in lower socio-economic groups, people born outside Western Europe, inner-city areas and in communities living in overcrowded conditions.

Incubation Period

3–6 weeks.

Infectious Period

This varies for different groups of people. In immunocompetent people, the virus is present for a few weeks in saliva, blood and some other body fluids after primary infection. In immunocompromised people, the infectious period may be prolonged after primary infection. Also, when people experience reactivation of CMV, the infection may last for weeks or months. Infected neonates can shed virus in urine for several weeks after birth.

CMV is a herpesvirus which becomes latent in humans once active infection has been resolved. The virus can reactivate to produce another infection later in life – this is much rarer in persons who are not immunocompromised.

At-Risk Groups

CMV can infect anyone who has saliva or sex contact with an actively infected person or who receives blood or organs from a CMV-positive person. Unborn children of mothers

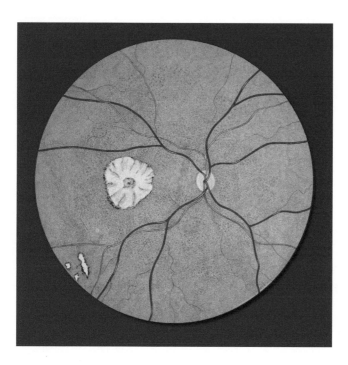

Figure 3.1 CMV retinitis (courtesy of CDC)

with active infection and immunocompromised persons are at increased risk of severe, life-threatening infection.

Clinical

Symptoms

CMV infection is usually mild or asymptomatic in immunocompetent persons. However, infection in pregnancy can lead to congenital infection and immunocompromised patients (HIV positive, transplant recipients) often experience severe or fatal infection.

Immunocompromised Persons

CMV symptoms vary in different groups of immunocompromised patients.

- In patients with HIV/AIDS, CMV disease is associated with retinitis, colitis, encephalitis and falling white blood cells. This occurs more frequently when the lymphocyte counts fall below 200. Primary infection is relatively uncommon and most infections are caused by a reactivation of latent CMV infection. Figure 3.1 shows CMV retinitis.
- In patients who have received solid organ transplants, the highest risk of severe or fatal CMV disease occurs with primary infection, when CMV infection is acquired with the donated organ. Of CMV antibody–negative recipients who receive organs from CMV antibody–positive donors, 80% will acquire CMV infection. The severity of disease associated with this infection will vary according to the amount of

immunosuppression given. In general, patients receiving kidney, liver and heart transplants will have less severe disease than those receiving bowel, heart-lung and lung transplants.

Reactivation of CMV is usually associated with less severe disease but can be fatal in severely immunocompromised patients.

- In patients who have received bone marrow transplants, severe infection can arise as a result of reactivated infection in the recipient or donor-acquired disease.

Immunocompetent Patients

Most infections are asymptomatic, but in those who develop symptoms, these most commonly present as fever, malaise, sweats, jaundice and raised liver function test values; symptoms can persist for several months.

Infection in Pregnancy

CMV infection at any stage of pregnancy can give rise to congenital infection even in women who have no symptoms. Of women with primary infection, 40% will transmit infection to their babies. Of those babies infected, 1% will have severe/fatal infection while 10% will have mild symptoms. Approximately 90% will be asymptomatic at birth, although they may develop signs and symptoms of congenital CMV disease (retinitis, deafness) early in life. Primary infection is associated with a higher risk of congenital infection than reactivation. Symptoms in newborn babies include chorioretinitis, deafness, brain damage, hepatosplenomegaly and petechial rash, and intrauterine and neonatal death.

Expert virological and obstetric advice should be sought in women with CMV infection in pregnancy.

Laboratory Diagnosis

Several laboratory methods and clinical specimens can be used to diagnose CMV infection (see Table 3.1).

Management

Treatment

Ganciclovir or valganciclovir are the drugs of choice for treating CMV infection. They are only licensed for use in severe/life-threatening CMV infection in immunocompromised patients. Regular monitoring for viral clearance is recommended, with treatment continuing until that is achieved.*

Treatment can be monitored by performing quantitative NAAT at the start of treatment and after 1 week of ganciclovir treatment. Falling CMV NAAT values indicate that treatment is being effective. If the patient's symptoms are not significantly improved by the end of the course of ganciclovir, and CMV NAAT values have not fallen by

---

* Note: Always check the latest nationally or locally agreed protocols and drug data sheets before prescribing antiviral drugs.

Table 3.1 Laboratory diagnosis of CMV

Patient category with CMV infection	Specimens	Test	Interpretation of positive result
HIV/AIDS	EDTA blood	Qualitative NAAT*	Indicates CMV infection
		Quantitative NAAT	Can indicate likely severity of disease and disease progression if done sequentially
Transplant/ Immunocompromised	EDTA blood	Qualitative NAAT	Indicates CMV infection
		Quantitative NAAT	Can indicate likely severity of disease and disease progression if done sequentially
	Urine, BAL	Qualitative NAAT	Indicates CMV infection
	Clotted blood	CMV IgM	Low-level positive results must be interpreted with extreme caution and a second confirmatory specimen sought. Strong positive results are a good indicator of recent infection if the laboratory has validated tests. CMV IgM can be detected up to 2 years after primary infection in solid organ transplant recipients.
		CMV IgG	Seroconversion indicates recent infection.
Immunocompetent**	Clotted blood	CMV IgM	Low-level positive results must be interpreted with extreme caution and a second confirmatory specimen sought. Strong positive results are a good indicator of recent infection if the laboratory has validated tests.
	Clotted blood	CMV IgG	Seroconversion indicates recent infection. Presence of low avidity CMV IgG confirms infection in previous 3–6 months.
	Urine/BAL	Qualitative NAAT	Indicates CMV infection
Neonates	Saliva/urine	Qualitative NAAT	Indicates congenital infection if specimen taken in first 3 weeks of life

Notes: * NAAT – nucleic acid amplification test; of which PCR is most commonly used.
** CMV DNA is rarely detected in EDTA blood in immunocompetent persons.

≥2 logs, ganciclovir-resistant CMV infection should be considered as a possibility and CMV ganciclovir resistance tests should be done.

Alternative antiviral drugs including cidofovir, foscarnet, letermovir and valaciclovir are available for treatment of patients with ganciclovir-resistant severe CMV infection.*

In babies born with severe congenital infection, including brain damage and deafness, valganciclovir treatment within the first month of life has been shown to be beneficial. Since valganciclovir is not licensed for this use, the benefits and side effects of treatment should be fully discussed with parents/carers before advocating treatment*.

Prophylaxis

CMV disease can be prevented or ameliorated in those patients at high risk of developing severe CMV disease.

- Solid organ transplant patients (especially CMV antibody–negative recipients of organs from CMV–positive donors) should be given post-transplant prophylaxis with IV ganciclovir or oral valganciclovir.*
- CMV antibody–positive bone marrow transplant recipients especially those with a CMV-positive donor should be considered for prophylaxis.* However, since valganciclovir can cause leucopaenia, weekly CMV DNA monitoring of EDTA blood and rapid treatment, if CMV DNA is detected, are frequently undertaken.
- HIV-positive patients with low white blood cell counts and/or evidence of recurrent eye/bowel symptoms should be considered for continuous prophylaxis.

Infection Control

CMV does not transmit easily between humans in the absence of sexual or intimate contact. It is very rarely transmitted between humans in hospitals. Special precautions are not recommended; normal hand washing and universal precautions (see Chapter 56) are sufficient to prevent transmission of infection in the hospital setting.

Enteroviruses

Chapter 4

The Viruses

Enteroviruses are small single-stranded RNA viruses belonging to the family Picornaviridae, divided into nine species of true enteroviruses (four human ones) and three species of rhinoviruses (which cause the common cold). More than 70 serotypes exist. Coxsackie A, Coxsackie B, echoviruses and polioviruses are all different serotypes of enteroviruses. Because of the similarity in viral genome, later serotypes were just called enterovirus followed by a sequential number, for example enterovirus 71 (EV71) and enterovirus 72 (EV72).

Epidemiology

Route of Spread

As the name implies these are spread by the enteric route via faecal-oral spread (e.g. by ingesting contaminated food or water) but different enteroviruses have different modes of spread. They can also be transmitted by the respiratory route and by direct contact (e.g. in haemorrhagic conjunctivitis).

Prevalence

Enteroviruses are endemic worldwide and a very common infection of childhood. Young children are often infected with more than one enterovirus at a given time. Enterovirus infections are more common in those countries with poor standards of hygiene. Polio, which is caused by an enterovirus, has been eradicated from most of the countries in the world following massive vaccination campaigns under the World Health Organization (WHO) expanded programme of immunisations. The countries where polio is still considered to be endemic by the WHO are Afghanistan and Pakistan, and, although not endemic, it has been reintroduced in a handful of other countries (from where it had been eradicated) by means of live vaccine strains reverting to the wild type virus.

Outbreaks of infections with different serotypes causing particular clinical manifestations (e.g. conjunctivitis and hand, foot and mouth disease) occur from time to time. There have been large outbreaks of hand, foot and mouth disease, some cases with severe neurological symptoms, caused by EV71, in the Asia- Pacific region in recent years.

Incubation Period

Variable: generally 3–7 days, with 7–14 days for polio.

Infectious Period

Enteroviruses are shed in the faeces for a long time. Polio virus can be shed in the faeces for many weeks after infection or live oral polio vaccination.

At-Risk Groups

Polio virus infection is common and can cause illness in all age groups; children generally tend to have asymptomatic infection.

Neonates are at particular risk as enteroviruses may cause disseminated infection involving multiple systems; such disseminated infections have a high mortality, especially in babies with a birthweight of less than 1500 g.

Clinical

Enteroviruses replicate in the gut but despite their name they do not cause extensive GI symptoms/illness or gastroenteritis.

Enteroviruses present with a wide spectrum of clinical illness, although the majority of infections, especially in children, are asymptomatic. Infection with one serotype does not offer cross-protection with others; therefore, multiple episodes of enterovirus can occur in an individual during their lifetime.

- *Non-specific illness*: Fever, malaise, fatigue, non-specific rash.
- *Rashes*:
  o Painful ulceration in the mouth is known as herpangina. Lesions typically involve the soft palate, uvula and tonsillar fossa.
  o Hand, foot and mouth disease (a different infection to foot and mouth disease in cattle). If the ulcers occur on hands and soles of feet in addition to those in the mouth then the disease is called hand, foot and mouth disease. There may be non-specific systemic symptoms associated with both.
- *Conjunctivitis*: Severe conjunctivitis, usually bilateral, may be haemorrhagic; outbreaks may occur.
- *Respiratory*: Upper respiratory symptoms may present as the common cold or pharyngitis. In small children enteroviruses can cause bronchiolitis and pneumonitis.
- *Central nervous system*:
  o Meningitis and meningoencephalitis: Headache, photophobia, fever, often preceded by a viral prodrome of upper respiratory symptoms, fever and malaise.
  o Flaccid paralysis: Polio viruses 1, 2 and 3 cause infection of motor neurons which results in the loss of lower motor function and flaccid muscle paralysis. This syndrome is called poliomyelitis. The paralysis is usually accompanied by a prodrome of fever and other signs of a non-specific viral illness. Only 0.1–1% of infections with polio viruses result in poliomyelitis, depending on the polio virus type and the social conditions; the rest are either asymptomatic or cause non-specific illness. Other enteroviruses (e.g. EV70, 71 and 72) may also cause flaccid paralysis or 'non-polio poliomyelitis'. The WHO has been effective in eliminating the dreaded condition from most of the world. Whole continents including Europe have been declared polio-free. An active surveillance programme to investigate and identify the cause of flaccid paralysis is in place to ensure that polio does not re-enter the polio-free areas.

- *Neonates*: Neonates may acquire infection from the mother at the time of delivery. Use of interventions such as scalp electrodes to measure fetal oxygen levels (PO2) increase the risk of such infections. Neonatal enterovirus has a relatively high mortality in preterm and low-birthweight children due to disseminated infection involving multiple systems.
- *Bornholm disease (epidemic myalgia)*: Severe chest pain due to infection of the upper abdominal and pectoral muscles.

Laboratory Diagnosis

Serology is of limited use. The mainstay of diagnosis is a nucleic acid amplification test (usually PCR) for detection of the virus in appropriate specimens depending on clinical presentation (see Table 4.1). Faeces is a useful, non-invasive specimen to send in all cases. However, a positive result, especially in children, should be interpreted with caution because asymptomatic enterovirus infection is common in children. Some diagnostic laboratories use primers targeting the highly conserved regions which will detect rhino-viruses, enteroviruses and parechoviruses; primers targeting the specific regions can distinguish species and identify virus genotype. Finding enterovirus RNA in CSF is a good indication of central nervous system infection.

Management

Treatment

There is no specific antiviral treatment.

Prophylaxis

There is no prophylaxis except for polio and EV71. Polio is a vaccine-preventable disease and vaccination has been one of the success stories in almost eradicating polio worldwide. The WHO has declared wild type polio 2 and 3 to be eradicated and currently wild type polio 1 to be endemic only in Afghanistan and Pakistan at present. There are enhanced vaccination programmes with active case findings going on in these countries with the ultimate aim to declare worldwide eradication of polio. Vaccine-derived polio infections have been detected via active surveillance schemes in some countries where the disease has been eradicated, as a result of travel from those countries where live polio vaccine is still administered. While polio is still endemic in some countries there is a danger that it may be reintroduced in countries from where it has been eradicated; therefore childhood vaccinations still remain the mainstay of prevention globally.

There are two types of polio vaccines, both of which are equally effective and are given as a primary course of three vaccines, followed by two boosters.

Live attenuated (Sabin vaccine) polio vaccine: Introduced in the UK in 1962, but not currently in use. It contains attenuated polio virus 1, 2 and 3 serotypes. Being an oral vaccine, it has ease of delivery. It is contraindicated in the immunosuppressed and those who are in contact with the immunosuppressed as the vaccine virus can be shed in the faeces for weeks and may revert to wild type. Vaccine-associated polio is a rare complication in both the vaccinee and their contacts.

Killed (Salk) polio vaccine: Introduced in the UK in 1956 and is the vaccine currently in use. UK polio vaccine schedule is 2, 3 and 4 months, 3–4 years and 14

Table 4.1 Clinical illnesses and associated enteroviruses

Clinical illness	Associated enteroviruses	Laboratory specimen
Herpangina	Coxsackie A ++	Mouth or throat swab
Hand, foot and mouth disease	Coxsackie A6 ++ Coxsackie A16 ++ EV71 ++	Throat swab, lesion swab, faeces
Conjunctivitis	EV70 ++ Coxsackie A24 +	Conjunctival swab
Respiratory	Echoviruses ++	NPA*, throat swab, faeces
Aseptic meningitis	Coxsackie A ++ Coxsackie B ++ Echoviruses ++ E69, E73 +	CSF, faeces, throat swab
Flaccid paralysis (polio and non-polio myelitis)	Polioviruses 1 ,2, 3 +++ EV71 ++, EV68, EV69 + Coxsackie A and B +	CSF, faeces, throat swab
Encephalitis	Coxsackie A ++ Coxsackie B ++ EV71 +	CSF, faeces, throat swab
Myocarditis/ pericarditis	Coxsackie B++ Coxsackie A + Echoviruses +	Muscle biopsy, faeces, throat swab
Bornholm disease	Coxsackie B +++ Coxsackie A + Echovirus +	Faeces, throat swab

Note: * NPA – nasopharyngeal aspirate.

years. It is as effective as the live vaccine and also contains poliovirus 1, 2 and 3 serotypes. It is given as an intramuscular injection in combination with other childhood vaccines. This is the vaccine used in most of the developed countries now because after eradication, the small risk of the vaccine strains reverting to wild virus and causing polio is prohibitive. In countries where the oral polio vaccine is still being used, the killed vaccine is recommended for immunosuppressed patients and their contacts.

There are several inactivated EV71 vaccines available in China, in use since 2017. They have proved to be more than 90% effective in preventing hand, foot and mouth disease and preventing severe neurological symptoms.

Infection Control

It is difficult to control the spread of enteroviruses in the community especially where small children congregate. In the hospital, enteric precautions (Chapter 56) with strict handwashing should be instituted to prevent transmission to those patients at risk of severe or fatal infection (e.g. neonates).

Chapter

5

Epstein–Barr Virus

The Virus

Epstein-Barr virus (EBV), also known as human herpesvirus 4, is a double-stranded DNA virus and belongs to the family Herpesviridae.

Epidemiology

Route of Spread

EBV is transmitted via saliva and close sexual contact, hence the name 'kissing disease'. Infection is common in younger children and sexually active adolescents.

Prevalence

EBV is a ubiquitous virus, which infects 95% of people in the UK before the age of 25.

Incubation Period

2–3 weeks.

Infectious Period

EBV is primarily shed in saliva and can be present in the saliva for many weeks or months. It can also be present in genital secretions, for example semen. Reactivation of latent infection can occur frequently in some people, especially if they are immunosuppressed, with prolonged shedding of infectious virus, often asymptomatically.

At-Risk Groups

Immunosuppressed persons.

Clinical

Symptoms

Most primary EBV infections are subclinical. Classical clinical EBV syndrome is infectious mononucleosis which is more commonly referred to as 'glandular fever', with symptoms of sore throat, hepatitis, lymphadenopathy, fever and malaise. Splenomegaly is common and occurs in about 50–70% of cases. Atypical lymphocytes are present in the peripheral blood, and liver function tests are usually deranged with mildly elevated alanine aminotransferase. Hepatomegaly and jaundice may occur but are less common.

Complications

EBV is a self-limiting illness and complications are rare.

- Morbilliform rash is associated with ampicillin administration.
- Chronic fatigue – some patients may suffer with tiredness and fatigue for weeks to months post acute EBV infection; this may or may not be accompanied with lymphadenopathy.
- Rarely, enlarged spleen may lead to splenic rupture therefore patients are advised to refrain from contact sports until acute symptoms have subsided.
- Guillain–Barré syndrome is a rare post-infectious complication of EBV infection and presents as an ascending motor paralysis due to an immune-mediated demyelination of the spinal cord.
- EBV is associated with malignancies, such as Burkitt's lymphoma (malaria is considered as a co-factor) and nasopharyngeal carcinoma, post-transplant lymphoproliferative disease (PTLD), Hodgkin's lymphoma and other associated lymphomas.
- Oral hairy leukoplakia occurs in HIV-positive persons.
- Haemophagocytic lymphohistiocytosis (HLH) – EBV is recognised as one of the initiating causes for HLH.
- X-linked lymphoproliferative syndrome (Duncan's syndrome) is due to a specific X chromosome–linked recessive genetic defect which leads to impaired antibody response to EBV alone. It affects the male members of the family who either die of an overwhelming EBV infection or develop lymphoproliferative malignancies.

Differential Diagnosis

CMV, *Toxoplasma gondii* and adenovirus infections should be considered in the differential diagnosis of EBV glandular fever–type illness (see Chapter 37 on glandular fever–type illness).

Laboratory Diagnosis

See Table 5.1.

Management

Treatment

There is no evidence that any antiviral drugs are useful in the treatment of EBV infections. In immunosuppressed patients, reducing the amounts of immunosuppression will reduce the severity of disease and the frequency of EBV reactivation. Rituximab is recommended for treatment of PTLD and may also be useful to treat other EBV proliferative syndromes in immunosuppressed patients.

Table 5.1 Laboratory diagnosis of EBV

Sample	Laboratory test	Result interpretation
Clotted blood (serum)	EBV IgM	Positive results indicate recent EBV infection. Interpret positive results with caution; some will be non-specific. Beware of rheumatoid factor interference.
	EBV virus capsid antigen (VCA) IgG antibody	Positive result indicates EBV infection at some time.
	EBV nuclear antigen (EBNA) IgG antibody	This antibody is produced about 6–12 weeks after infection. If positive, indicates EBV infection more than 6–12 weeks.
	EBNA IgG antibody negative, VCA IgG antibody positive	Suggests recent EBV infection but false negative EBNA results, especially in patients >60 years old and immunosuppressed persons, may occur.
	Paul–Bunnell/Monospot test	Provides a quick diagnosis but can be false positive and false negative. Not useful for persons under the age of 16 years.
EDTA blood	EBV DNA NAAT* (e.g. PCR) assays	The presence of EBV DNA indicates current infection. Quantitative PCR is a guide to the severity of infection in immunocompromised patients and a guide to management.

Note: * NAAT – nucleic acid amplification test; of which PCR is most commonly used.

Infection Control

EBV does not pose any infection control risks, although sharing drinking vessels and bottles can transmit infection via saliva. For certain high-risk patients such as bone marrow transplant patients, a baseline donor/recipient EBV serological status with EBV PCR surveillance post-transplant for high-risk patients is recommended for early detection and control.

Hepatitis A Virus

The Virus

Hepatitis A virus (HAV) is a single-stranded RNA virus belonging to the genus *Hepatovirus* in the family Picornaviridae.

Epidemiology

Route of Spread

Hepatitis A is spread by the faecal-oral route through eating and drinking contaminated food and water and by person-to-person spread. Water-borne outbreaks have been described in countries where infection is endemic. Outbreaks have also occurred in persons who inject drugs (PWIDs) by injecting substances reconstituted in contaminated water and through oro-anal sex. Rarely it may be transmitted through blood transfusion through a viraemic donor.

Prevalence

Infection occurs worldwide. Globally it is estimated that 1.4 million cases occur every year. In developed countries, because of good hygiene, the majority of adults have not acquired the infection as compared to developing countries where >90% of infection occurs in childhood. People travelling to countries with high prevalence are therefore at risk of acquiring infection during their travel and this is the major risk factor for acquisition of infection in developed countries, most commonly by eating uncooked food, for example salad washed in contaminated water. Shellfish grown in contaminated water are another source of hepatitis A infection as they concentrate the virus. In Europe the prevalence of antibody in adults varies from 10% to 50%. People from lower socio-economic groups are more likely to have had infection.

Incubation Period

Average incubation period is 2–6 weeks.

Infectious Period

Virus is shed in the faeces of the infected individual from 2 weeks before jaundice develops to about 1 week after the jaundice. The maximum amount of virus is shed before the jaundice develops; therefore, patients are most infectious in the late incubation period.

At-Risk Groups

Those travelling to countries where infection is endemic; people from lower socio-economic groups (due to poor hygiene); those occupationally exposed, for example healthcare workers and sewage workers; men who have sex with men (due to sexual practices); and PWIDs.

Clinical

Acute Hepatitis

Infection in children, especially under 5 years, is usually asymptomatic. In adults, about 50% of infection is asymptomatic.

A prodrome of nausea, myalgia, malaise, fever and joint pains may occur followed by development of jaundice, dark urine, pale stools and tenderness in the right upper quadrant of the abdomen. Symptoms may last up to a few weeks but normally clear in a couple of weeks. Investigations reveal abnormal liver function tests with alanine aminotransferase in the thousands. Clinically, hepatitis A infection may be difficult to distinguish from hepatitis caused by hepatitis B and C virus or that by Epstein–Barr virus or cytomegalovirus. There may be epidemiological clues, that is, history of contact with a case or travel to an endemic country. For definite diagnosis confirmation, specific virological tests are required.

Unlike hepatitis B or C infection, hepatitis A infection does not give rise to chronic infection and full clinical and biochemical recovery occurs after acute infection.

Complications

Infection is almost always self-limiting. Fulminant hepatitis and death may occur in a very small minority (<1% of cases), generally in older individuals and those with an underlying liver disease or hepatitis B and C infection. Fulminant hepatitis is a clinical emergency and is an urgent reason for liver transplant without which the mortality is high.

Laboratory Diagnosis

See Table 6.1.

Other Laboratory Investigations

Other laboratory investigations include liver function tests and liver ultrasound.

Management

Treatment

There is no specific treatment; treatment is supportive. If fulminant hepatitis develops, liver transplantation may be indicated.

Prophylaxis

Pre-exposure

Killed hepatitis A virus vaccine is available. Combined hepatitis A and B vaccine and a combined hepatitis A and typhoid vaccine are also available. All of these vaccines offer

Table 6.1 Laboratory diagnosis of hepatitis A

Clinical indication	Specimen	Test	Significance	Essential information for laboratory
Acute hepatitis	Clotted venous blood, 5–10 ml	Hepatitis A IgM	Becomes positive about 5 days after the onset of symptoms and remains positive for up to 3 months, sometimes for longer. Signifies acute infection.	Clinical symptoms, relevant epidemiology, date of onset of illness.
Check immune status	As above	Hepatitis A IgG	Becomes positive from a week after onset of illness or receiving hepatitis A vaccination and persists throughout life. When detected alone, for example without IgM, signifies immunity to infection due to either past infection or vaccination.	Must state if the test is to check immune status or to rule out acute infection, for later see above.
Research or epidemiology	Faeces	NAAT* for hepatitis A virus RNA	Virus present from a couple of weeks before onset of acute hepatitis to a couple of weeks after. Not used for routine diagnosis. Research and epidemiological tool.	Same as for IgM

Note: * NAAT – nucleic acid amplification test; of which PCR is most commonly used.

equal protection. Two doses of hepatitis A vaccine given 1 year apart offer protection for up to 10 years. A booster may be required at 10 years but recent evidence suggests that the two doses will give lifelong protection. Pre-exposure prophylaxis is indicated for at-risk groups and those travelling abroad to endemic countries and food handlers. Depending upon the cost-effectiveness there is a case for instituting childhood vaccination programmes in countries where the virus is endemic.

Post-exposure

Normal human immunoglobulin (HNIG) should be given to household contacts as soon as possible but within 14 days of exposure. There is good evidence that post-exposure vaccination (as the antibody response occurs in 7–10 days) given within a week of exposure is effective in preventing or attenuating infection in exposed individuals and effective in interrupting outbreaks.

Depending upon the risk factors, vaccination with or without HNIG should be offered to all susceptible contacts. HNIG is recommended, in addition, for those less able to respond to the vaccine, for example the immunosuppressed. For those exposed between 2 and 4 weeks, HNIG may still be given to modify disease in those at high risk of complications. Consult the latest UK Health Security Agency guidance on post-exposure prophylaxis.

Infection Control

Enteric infection control precautions should be instituted (see Chapter 56). Where possible patients should be put in a single room and strict hand washing should be adhered to. Ensure that healthcare workers providing nursing care are immunised against hepatitis A.

Pre- and post-exposure vaccination should also be used as appropriate.

Useful Website

Public Health England: Public health control and management of hepatitis A: 2017 guidelines: https://assets.publishing.service.gov.uk/government/uploads/system/uploads/attachment_data/file/727411/Public_health_control_and_management_of_hepatitis_A_2017.pdf

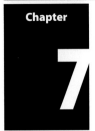
Hepatitis B and D Viruses

The Viruses

Hepatitis B virus (HBV) is a member of the Hepadnaviridae family of viruses and has a double-stranded circular DNA and a DNA polymerase enzyme. It has two major proteins, hepatitis B surface antigen (HBsAg) which is an outer protein expressed in excess when the virus replicates in the liver, and hepatitis B core antigen, an inner protein which is expressed only within the hepatocytes in the liver. A third protein, hepatitis B e antigen (HBeAg), is also shed in the blood when the virus replicates and its presence is associated with high infectivity. Figure 7.1 shows an electron micrograph of HBV.

Hepatitis D virus (HDV) is a defective RNA virus which cannot replicate in humans in the absence of HBV. Persons can be co-infected with HBV and HDV, or HBV-infected persons can be superinfected with HDV.

Hepatitis B Virus

Epidemiology
Route of Spread

The routes of transmission are:
- parenteral (blood exposure)
- sexual
- vertical (from mother to baby).

Prevalence

Worldwide, almost 300 million people are infected with HBV (4% of the world's population); prevalence across the globe ranges from around 7.5% in Africa to 0.3–2% in Europe, Australasia and the Americas. This prevalence used to be much higher, but has been reduced due to extensive deployment of HBV vaccines in many countries. The UK is a very low-prevalence country, but prevalence of HBsAg varies across the country and is higher in those born in high-endemicity countries, many of whom will have acquired infection at birth or in early childhood. In countries with high prevalence, vertical transmission (usually occurring during birth) and in early childhood are the most significant routes of transmission, with some sexual spread. In lower prevalence areas, the disease is predominantly spread sexually or via drug usage, with fewer vertically transmitted infections.

Incubation Period

Infection can develop from 30 to 180 days after exposure to the virus.

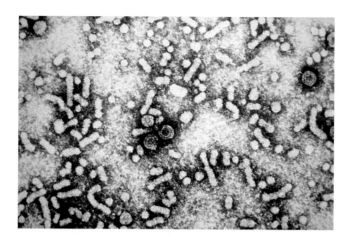

Figure 7.1 An electron micrograph of negatively stained HBV (courtesy of CDC)

Infectivity

Infectivity is related to the presence of HBsAg in the blood. Persons are infectious as long as HBsAg or HBV DNA are detectable in peripheral blood. The infectivity can be high (up to 90%) or low (1–3%) depending upon the presence of HBeAg in the blood. HBeAg is a marker of high infectivity, whereas the presence of antibody to HBeAg (anti-HBe) denotes absent or low infectivity (if not found alongside HBeAg). The presence or absence of HBV DNA in the blood is a more accurate marker of infectivity. This is partly because HBV mutants exist that either do not express HBeAg (core mutants) or that produce altered HBeAg (pre-core mutants); persons infected with these mutants usually have a high level of HBV DNA in their blood and are highly infectious. Absence of HBV DNA in the blood signifies absence of infectivity. The exception to this is in organ transplantation, where organ donors who transmit HBV infection to recipients can have no detectable HBsAg or HBV DNA detectable in peripheral blood, but can have circulating anti-HBc (denoting previous HBV infection) and can have small undetectable amounts of HBV DNA in the donated organ.

At-Risk Groups

The groups most at risk of HBV infection are shown in Table 7.1 along with the potential route of transmission.

Clinical

Acute Hepatitis B

The percentage of patients exhibiting symptoms increases with age with only 10% of infections in children being symptomatic compared to about 50% of infections in young adults. Acute infection is accompanied by a rise in alanine transaminase (ALT) of >500 IU/L and jaundice. The hepatitis is immune-mediated and liver damage occurs due to cytotoxic T-cells attacking the infected hepatocytes. Fulminant hepatitis and death may occur in <1%.

Of immunocompetent adults, 95% clear the virus within 6 months after an acute infection. Failure to clear the virus and progress to chronic infection or carriage is

Table 7.1 At-risk groups for HBV infection

Mode of transmission	At-risk groups	Preventive measures
Parenteral Percutaneous or mucous membrane exposure to blood or blood-contaminated secretions.	Persons who inject drugs. Healthcare workers. Blood, organ and blood product recipients. Persons undergoing tattoos/body piercing/acupuncture. Patients undergoing dental or surgical treatment.	Do not share injecting equipment. Avoid needle-stick injuries. Screening of blood and organ donors. Clean fresh equipment for each patient. Vaccinate at-risk people. Exclusion of infected healthcare workers from performing exposure-prone procedures. Use a barrier method (condoms) during sexual intercourse. Vaccinate at-risk people.
Sexual Increased risk of transmission if genital ulcers due to other sexually transmitted infections present.	Multiple sexual partners. Men who have sex with men. Sex workers.	Use of barrier method (condoms) during sexual intercourse. Vaccinate at-risk people.
Vertical (from mother to baby) Transmission is in the perinatal period due to feto-maternal mixing of blood and mucous membrane exposure to infected maternal secretions at the time of vaginal delivery.	Babies born to mothers who are chronic carriers of HBV or who have acute HBV infection in pregnancy.	Avoid scalp electrodes or use of other sharp instruments on the fetus at delivery. Treat mother with antivirals (e.g. tenofovir) from 28 weeks gestation, to reduce the viral load at birth. Vaccinate baby at birth and give hepatitis B immunoglobulin for low birthweight babies <1500 g and those whose mothers are negative for anti-HBe. Breastfeeding is not contra-indicated (unless cracked nipples, etc.).

associated with an inadequate immune response to the virus in the very young, the chronically ill or those who are immunocompromised.

The serological markers of acute hepatitis B infection are shown in Figure 7.2.

Chronic Hepatitis B

Chronic infection is defined as persistence of HBsAg or HBV DNA in the blood beyond a period of 6 months following acute hepatitis B infection. Figure 7.3 shows the hepatitis B virus serological markers of chronic HBV infection. Figures 7.4 and 7.5 show clinical interpretation of HBV markers in hepatitis B surface antigen positive and negative patients. Failure to clear the virus may lead (after a period of several years) to progressive liver damage with persistent hepatitis→chronic hepatitis→cirrhosis→hepatocellular carcinoma. HBV is the single most important risk factor (with HCV) for the development of hepatocellular carcinoma.

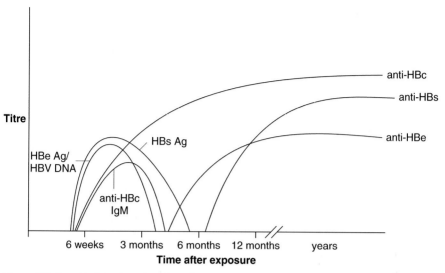

Figure 7.2 Hepatitis B serological markers of acute infection

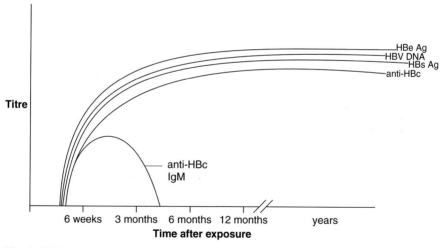

Figure 7.3 Hepatitis B serological markers of HBeAg chronic infection

Neonatal Hepatitis B

Infection is acquired from the mother at the time of birth and commonly leads to chronic infection in the baby, especially if the mother is HBeAg positive. To prevent neonatal hepatitis B infection, in the UK, there is a programme for universal hepatitis B screening of pregnant women to identify and vaccinate babies born to infected mothers. Many countries, especially those with a high prevalence of HBV infection, have opted to vaccinate all neonates against hepatitis B. Since 1987, the World Health Organization has recommended universal infant or adolescent hepatitis B immunisation. Most countries have incorporated hepatitis B vaccine as an integral part of their national infant immunisation programmes. The UK incorporated HBV vaccine into its childhood vaccine

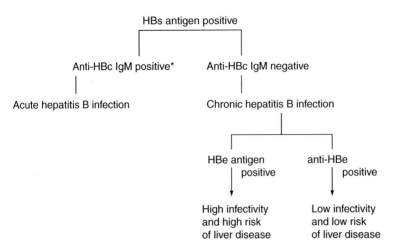

* Strongly positive anti-HBc IgM is consistent with acute hepatitis B infection.
Weakly positive anti-HBc IgM can be found in patients with chronic hepatitis B infection.

Figure 7.4 The clinical interpretation of HBV markers in hepatitis B surface antigen–positive patients

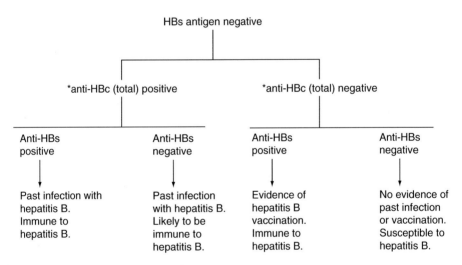

* There are no specific tests to measure anti-HBc IgG, positive anti-HBc total antibody in the absence of anti-HBc IgM indicates that antibody is of IgG class.

Figure 7.5 The clinical interpretation of HBV markers in hepatitis B surface antigen–negative patients

programme in 2017, with HBV vaccine being given at 8, 12 and 16 weeks of age. Antiviral drugs (e.g. tenofovir) should be considered for mothers with HBV infection during pregnancy from 28 weeks gestation, to reduce the viral load at the time of delivery.

Laboratory Diagnosis

Hepatitis B infection is diagnosed by testing a clotted blood sample for HBsAg; 5–10 ml of clotted blood should be sent to the laboratory. Acute or chronic infection can be

Table 7.2 Hepatitis B serological markers in the blood at different stages of infection

Hepatitis B surface antigen (HBsAg)	Outer protein coat of virus	Detected in blood in both acute and chronic hepatitis B infection. Marker of infection and used as the primary screening test for hepatitis B.
HBV DNA	Viral DNA	Present in hepatocytes and also in the blood of infected patients. Level can be quantified and used to monitor treatment response and risk of infection to others in certain circumstances (e.g. healthcare worker to patient if undertaking exposure-prone procedures).
Hepatitis B e antigen (HBeAg)	Part of inner viral protein	Present in early phase of acute infection. May persist if the virus is not cleared. Presence in blood signifies a high HBV DNA level and high infectivity. About 10–15% of chronic carriers clear the HBeAg spontaneously every year and seroconvert to anti-HBe positivity.
Hepatitis B e antibody (anti-HBe)	Antibody to HBe antigen	Anti-HBe appears when HBeAg is cleared. Its presence normally indicates an inert hepatitis B infection accompanied with low or absent HBV DNA in blood but up to 20% of patients may have a mutant virus and a high level of DNA even in the presence of anti-HBe.
Hepatitis B core antibody (anti-HBc)	Antibody to the hepatitis B core antigen. The core antigen is present only in the hepatocytes and NOT in the blood	Anti-HBc is detected once the body mounts an immune response to the virus. Anti-HBc of the IgM class (anti-HBc IgM) signifies and is diagnostic of acute HBV infection. It is the only marker which can distinguish between acute and chronic infection (provided that the anti-HBc IgM result is reliable and interpreted correctly). Anti-HBc of the IgG class (as measured by anti-HBc total antibody) persists for life. The presence of low avidity anti-HBc IgG antibody is an indication of recent primary HBV infection.
Hepatitis B surface antibody (anti-HBs)	Antibody to hepatitis B surface antigen	HBsAg is replaced by anti-HBs once the virus is cleared. Anti-HBs is the protective antibody and denotes immunity to further infections. This is also the antibody that is produced in response to hepatitis B vaccination.

differentiated by testing for a combination of different serological markers for hepatitis B. See Tables 7.2, 7.3 and 7.4.

Management
Treatment
Acute Hepatitis B

Acute infection is self-limiting, with 95% of immunocompetent adults clearing the virus within 6 months of onset acute hepatitis. Fulminant hepatitis may occur in <1% and may require a liver transplant.

Table 7.3 Clinical interpretation of HBV markers in hepatitis B surface antigen–positive persons

HBV laboratory test results	Clinical interpretation
HBsAg positive Anti-HBc IgM positive* Anti-HBc (total) positive	Indicates acute HBV infection.
HBsAg positive HBeAg positive Anti-HBe negative Anti-HBc IgM negative Anti-HBc (total) positive	Indicates HBV infection more than 3–6 months ago (probably chronic HBV infection) with high infectivity.
HBsAg positive HBeAg negative Anti-HBe positive Anti-HBc IgM negative Anti-HBc (total) positive	Indicates HBV infection more than 3–6 months ago (probably chronic HBV infection) with low infectivity.
HBsAg positive HBeAg negative Anti-HBe negative Anti-HBc IgM negative Anti-HBc (total) positive	Indicates HBV infection more than 3–6 months ago (probably chronic HBV infection) with high infectivity.

Note: * Strong positive anti-HBc IgM results would be consistent with recent acute HBV infection. Weakly positive anti-HBc IgM results may be non-specific or consistent with a recent flare in persons with chronic HBV infection. Anti-HBc IgM results should be interpreted with caution.

Chronic Infection

A small number of patients will spontaneously clear the virus, with 10–15% of HBeAg-positive patients per year naturally seroconverting to anti-HBe-positive status and then, over a period of time, clearing the virus altogether.

The management of uncomplicated acute viral hepatitis usually involves symptomatic supportive care.

Treatment for chronic hepatitis B infection should be initiated by a specialist. The main goal of treatment is to improve survival and quality of life by preventing disease progression, and consequently hepatocellular carcinoma development. The long-term suppression of HBV replication represents the main aims of current treatment strategies which are either to convert the patient's status from HBsAg positive to anti-HBs status, from HBeAg positive to anti-HBe positive or to significantly lower the HBV DNA viral load. The typical indication for treatment would typically be HBV DNA >2,000|IU/ml, elevated ALT and/or at least moderate histological lesions.

According to current medical advice, entecavir, peginterferon alfa, tenofovir alafenamide and tenofovir disoproxil are options for the treatment of chronic hepatitis B infection. Entecavir and tenofovir disoproxil can be used in patients with decompensated liver disease. Other drugs licensed for the treatment of chronic hepatitis B infection include adefovir dipivoxil and lamivudine. If drug resistance emerges during treatment, consider switching to or adding another antiviral drug to which the virus is sensitive;

Table 7.4 Clinical interpretation of HBV markers in hepatitis B surface antigen–negative persons

HBV laboratory test results	Clinical interpretation
HBsAg negative Anti-HBc (total) positive Anti-HBs positive	Indicates past, resolved HBV infection. Immune to Hepatitis B.
HBsAg negative Anti-HBc (total) positive Ant-HBs negative	Indicates past, resolved HBV infection. Likely to be immune to Hepatitis B.
HBsAg negative Anti-HBc (total) negative Anti-HBs positive	Evidence of HBV vaccination. Immune to Hepatitis B.
HBsAg negative Anti-HBc (total) negative Anti-HBs negative	No evidence of past HBV infection or vaccination. Susceptible to Hepatitis B.

ensure the antiviral drug does not share cross-resistance. Hepatitis B viruses with reduced susceptibility to lamivudine have emerged following extended therapy. Duration of treatment is dependent on several factors including response (e.g. viral suppression, antigen loss and seroconversion), patient characteristics (e.g. liver disease) and treatment tolerability. Treatment is usually continued long term in patients with decompensated liver disease. Website addresses are given at the end of this chapter to facilitate up-to-date treatment advice. Liver transplantation may be the last resort in case of liver failure.

In 2017, the European Association for the Study of the Liver (EASL) reported that the best results reported in treatment trials for treating HBeAg-positive patients with chronic HBV infection with pegylated interferon alpha and nucleoside analogues were 7% (HBsAg loss), 32% (HBeAg to anti-HBe conversion) and 76% (reducing HBV DNA to <60IU/ml).

Prophylaxis

An effective recombinant vaccine is available for both pre- and post-exposure prophylaxis for hepatitis B. Hepatitis B vaccines contain HBsAg prepared from yeast cells using recombinant DNA technology.

Pre-exposure Prophylaxis

For current advice on doses and vaccination schedules in different categories of patients, consult the latest Green Book Hepatitis B chapter (the website address is given at the end of this chapter).

The following groups have a poorer response to the vaccine:

- males
- persons >40 years old
- obese persons
- smokers
- persons with alcohol dependency
- immunocompromised persons
- patients undergoing regular renal dialysis.

Priority groups in the UK for receiving pre-exposure vaccination include:

- healthcare workers;
- those in close contact including household and sexual partners of patients with acute and chronic hepatitis B infection;
- babies born to mother who have acute hepatitis B in pregnancy or who are chronic carriers;
- those whose lifestyle puts them at risk of hepatitis B (e.g. intravenous drug users and sex workers);
- frequent or long-term travellers to endemic countries.

Post-exposure Prophylaxis

Post-exposure prophylaxis should be initiated rapidly to protect the following groups:

- babies born to hepatitis B–infected mothers
- other groups potentially exposed to hepatitis B:
  - ○ sexual partners
  - ○ persons who are accidentally inoculated or contaminated.

This is usually achieved by giving the HBV vaccine, but hepatitis B immunoglobulin is also recommended in the highest risk situations (e.g. babies born to HBeAg–positive mothers and persons who have failed to respond to HBV vaccination receiving a significant exposure from a known HBsAg–positive person). Consult the latest version of the Green Book Hepatitis B chapter for up-to-date advice (the website is given at the end of this chapter) .

Hepatitis D

Hepatitis D or delta virus is a defective RNA virus that requires HBV DNA to replicate and infect. Globally, Hepatitis D virus affects nearly 5% of people who have a chronic infection with HBV.

Two types of infection are described:

Co-infection: Where a person who is susceptible to HBV is exposed to someone who is co-infected with HBV and delta virus. This results in acute co-infection with both the viruses at the same time.

Superinfection: When an HBV carrier is exposed to infected blood from a co-infected person, then the exposure results in superinfection of the existing HBV infection with delta virus; this may result in development of acute hepatitis (due to delta) in an HBV chronic carrier. Superinfection is the most serious type of viral hepatitis due to its severity of complications. These include a greater risk of developing liver failure in acute infections and a rapid progression to liver cirrhosis, with an increased risk of developing liver cancer in chronic infections. In combination with hepatitis B virus, hepatitis D has the highest fatality rate of all the hepatitis infections (20%).

Infection is diagnosed by screening blood for delta virus IgG. Although delta IgM is not always present in acute infection, a positive result is useful in confirming acute delta infection.

In the UK delta infection is usually seen only in those who are recreational intravenous drug users (IVDUs). It has a higher prevalence in Mongolia, the Republic of Moldova and countries in western and central Africa.

Fortunately, as delta requires HBV to replicate and infect, protecting individuals from HBV through vaccination is effective in protecting against delta virus infection as well.

Infection Control

Infection control is achieved by implementing appropriate controls to prevent iatrogenic transmission. These include use of blood-borne virus nursing precautions, proper sterilisation of instruments before reuse, exclusion of infected healthcare workers from performing exposure-prone procedures, and taking appropriate measures in renal dialysis units. Screening and testing of blood and organ donors to exclude those who are infected and heat-treating products to inactivate the virus are also implemented. Other strategies include education of people at risk (e.g. IVDUs) for risk reduction, including needle exchange programmes.

Useful Websites

Hepatitis B, *The Green Book on Immunisation*, chapter 18 (Public Health England): https://assets.publishing.service.gov.uk/media/6200f92ad3bf7f78df30b3d3/Greenbook-chapter-18-4Feb22.pdf

National Institute for Health and Care Excellence/British National Formulary treatment summaries: https://bnf.nice.org.uk/treatment-summaries/hepatitis/#:~:text=Entecavir%2C%20peginterferon%20alfa%2C%20tenofovir%20alafenamide%2C%20and%20tenofovir%20disoproxil,be%20used%20in%20patients%20with%20decompensated%20liver%20disease

EASL: 2017 clinical practice guidelines on the management of hepatitis B virus infection: https://easl.eu/wp-content/uploads/2018/10/HepB-English-report.pdf

British Association for the Study of the Liver: www.basl.org.uk/

American Association for the Study of Liver Diseases: Practice guidelines on chronic hepatitis B: www.aasld.org/practice-guidelines/chronic-hepatitis-b

Public Health England: Interim guidance on the public health management and control of acute hepatitis B: https://assets.publishing.service.gov.uk/government/uploads/system/uploads/attachment_data/file/843970/Interim_guidance_on_the_public_health_management_control_of_acute_hepatitis_B.pdf

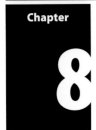

Chapter

8

Hepatitis C Virus

The Virus

Hepatitis C virus (HCV) is a single-stranded RNA virus belonging to the family Flaviviridae to which flaviruses like dengue and yellow fever viruses also belong. There is one serotype but up to eight different genotypes (1–8) have been described so far. Some of the genotypes are further divided into subtypes. For example, there are two subtypes to HCV genotypes 1 and 3 (e.g. 1a, 1b and 3a, 3b).

The genotypes were important because initially the treatment response depended upon the infecting genotype; however, now there are many direct acting antivirals (DAA) which are equally effective against all HCV genotypes. Genotypes and subtypes are still important epidemiological tools, as some are geographically limited in their distribution. In the UK most of the infections are due to genotypes 1a, 1b, 2 and 3. In Egypt and Central and West Africa genotype 4 predominates. Genotype 5 is most common in South Africa and genotype 6 is predominant in China and Southeast Asia.

Epidemiology

Prevalence

The World Health Organization (WHO) estimates that there are about 58 million people worldwide living with HCV infection. There are approximately 1.5 million new infections and 290,000 deaths every year globally. The HCV prevalence is not uniform throughout the population and varies according to risk and lifestyle.

In the UK in 2020, 81,000 were living with chronic HCV infection of which 27% were current or recent persons who inject drugs (PWIDs), 62% were past PWIDs and 11% constituted others who did not have a history of recent or past drug use. Therefore, in total, 89% of cases are in past or present PWIDs.

Route of Spread

As for hepatitis B, exposure to infected blood and secretions contaminated with infected blood is the main route of transmission through:

- *Blood and blood product transfusion*
  In the UK, the virus was transmitted to >90% of haemophiliacs through contaminated factor VIII prior to the introduction of screening of blood for HCV. An outbreak of HCV also occurred in Ireland related to a batch of contaminated immunoglobulin.

- *PWIDs*

  In the UK intravenous substance use (drug use) accounts for most of the infected cases and the prevalence of chronic HCV infection in PWIDs in 2020 was reported as 17.3%; this reduction in the past decade has been due to effective treatment rather than harm reduction. Sharing of contaminated equipment is the main cause.
- *Iatrogenic (through medical treatment)*

  Reuse of needles, syringes and sharp instruments without proper sterilisation for medical treatment in developing countries has been responsible for the spread of the virus. Egypt had a high rate of HCV infection because of the reported reuse of needles during the national vaccination campaign to eliminate shistosomiasis (bilharzia), a parasitic infection.

There are case reports of infection being passed on to patients from:

- Infected healthcare workers during surgical treatment (performance of exposure-prone procedures).
- Organ and tissue donation from infected donors prior to HCV screening being introduced resulted infection in the recipient.
- Renal dialysis if proper precautions are not followed. Outbreaks and high HCV prevalence in dialysed patients have been reported, but transmission in UK units is rare.
- *Occupational, for example healthcare workers (HCWs)*

  Infection can be transmitted after a sharps or needle stick injury from a source patient to an HCW. The risk of transmission after exposure to HCV-positive blood is approximately 3% and depends upon the level of viraemia, that is, the HCV viral load in the blood of the source patient.
- *Ear and body piercing, tattooing*

  Due to use of contaminated equipment.
- *Sexual* and *vertical (from mother to baby)* transmission may also occur but to a much lesser degree than hepatitis B. Babies born to HCV RNA–positive mothers have a 5% risk of being infected.

Incubation Period

The average incubation period from exposure to development of infection is 2–6 weeks, but may be as long as 3 months.

Infectious Period

About 80% of patients who acquire HCV infection go on to become chronically infected and infectious throughout their lifetime if untreated.

At-Risk Groups

PWIDs, HCWs, people who have received blood and blood products (although in developed countries where blood is now routinely screened for HCV this is no longer a risk), hospitalised patients (because of iatrogenic spread), patients at risk due to their lifestyle (body piercing, tattooing, multiple sexual partners) and babies born to HCV-infected mothers.

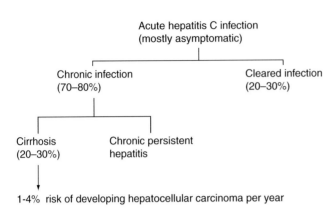

Figure 8.1 Clinical course of hepatitis C infection

Clinical

Symptoms

The vast majority of acute infections are asymptomatic; symptoms when they do occur are malaise, fatigue, nausea and jaundice. Only 20% of patients clear the virus after an acute infection and the majority (about 70–80%) will go on to develop chronic HCV infection. Patients with chronic HCV infection do not have specific symptoms but ongoing malaise and fatigue may occur many years after infection. About 20–30% of those with chronic infection will go on to develop cirrhosis of the liver after 20–30 years, a small proportion of whom will develop hepatocellular carcinoma (see Figure 8.1).

Older age at infection, male sex and associated liver damage due to alcohol and co-infection with other hepatitis viruses are factors leading to a poor prognosis.

Laboratory Diagnosis

See Table 8.1.

As most infections are asymptomatic, diagnosis of acute infection is not normally made and the majority of 'new' infections that are diagnosed are in those who have chronic infection. The HCV antibody test is used for screening of infection; a positive result denotes HCV infection but cannot distinguish between an acute or chronic HCV infection. Seroconversion from negative to positive HCV antibody is the only way to confirm an acute hepatitis C infection.

Management

Pegylated interferon and ribavirin were the first two drugs to be used for treatment of HCV infection and had response rates of 50–80% depending on the infecting HCV genotype. With the availability of numerous direct-acting antivirals (DAAs), which have come on the market in the last decade, the treatment of HCV has advanced tremendously from the initial two-drug treatment. The DAAs can be classified into those that:

- act on RNA-dependent RNA polymerase non-structural protein NS5B protein (examples are sofosbuvir and dasabuvir);
- act on non-structural protein NS5A (examples are pibfentasvir, ombitasvir, elbasvir, velapatasvir, ledispasvir); and

Table 8.1 Laboratory diagnosis of HCV infection

Clinical indication	Specimen	Test	Significance	Essential information for laboratory
Screening for acute or chronic HCV infection	5–10 ml of clotted venous blood or dried blood spot	Hepatitis C antibody and HCV NAAT* if antibody positive	Positive result indicates infection, initial screen MUST be confirmed by repeat testing. There is no HCV-specific IgM test available to distinguish acute from chronic infection.	Risk factors for infection, history of recent exposure to hepatitis C if any, clinical symptoms if present.
For establishing infection status of HCV antibody–positive patient	5–10 ml of clotted blood sample	Hepatitis C NAAT for HCV RNA. Mostly quantitative PCR (viral load) assay with a limit of detection of <15 IU/ml.	Positive result indicates either acute or chronic infection. Negative result indicates clearance of infection either naturally or post treatment.	As above + any history of treatment
Clinical follow-up of infected patient for treatment	5–10 ml of clotted blood sample	Hepatitis C genotype determination	In some settings HCV genotype will guide treatment decisions. However, due to availability of pan-genotype direct-acting antivirals, pre-treatment genotype analysis is not always required if these drugs are being used.	As above
Monitoring treatment response	5–10 ml of clotted blood sample	Quantitative hepatitis C PCR (viral load)	Negative PCR at week post treatment indicates sustained virus response (SVR)	Treatment history with date of start of treatment

Note: * NAAT – nucleic acid amplification test; of which PCR is most commonly used.

- are non-structural protein 3/4A protease inhibitors (examples are glecaprevir, paritaprevir, voxilaprevir and grazoprevir).

Treatment is recommended for all infected patients, whether treatment-naïve, with previous history of failed treatment or those who got reinfected. Patients should be referred to a specialist or a specialist centre for treatment of HCV infection as the treatment regime and follow-up are complicated and depend upon the infecting HCV genotype, presence of clinical liver disease, renal impairment, HIV co-infection and whether the patient is treatment-naïve or with history of previous failed treatment.

The goal of many treatment regimens is to increase the sustained virological response (SVR) rate, improve drug tolerability and shorten the duration of treatment. Combination treatment with two or more differently acting DAAs have shown SVR rates of up to >90% for HCV genotypes. Of those who achieve an SVR at week 12 of treatment, 99% will clear the virus. Pan-genotypic regimens (effective against all six HCV 1–6 genotypes) are available and deploy combination of differently acting DAAs in a single pill, achieving a 100% SVR rate for some of the genotypes. Chronic HCV infection therefore has become potentially eradicable, especially with recent drug trials starting in paediatric HCV-infected patients. The WHO has a global elimination target for HCV infection by 2030. HCV genotype determination may not necessarily be required if using pan-genotypic treatment regimens. However, genotype determination may be required in some patients because about 10–15% of HCV genotype 1 infected patients have resistance to NS5A inhibitors; this is particularly an issue with HCV 1a. Treatment regimens using NS5A inhibitors alone or in combination may not be as effective in this group of patients, therefore genotyping and resistance testing is recommended.

Older age at treatment, male sex, continuing alcohol consumption, high HCV viral load at initiation of treatment and infection with HCV genotype 1 are all poor prognostic factors for treatment response. However, with combination treatments these have become less of an issue.

The reader should refer to guidelines by the American Association for the Study of Liver Diseases (AASLD), the European Association for Study of Liver Disease (EASL), the British Association for Study of Liver Disease (BASL) and WHO guidelines for up-to-date treatment regimens recommended.

Prophylaxis

There is no vaccination available for hepatitis C despite active research going on in this area for the past 10–15 years. There is no passive prophylaxis in the form of specific immunoglobulin available either.

Infection Control

Infection control is the key to prevention and depends on:

- Screening and testing of blood and organ donors to exclude those who are infected and heat-treating blood products (plasma) to inactivate the virus.
- Implementing appropriate controls to prevent iatrogenic transmission. These include proper sterilisation of instruments before reuse, exclusion of infected HCWs from performing exposure-prone procedures and appropriate control measures in the renal dialysis units.
- Education of people at risk (e.g. PWIDs) for risk reduction including detoxification and needle exchange programmes. Reinfection rates of up to 8% have been described in PWIDs where risk behaviour continues.

Useful Websites

Hepatitis C Guidance 2019 Update: American Association for the Study of Liver Diseases–Infectious Diseases Society of America recommendations for testing, managing, and treating hepatitis C virus infection: https://doi.org/10.1002/hep.31060

EASL recommendations on treatment of hepatitis C: Final update of the series – *Journal of Hepatology*: https://doi.org/10.1016/j.jhep.2020.08.018

BASL: www.basl.org.uk/index.cfm/content/page/cid/3

WHO updated recommendations on treatment of adolescents and children with chronic HCV infection, and HCV simplified service delivery and diagnostics: www.who.int/publications/i/item/9789240052734

Chapter

9

Hepatitis E Virus

The Virus

Hepatitis E virus (HEV) is an RNA virus that is classified into the family Hepesviridae. There are at least four genotypes of the virus that can infect humans. Genotypes 1 and 2 only infect humans and genotypes 3 and 4 have animals as their reservoir and therefore are zoonotic infections.

Epidemiology

Route of Spread

HEV genotypes 1 and 2 are endemic and cause outbreaks in Southeast Asia, northern and central Africa, India and Central America, usually transmitted by the faecal-oral route due to faecal contamination of water or food. Outbreaks of epidemic hepatitis E commonly occur after heavy rainfalls, especially monsoons, because flooding can cause sewage to contaminate water supplies. Direct person-to-person transmission is uncommon. By contrast, genotypes 3 and 4 cause sporadic cases acquired zoonotically either from direct contact with animals (usually pigs) or indirectly from contaminated water or undercooked or raw pig and game meat, processed pork and shellfish.

Prevalence

Hepatitis E virus occurs worldwide and causes around 20 million infections a year. These result in around 3 million acute illnesses and 40,000 deaths. Most infections are asymptomatic, especially in children; symptomatic HEV infection is most commonly seen in men aged 15–35 years of age. HEV is a major cause of illness and death in the developing world and is a disproportionate cause of deaths among pregnant women.

The infection was first reported from the Indian subcontinent and subsequently from other parts of Asia, the Middle East, Central and South America, Africa, Central Europe and Russia. Increasingly, hepatitis E is being seen in developed nations. All the cases reported from the West have been due to genotype 3 of HEV for which pigs are the main reservoir. People travelling to countries with high prevalence are at risk of acquiring infection during their travel.

Genotype 1 has been isolated from many countries in Asia and Africa and genotype 2 has been isolated from Mexico, Nigeria and Chad and often associated with large outbreaks and epidemics in developing countries with poor sanitation conditions. Genotype 3 has been isolated almost worldwide including Asia, Europe, Oceania and North and South America and genotype 4 is found in Asia and indigenous cases from Europe. Genotypes 3 and 4 infect humans, pigs, and other animal species and have been responsible for sporadic cases of hepatitis E.

An increase in the number of non-travel cases of hepatitis E was detected in England and Wales in 2010. An epidemiological study implicated the consumption of processed pork products. A 2014 study found that more than 90% of British pigs were anti-HEV antibody positive. A 10-year retrospective surveillance study looked at data from 2008 to 2017 and found that non-travel-associated cases are likely to be older men, infected with HEV genotype 3 strain (related to the pig strain). Consumption of pork and pork products was significantly higher among patients with hepatitis E than in the general population.

Incubation Period

The average incubation period of hepatitis E is 40 days, ranging from 2 to 8 weeks.

Infectious Period

Virus has been detected in the faeces during the acute phase of disease but the exact infectivity period is not known.

At-Risk Groups

Travellers to countries where infection is endemic are at risk. Pregnant women and their unborn children are particularly at risk of complications due to HEV infection, who can develop an acute form of the disease that is fatal in 20% of cases or more in late pregnancy. Persons with chronic liver disease are also at risk of more severe symptoms if they acquire HEV infection.

Clinical

Acute Hepatitis

Clinical presentation is indistinguishable from other viral hepatitis and comprises of nausea, tiredness, myalgia, malaise, fever and occasionally joint pains accompanied by jaundice, dark urine and pale stools and tenderness in the right upper quadrant of the abdomen. The symptomatic phase coincides with raised levels of hepatic aminotransferase enzymes. Like hepatitis A, HEV is usually an acute and self-limiting infection with low death rates in more economically developed countries. Most infections are asymptomatic. However, it can be more severe in pregnant women and immunosuppressed people with substantially higher death rates. In pregnant women, especially in the third trimester, the disease is more often severe and is associated with fulminant liver failure, with maternal death rates around 20%, with other complications such as preterm delivery, abortion, stillbirth and neonatal death.

Chronic Hepatitis

Chronic HEV hepatitis occurs in immunocompromised persons, especially organ transplant recipients, which can be diagnosed after 3 months of continuous viremia. Chronic infection may result in a life-threatening illness such as fulminant liver failure or liver cirrhosis.

Table 9.1 Laboratory diagnosis of hepatitis E infection

Clinical indication	Specimen	Test	Significance	Essential information for laboratory
Acute hepatitis	Clotted venous blood, 5–10 ml	Hepatitis E IgM	Becomes positive within first week of acute hepatitis and remains positive for up to 3 months, sometimes for longer. Signifies acute infection.*	Clinical symptoms, relevant epidemiology, date of onset of illness.
		NAAT**	Finding HEV RNA confirms recent infection (except in immunocompromised persons who can have prolonged carriage)	
Check immune status	As above	Hepatitis E IgG	Becomes positive from a week to 2 weeks after onset of illness. When detected alone, for example without IgM, signifies immunity to infection due to past infection.	Must state if the test is to check immune status or to rule out acute infection, for latter see above.

Notes: * If HEV IgM is the only positive laboratory finding, it should be interpreted with caution unless the result value is high and/or accompanied by HEV IgG.
** NAAT – nucleic acid amplification test; of which PCR is most commonly used.

Laboratory Diagnosis

HEV RNA becomes detectable in faeces and blood during the incubation period. Serum HEV IgM and IgG antibodies appear just before the onset of clinical symptoms. Recovery leads to virus clearance from the blood, while the virus may persist in faeces much longer. IgM antibodies persist for several weeks after the acute infection, when increased levels of IgG antibodies are found.

See Table 9.1.

Other laboratory investigations include liver function tests and liver ultrasound.

Management

Treatment

There is no specific treatment in immunocompetent persons. Ribavirin, along with reduction in dose of immunosuppressive drugs, can be used to treat chronic infection in solid organ transplant recipients.

Prophylaxis

There is no vaccine or passive prophylaxis available; avoidance of infection is the only preventative measure.

Infection Control

In hospital, strict hand washing should be adhered to and where possible patients should be put in a single room. During the first 2 weeks of hepatitis E illness, infected persons should avoid preparing food for and limit contact with others if possible, especially pregnant women, or people with chronic liver disease. Close contacts should wash hands thoroughly with soap and warm water and then dry properly after contact with an infected person and wash hands after going to the toilet and before preparing, serving and eating food.

Herpes Simplex Virus

The Virus

Herpes simplex virus (HSV) is a double-stranded DNA virus and a member of the Herpesviridae family of viruses. There are two types of HSV, HSV type 1 and HSV type 2. HSV-2 is associated with genital infection, whereas HSV-1 causes infection in other sites.

Epidemiology

Route of Spread

HSV is transmitted by sexual contact and skin/genital/eye contact with infected secretions or HSV skin lesions. Transmission can occur from asymptomatic or symptomatic persons with primary or recurrent HSV infection or reactivation.

Prevalence

HSV infection occurs worldwide and the prevalence of infection varies considerably. According to the World Health Organization globally 3.7 billion people under the age of 50 years have HSV-1 infection. Prevalence is highest in low- and middle-income countries, HSV seroprevalence being >90% in many of those populations. In the high-income countries the prevalence has declined especially in young adults and adolescents, hence putting them at risk of primary HSV infection later in life.

Incubation Period

2–12 days (mean 4 days).

Infectious Period

From the onset of symptoms until the lesions are fully crusted or resolved.

At-Risk Groups

- Immunocompromised persons
- Neonates
- Pregnant women
- Sexually active adults

- Those who participate in contact sport
- Patients with atopic dermatitis are at risk of disseminated skin lesions called eczema herpeticum

Clinical

Symptoms

Primary HSV infection occurs when a person first encounters the virus. It first infects an area of skin, then the virus travels down a sensory nerve and establishes a latent infection in the dorsal route ganglia and becomes dormant. Primary HSV infection is generally asymptomatic, especially if acquired in childhood but may present as mucocutaneous skin lesions.

Most infected persons do not experience a reactivated infection, where the virus reactivates and causes another clinical episode at the site of the primary infection. However, many do and some experience frequent recurrences (e.g. cold sores on the lip).

HSV can infect various sites in the body. The most severe infection is HSV encephalitis which has a 70% mortality if untreated. Infection in immunocompromised patients can be severe or fatal.

- *Skin*
  HSV causes fluid-filled skin blisters (vesicles) which can sometimes be difficult to distinguish from varicella-zoster virus (VZV) infection.
- *Mouth and lips*
  Primary infection in children often occurs in the mouth and on the lips. Infection can be missed unless severe gingivostomatitis is present. Reactivated infection is usually seen as a cold sore on the lip.
- *Genitals*
  HSV causes vesicles and shallow ulcers on the labia, cervix, penis and perianally. Genital HSV-1 infection in the West is now as common as HSV-2 infection, primary HSV-1 infection being transmitted mainly through oral genital sex.
- *Encephalitis*
  This is the most severe HSV infection, which is often severe or fatal and requires prompt treatment and diagnosis.
- *Meningitis*
  Usually associated with HSV-2.
- *Eye infection*
  HSV causes keratoconjunctivitis in the eye, which is mainly as a result of reactivation of latent infection. Repeated reactivated infection of the cornea can cause corneal scarring and blindness.
- *Pneumonitis*
  This is rarely seen in immunocompetent persons. It is usually a reactivation of latent infection in immunocompromised patients (e.g. after lung transplantation).
- *Neonatal herpes*
  Babies who acquire HSV infection from the mother's genital tract at the time of delivery (vertical transmission from mother to baby) are at risk of severe or fatal

Table 10.1 Laboratory diagnosis of HSV infection

Clinical indication	Specimens	Test	Interpretation of positive result
Skin lesion	Vesicle fluid	NAAT	Indicates HSV-1 or HSV-2 infection
Encephalitis or meningitis	Cerebrospinal fluid (CSF)	NAAT	Indicates HSV-1 or HSV-2 infection
Eye lesions	Corneal swab	NAAT	Indicates HSV-1 or HSV-2 infection
Pneumonitis	Bronchoalveolar lavage	NAAT	Indicates HSV-1 or HSV-2 infection
Neonatal herpes	Skin swab, mouth, nose and eye swab and CSF	NAAT	Indicates HSV-1 or HSV-2 infection
Has the patient had HSV infection before?	Clotted blood	HSV-2 – and HSV-2-specific IgG test	Indicates previous HSV-1 or HSV-2 infection

neonatal HSV infection. Most neonatal infection is acquired perinatally but postnatal and intrauterine transmission can also occur. Babies delivered vaginally to mothers who have primary HSV genital lesions at the time of delivery are at the highest risk; however, HSV reinfection or asymptomatic viral shedding from the genital tract poses a risk of vertical transmission as well. For this reason, caesarean delivery should be considered.

Expert specialist advice on the mode of delivery, treatment and prophylaxis should be sought as soon as possible, as management depends upon risk assessment of vertical transmission.

Differential Diagnosis

Vesicular skin lesions caused by HSV can be mistaken as VZV infection. HSV lesions are usually all at the same stage of development in the same cluster.

Chickenpox usually causes widespread lesions, especially on the body, with vesicles at various stages of development in one cluster. Shingles vesicles are usually confined to an area of skin (dermatome) on one side of the body served by a sensory nerve (although immunosuppressed patients can have much more extensive lesions).

Laboratory Diagnosis

See Table 10.1.

NAAT (nucleic acid amplification test; of which PCR is most commonly used) for detection of HSV-1 and HSV-2 is the mainstay of diagnosis.

Herpes encephalitis and neonatal HSV infection are medical emergencies and an urgent NAAT should be requested for rapid diagnosis; however, initiation of treatment should not wait for the result of the NAAT.

Table 10.2 Antiviral treatment for HSV infection*

Clinical indication	Drug
HSV skin or genital infection in immunocompetent patients	Oral aciclovir, valaciclovir or famciclovir
	Aciclovir cream
HSV skin infection in immunocompromised patients	Oral aciclovir, valaciclovir or famciclovir
Severe HSV skin infection in immunocompromised and immunocompetent patients	IV Aciclovir
HSV encephalitis	IV Aciclovir
Genital HSV infection in pregnancy. Treatment and suppression of genital HSV infection in pregnancy	Oral aciclovir or valaciclovir
Neonatal herpes simplex infection	IV aciclovir
HSV corneal infection	Aciclovir Eye ointment
Prevention of HSV recurrence (including genital herpes) in immunocompetent patients with frequent recurrences	Oral aciclovir or valaciclovir
Prevention of HSV recurrence in immunocompromised patients and neonates at high risk of severe infection	IV/oral aciclovir or valaciclovir

Clotted blood/HSV antibody tests are not useful in the diagnosis of acute HSV infection.

Management

Treatment

See Table 10.2.

Oral aciclovir is cheaper than other oral forms of treatment as it is available in generic formulation. Rarely, other antivirals (e.g. foscarnet or adefovir) may be useful, especially in immunocompromised patients with aciclovir-resistant HSV infection (see Chapter 54).

Prophylaxis*

Some HSV antibody–positive groups of patients (e.g. lung transplant, bone marrow transplant and HIV-positive patients) will require antiviral prophylaxis to prevent severe or potentially fatal HSV reactivation disease.

---

* Note: Check nationally agreed protocols or drug data sheets before initiating treatment or prophylaxis.

Infection Control

HSV is transmitted by close personal contact and is rarely associated with infection control problems. However, healthcare staff who have HSV skin lesions on their hands should cover them with a waterproof dressing to avoid transmitting infection to patients and those with severe lesions should seek Infection Control/Occupational Health advice before working in direct patient contact, especially with immunocompromised patients.

HIV and AIDS

The Virus

HIV (human immunodeficiency virus) is an RNA virus and belongs to the genus *lentivirus* (*lenti*: slow) within the family Retroviridae (*retro*: backwards), so called because viruses (including HIV) in the family possess a reverse transcriptase enzyme to convert the viral RNA template into DNA which integrates in the cellular DNA to cause persistent infection. The other virus in the genus *lentivirus* is simian immunodeficiency virus (SIV) which infects monkeys.

There are two known HIV viruses which cause human infection: HIV-1 and HIV-2. Three groups of HIV-1 have been identified on the basis of differences in the envelope region: M, N and O. Group M is the most prevalent and is subdivided into eight subtypes (or clades), based on the whole genome, and which are geographically distinct. The most prevalent are subtypes B (found mainly in North America and Europe), A and D (found mainly in Africa) and C (found mainly in Africa and Asia); these subtypes form branches in the phylogenetic tree representing the lineage of the M group of HIV-1.

For practical purposes these viruses are collectively referred to as HIV as the mode of spread and clinical manifestations are indistinguishable.

Epidemiology

Route of Spread

HIV is closely related to SIV which has evolved into many strains, classified by the natural host species. SIV infects African green monkeys (SIVagm) and sooty mangabeys (SIVsmm) which have a long evolutionary history with their hosts. See Table 11.1 for the three main routes of spread of HIV.

Prevalence

HIV has a worldwide prevalence, although some regions (e.g. Africa and Asia) are more heavily affected than others. In 2021, 38.4 million people worldwide were living with HIV, including 2 million children. Acquired immunodeficiency syndrome (AIDS)–related deaths have reduced by 68% since the peak of 2004, as a result of better availability of antiretroviral therapy (ART) and other targeted interventions. There were 1.5 million new infections in 2021, with 28.7 million accessing ART. There were 2,630 new HIV diagnoses in the UK in 2020, 45% in gay/bisexual men and 26% in women.

HIV-2 is confined to small numbers, mainly in West Africa and a lower prevalence of infection in European countries with links to western Africa (e.g. Portugal and Belgium).

Table 11.1 Three main routes of spread of HIV

Mode of spread	Risk groups
Sexual: HIV is a sexually transmitted infection (STI). Virus is present in semen and cervical secretions. Unprotected penetration sexual intercourse has a high risk of transmission. Coexistent ulcerative STIs like herpes increase risk of transmission.	Globally, the most common mode of HIV transmission is via sexual contacts between people of the opposite sex; however, the pattern of transmission varies among countries. Men who have sex with men has been by far the major route of transmission in the Western world. For heterosexuals the main source of transmission is Central Sub-Saharan Africa, and Southeast Asia and the Indian subcontinent.
Vertical (mother to child): 25% rate of transmission, but with intervention (see management section) risk can be reduced to <1%. Risk is highest if mother has high HIV viral load.	In utero – transmission may occur but this can be reduced with antenatal antiretroviral therapy. Perinatal – the majority of infections are transmitted at the time of delivery due to exposure of the fetus to contaminated maternal secretions. Premature or prolonged rupture of membranes increases the risk. Postnatal – via breast milk. Breastfeeding increases the risk of transmission by up to 28%.
Blood-borne	Blood and blood products and organ donation. Blood transfusion with contaminated material has a high risk of transmission. This route has been virtually eliminated from developed countries by HIV screening of all donors. Persons who inject drugs, persons having tattoos and body piercing and using unsterile and contaminated equipment. Needlestick injuries to healthcare workers. Healthcare-associated HIV infection has been transmitted in the healthcare setting from both healthcare workers to patients and vice versa. Overall risk of transmission after a needlestick injury is 0.3%, risk being highest if injury is with a hollow needle used to withdraw blood from an infected patient with a high viral load.

Incubation Period

2–4 weeks, but may be as long as 3 months.

Pathogenesis

HIV infects cells in the human immune system, such as helper T-cells (specifically $CD4^+$ T-cells), macrophages and dendritic cells by the interaction of the virion envelope glycoproteins (gp120) with the CD4 molecule on the target cells' membrane and also with chemokine co-receptors (CCR5 and CXCR4) which are required to gain entry to these cells. Once inside the cell, the RNA is transcribed into DNA which integrates in the cellular DNA. HIV infection leads to low levels of $CD4^+$ T-cells through a number of mechanisms, including pyroptosis of abortively infected T-cells, apoptosis of uninfected bystander cells, direct viral killing of infected cells and killing of infected $CD4^+$ T-cells by $CD8^+$ cytotoxic lymphocytes that recognize infected cells. When CD4$^+$ T-cell numbers decline below a critical level cell-mediated immunity is lost, and the body becomes progressively more susceptible to opportunistic infections, leading to the development of AIDS.

Infectious Period

Infectivity is highest during the acute illness or seroconversion phase and once full-blown AIDS develops, for example at times when there is high HIV viral load in the blood. Patients are infectious throughout life, but as infectivity is related to the level of viraemia those with undetectable viral load are not infectious.

At-Risk Groups

These depend on the likely mode of transmission:

- *Sexual*: those engaging in either homosexual or heterosexual unprotected intercourse with frequent and casual sexual partners.
- *Vertical*: babies born to infected mothers.
- *Blood/blood borne*: persons who inject drugs (PWIDs), those undergoing tattoos and body piercing, iatrogenic through unscreened blood or blood products and from infected healthcare workers to patients or vice versa during exposure-prone procedures.

Clinical

Both HIV-1 and HIV-2 cause clinically indistinguishable illness; however, HIV-2 progresses far more slowly to AIDS.

Acute HIV Seroconversion Illness

Acute HIV infection is the earliest stage of HIV infection. During this time, some people have flu-like or glandular fever–like symptoms, such as fever, headache and rash (seroconversion illness) and HIV multiplies rapidly and spreads throughout the body. During the acute HIV infection stage, the level of HIV in the blood is very high, which greatly increases the risk of HIV transmission. A person may experience significant health benefits if they start ART during this stage.

Chronic HIV Infection

The second phase of HIV infection is chronic HIV infection (also called clinical latency), where HIV continues to multiply in the body, but at very low levels. People with chronic infection may not have any HIV-related symptoms and they usually have a normal CD4 lymphocyte count. Without ART, chronic HIV infection usually progresses to AIDS in about 10 years. People who are taking ART may have their HIV infection stabilised in this phase for many years and if they have an undetectable viral load at this time, the risk of transmission to others is extremely low.

AIDS

AIDS is the most severe and final phase of HIV infection, when HIV has severely damaged the immune system, leading to opportunistic infections (e.g. *Pneumocystis jiroveci* pneumonia, *Toxoplasma gondii*, cytomegalovirus) and other AIDS-defining illnesses taking hold. People with HIV are diagnosed with AIDS if they have a CD4 count of fewer than 200 cells per mm^3 or if they have certain AIDS-defining illnesses. At this stage, people usually have a very high viral load and can transmit to others.

AIDS-defining illnesses can be grouped under:

Viral

- Cytomegalovirus – retinitis, gastrointestinal infection, central nervous system (CNS) infection
- Varicella zoster virus – shingles
- Progressive multifocal leukoencephalopathy
- Herpes simplex virus: chronic ulcer(s) (more than 1 month in duration), bronchitis, pneumonitis or esophagitis
- Epstein–Barr virus (EBV) – lymphadenopathy, hairy oral leukoplakia

Bacterial

- *Mycobacterium avium* complex or *M kansasii*, disseminated or extrapulmonary
- *Mycobacterium tuberculosis*, any site (pulmonary or extrapulmonary)
- Mycobacterium, other species or unidentified species, disseminated or extrapulmonary

Fungal

- *Pneumocystis jiroveci* pneumonia
- *Candia albicans* – oral, oesophageal thrush
- *Cryptococcus neoformans* – meningitis
- Coccidioidomycosis, disseminated or extrapulmonary
- Histoplasmosis, disseminated or extrapulmonary

Parasites

- *Toxoplasma gondii* – CNS infection, lymphadenopathy
- *Cryptosporidium* – chronic gastrointestinal infection
- Isosporiasis, chronic intestinal (more than 1 month in duration)

Malignancies

- Kaposi's sarcoma – endothelial sarcoma driven by human herpes virus 8
- EBV-driven lymphomas
- Non-Hodgkin's lymphoma
- Carcinoma of the uterus or cervix

Laboratory Diagnosis

HIV antibody: HIV is a chronic infection in 100% of cases and the virus persists in the presence of antibodies so antibody positivity is indicative of infection and HIV antibody tests are used as the screening test for infection. Most current screening tests also detect an antigen, p24, which greatly reduces the window period following infection when the virus cannot be detected using antibody tests alone. Because no test is 100% specific

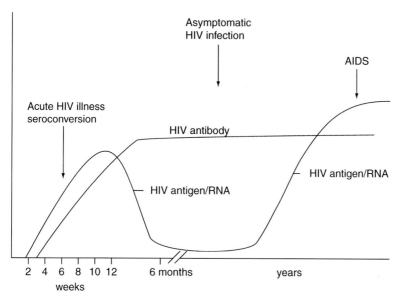

Figure 11.1 Diagrammatic representation of HIV serological markers in acute and chronic infection

positive, results MUST be confirmed by a battery of tests and by testing a repeat follow-up sample.

HIV p24 antigen: Appears 3–7 days before the antibody and is therefore helpful in making an early diagnosis in acute HIV infection (Figure 11.1). Testing for HIV antigen reduces the so-called window period which is the time from infection to a positive HIV antibody test (Figure 11.1).

HIV RNA nucleic acid amplification test (NAAT) (usually PCR): Used to diagnose acute infection and then to monitor the progression of disease and treatment response. The goal of treatment is complete suppression of viral replication (as denoted by negative PCR); a positive HIV RNA PCR in patients on treatment may indicate non-compliance to therapy or drug resistance and change of drug regimen.

HIV RNA PCR is done on EDTA blood sample. The plasma must be separated within 6 hours for testing so inform the laboratory before taking samples.

HIV RNA viral load: Used to quantitate how much HIV RNA is circulating in an infected person's bloodstream. This test should be done soon after the initial HIV diagnosis and at intervals to reveal the response to ART. Persons with HIV should have their viral load assessed within 6 weeks of commencing ART.

Genotypic resistance test: Detects the presence of specific genetic mutations that are known to cause resistance to drugs to treat HIV.

Persons newly diagnosed with HIV should have a genotypic resistance test performed within 3 months of first diagnosis.

Table 11.2 summarises the laboratory diagnosis of HIV.

Diagnosis of Congenital/Vertical HIV Infection in Neonates
Diagnosis of congenital/vertical HIV infection requires testing for HIV RNA or DNA NAAT (PCR) at birth, 6 weeks and 12 weeks followed by an antibody test at 18 months

Table 11.2 Laboratory diagnosis of HIV infection

Clinical indication	Test	Significance
Acute HIV infection or suspected seroconversion	HIV antibody and antigen HIV NAAT (RNA)	Positive result indicates infection. Result must be confirmed by testing a repeat follow-up specimen.
HIV screening	HIV antibody (must use the most sensitive available assay)	The initial positive assay result must be confirmed by other tests and by testing a repeat follow-up specimen.
Neonatal HIV infection	NAAT for HIV viral DNA or HIV RNA	HIV RNA or HIV DNA nucleic acid tests that directly detect HIV must be used to diagnose HIV in infants and children aged <18 months with perinatal and postnatal HIV exposure; HIV antibody and HIV antigen/antibody tests should also be used (see current guidance for test timings). Plasma HIV RNA or cell-associated HIV DNA PCRs are generally equally recommended. However, the results of plasma HIV RNA or plasma HIV RNA/DNA PCR can be affected by ART drugs administered to the infant as prophylaxis or presumptive HIV therapy.
Follow-up of infected patients	Quantitative HIV RNA NAAT (PCR) (viral load)	High level is indication for treatment. Positive PCR in patients on treatment and with previously undetectable virus may indicate viral drug resistance or non-compliance to therapy.
	Genotypic resistance test	Detects the presence of specific genetic mutations that are known to cause resistance to drugs to treat HIV.

to show clearance of maternal antibody. A positive PCR or persistent of antibody beyond 18 months is indicative of vertically transmitted infection.

Management

Treatment

All people living with HIV should be on ART and those with newly diagnosed infection should be urgently assessed by an HIV specialist and offered treatment. Newly diagnosed persons should be offered a baseline genotypic resistance test and there should not be treatment interruptions. There are many antiretroviral drugs (and combinations of drugs) available now for treatment of HIV (Chapter 54). Current treatment guidelines (e.g. British HIV Association (BHIVA) antiretroviral treatment guidelines) should be consulted before treating HIV. As the virus develops drug resistance rapidly to single drugs these drugs are used in combination, referred to as ART. The treatment should be discussed in detail with the patient and drugs chosen to maximise compliance and minimise drug toxicity so as to avoid development of drug resistance.

Patients are monitored for response to therapy by regular testing for HIV RNA (viral load). Viral load falls rapidly, within 4–6 weeks of start of treatment, and the aim of the therapy is to maintain the viral load at an undetectable level. The fall in viral load is accompanied by a consequent improvement in immune system due to rise in CD4 cell count. Drug resistance due to viral mutations is heralded by a rise in viral load and calls for a change in drugs being used.

Patients need to be on the antiretroviral drugs lifelong but their use has changed the clinical outcome of infection with most patients living a normal life.

Treatment of HIV-Positive Pregnant Women and Their Babies

Antiretroviral therapy of pregnant mothers, followed by prophylactic treatment of the newborn, has reduced the incidence of vertical infection from about 25% to <3% provided that breastfeeding is also avoided.

All HIV-positive pregnant women, if not already on ART, should commence ART by week 24 of pregnancy (and sooner if they have a high viral load). Consult current guidelines.

Women with undetectable HIV viral load results should be supported in having a vaginal delivery and breastfeeding but Caesarean section should be the preferred option for those mothers with detectable HIV RNA (see current guidelines).

ART should be given to all babies born to HIV-positive mothers, with the drug regimen and length of treatment determined by the mother's viral load results (see current guidelines).

Intercurrent Infection/Disease

Treatment of opportunistic infections and malignancies is equally important and depends upon the presenting infection/disease.

Prophylaxis

There is no effective HIV vaccine. Vaccine research has been going on for many years but the biggest barrier to development of a successful vaccine is the inability of the host to develop protective antibody to the virus and the genetic variability of the virus and its ability to rapidly mutate.

Pre-exposure Prophylaxis

Pre-exposure prophylaxis (PrEP) is recommended for those individuals at increased risk of acquiring HIV (e.g. HIV-negative males who have sex with men (MSM) who participate in condomless sex, and HIV-negative people who have condomless heterosexual sex with HIV-positive partners). See latest guidelines.

Post-exposure Prophylaxis

Antiretroviral drugs are used for post-exposure prophylaxis (PEP) for:

- MSM who have had receptive anal sexual intercourse with a person known to be HIV positive or of unknown status;
- people who have had receptive vaginal intercourse with an index HIV-positive partner;

- healthcare workers sustaining accidental exposure or needlestick injuries from HIV-infected patients; and
- PWIDs with recent exposure to an HIV-positive index injecting partner.

Consult the latest guidance for ART and testing regimens.

Infection Control

The mainstays of prevention are:

- screening of all blood, organ and tissue donors and excluding the infected from donating;
- 'safe sex' and use of the barrier method for sexual intercourse;
- needle exchange schemes for PWIDs;
- PrEP for those at high risk of acquiring infection;
- PEP for those people at greatest risk of acquiring infection; and
- medical practices to reduce the risk of transmission.

Useful Websites

BHIVA/BASHH/BIA adult HIV testing guidelines 2020: https://doi.org/10.1111/hiv.13015

BHIVA current guidelines: www.bhiva.org/guidelines

BHIVA/BASHH guidelines on the use of HIV pre-exposure prophylaxis (PrEP) 2018: www.bhiva.org/PrEP-guidelines

BHIVA guidelines for the management of HIV in pregnancy and postpartum 2018 (2020 third interim update): www.bhiva.org/file/5f1aab1ab9aba/BHIVA-Pregnancy-guidelines-2020-3rd-interim-update.pdf

BASHH UK guidelines for the use of HIV post-exposure prophylaxis 2021: www.bashhguidelines.org/media/1265/pep-21.pdf

12

Human Coronaviruses (Including Covid-19, SARS and MERS)

The Viruses

Coronaviruses are single-stranded RNA viruses and belong to the family Coronaviridae. The outer surface protein of the virus projects from the virus surface as spikes (spike protein) giving the virus a crown-like appearance, hence the name coronavirus (see Figure 12.1, which shows an electron microscopic image of coronavirus). Coronaviruses fall into four distinct genera: alpha, beta, gamma and delta. Human coronaviruses (HCoV) are in two of these genera.

- Alpha coronaviruses include HCoV-229E and HCoV-NL63.
- Beta coronaviruses include HCoV-HKU1, HCoV-OC43, Middle East respiratory syndrome coronavirus (MERS-CoV), severe acute respiratory syndrome virus (SARS-CoV) and SARS-CoV-2, the etiological agent of the recent Covid-19 pandemic.

Coronaviruses are widespread among birds and mammals with bats being host to the largest variety. All human coronaviruses are likely to have animal origins, probably bats.

Coronaviruses cause respiratory illness but can be found in the human gut, although there is no clear disease association.

Route of Spread

Coronaviruses are spread by the respiratory route, by direct contact with large aerosol droplets and by small aerosol particle inhalation. Virus is also spread by touching contaminated surfaces and fomites and then touching eyes/mouth to provide a route of entry through the mucous membrane. In addition, SARS-CoV was shown to be spread by the faecal-oral route, probably through aerosolisation of infected faecal material.

Seasonal Human Coronaviruses (HCoV-229E, HCoV-NL63, HCoV-HKU1, HCoV-OC43)

Seasonal human coronaviruses (seasonal HCoV) have been around for decades and have a worldwide distribution. Almost all adults in the UK have been infected by at least one type of coronavirus. The incubation period is 2–5 days and patients are most infectious while symptomatic. Infection usually occurs in winter or spring and is associated with upper respiratory tract infection. These coronaviruses produce a range of symptoms from asymptomatic infection to upper respiratory symptoms (a 'cold'), malaise and fever. It is suggested that they are responsible for 5–10% of all colds in adults. They are also associated with lower respiratory tract infections (LRTIs) like bronchiolitis and

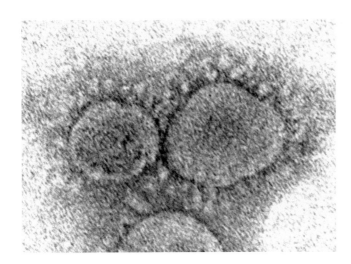

Figure 12.1 Electron microscopic image of a negatively stained particle of SARS-CoV-2 (courtesy of CDC)

pneumonitis in patients of all ages, but their role in pathogenesis of LRTIs is not clear as they are frequently found as co-pathogens rather than on their own.

The severity of illness is similar to that of rhinovirus infection but less severe than infection with respiratory syncytial virus or influenza viruses. Symptoms are usually more severe in elderly persons. Reinfection is common.

Parainfluenza, respiratory syncytial virus (RSV), adenovirus and HCoV and other respiratory viral infections should be considered in the differential diagnosis of all human respiratory infections. Laboratory diagnosis is by polymerase chain reaction (PCR) in respiratory samples/secretions and many laboratories now include PCR primers for testing these viruses in their respiratory PCR panel.

SARS-CoV

SARS stands for severe acute respiratory syndrome and is caused by SARS coronavirus (SARS-CoV). SARS-CoV caused a worldwide outbreak between March and July 2003; most cases occurred in hospital workers or family members in contact with cases. SARS-CoV had an incubation period of 2–7 days. There were over 8,000 cases reported from 32 countries. There was a smaller outbreak, probably associated with laboratory-released SARS-CoV, in 2004. There have been no more cases since then. The 2003 outbreak originated in Guangdong Province in China and is thought to have transmitted from the civet cat (a variety of wild cat) to humans with subsequent human-to-human spread. SARS-CoV causes high fever (>38°C), dry cough, shortness of breath, myalgia, headache and diarrhoea. Chest X-rays showed pneumonia or an acute respiratory distress syndrome–like picture. Symptoms were usually severe enough to warrant hospital admission. The overall fatality rate was 15% in outbreaks, higher in elderly patients and those with other respiratory conditions; less than 1% in persons less than 24 years of age, 6% in those aged 25–44 years, 15% in those aged 45–64 years and greater than 50% in persons aged 65 years or older.

SARS patients should be nursed inside rooms, preferably negative pressure rooms, with gloves, aprons and a respirator mask conforming to at least European standard EN149:2001 FFP3.

Diagnostic tests should be done in specialist reference laboratories with Category 4 diagnostic facilities. Lower respiratory tract secretions (e.g. bronchioalveolar lavage/ endotracheal secretions and a combined oropharyngeal/nasopharyngeal swab) should be tested by PCR. Serology on acute and convalescent sample can also be done.

MERS-CoV

The first case was described in 2012 from a man in Saudi Arabia who was admitted to hospital with pneumonia and acute kidney injury. Soon afterwards more cases were identified; all patients had a link to the Middle East. The etiological agent was identified as a novel coronavirus and the disease was named as Middle East respiratory syndrome (MERS) and the virus as MERS-CoV. An African variant of MERS-CoV has also been described. Dromedary camels are the natural host and humans get infected by close contacts with camels and drinking camel milk. Since 2012 several thousands of cases of MERS have been reported to the World Health Organization (WHO). Most cases have been reported from the Arabian Peninsula, especially Saudi Arabia, but cases have been reported from North Africa, Asia, Europe, the UK and North America. In countries outside of the Arabian Peninsula the cases occur in returning travellers or those with close contact with infected patients as human-to-human spread is well described with many case clusters and small outbreaks. As with other coronavirus MERS-CoV is spread by the respiratory route and can be shed in the respiratory secretions for weeks after infection. Clinically, MERS presents as severe pneumonia and acute respiratory distress syndrome, requiring mechanical ventilation. The mortality rate is around 30%. Symptoms include fever and chills, sore throat, cough, shortness of breath and myalgia. In addition, diarrhoea, vomiting and abdominal pain might also occur and some patients may show signs of acute kidney injury. The incubation period is between 2 and 7 days, but longer incubation periods of up to 12 days have been reported. The WHO recommends that MERS should be suspected and excluded in anyone who presents with respiratory illness within 14 days of return from the Arabian Peninsula and neighbouring countries.

MERS patients should be nursed in side rooms, preferably negative pressure rooms, with gloves, aprons and a respirator mask conforming to at least European standard EN149:2001 FFP3.

Diagnostic tests should be done in specialist reference laboratories with Category 4 diagnostic facilities. Lower respiratory tract secretions (e.g. bronchioalveolar lavage/ endotracheal secretions and a combined oropharyngeal/nasopharyngeal swab) should be tested by PCR. Serology on acute and convalescent samples can also be done.

SARS-CoV-2/Covid-19

Epidemiology

At the end of 2019, a novel coronavirus was identified as the causative agent of a cluster of cases of respiratory illness in Wuhan, China. The virus rapidly spread, causing a global pandemic in 2020. Viral sequencing identified the virus as a coronavirus, belonging to the genus betacoronavirus and in the same subgenus as SARS-CoV but in a different clade. It was subsequently designated as SARS-CoV-2 and the illness it caused as Covid-19 (an acronym for coronavirus disease 2019). Up to the first quarter of 2023, >600 million cases had occurred worldwide with >6 million reported deaths. Seroprevalence studies from the USA and Europe, however, suggest that case reports underestimate the disease incidence by almost tenfold. One study estimated that >3 billion, that is, 44% of the world's population, had been infected by SARS-CoV-2 at least once by 2023.

Since its introduction in humans in 2019, many variants of the virus have appeared (due to mutations), notably alpha, beta, delta and omicron.

The virus is constantly mutating and sublineage of these variants also appears. There is a programme of worldwide surveillance to monitor the appearance of these variants which are designated as 'variants of interest' if they possess genetic markers that predict their transmission capability or how well diagnostics/treatment/vaccines will work. In addition, a 'variant of concern' shows evidence of increased infectiousness or virulence or is divergent enough so that the existing vaccines are no longer protective.

As the virus is constantly mutating with emergence of new variants, reinfections are common but usually individuals are protected for the first 6–9 months after the initial infection. This though, is dependent upon the circulating variant, as it is not clear how much cross-protection may exist after infection by a previous variant. Reinfections are generally milder than initial infections but severe reinfections have been reported, especially in those with risk factors.

Route of Spread

The virus is shed in the respiratory secretions and the main route of transmission is by large aerosol droplets which have been shown not to travel beyond 2 metres. Airborne transmission also occurs via small aerosolised particles which are inhaled. In addition, transmission through infected fomites and environmental contamination occurs when these surfaces are touched by hand; the virus is then carried by touch to nose, mouth or eyes.

The virus gains entry into cells by host receptor angiotensin-converting enzyme 2 (ACE2) to which the virus spike protein binds.

Incubation Period

The incubation period can be variable, depending upon the infecting variant.

The average incubation period is 2–7 days. Most cases occur within 3–5 days, but may be as long as 10 days in some cases.

Infectivity Period

SARS-CoV-2 patients are infectious for up to 2 days before the onset of symptoms. The infectivity is highest at the peak of the symptoms. Most patients clear the virus by day 5–10 of illness but infectivity persists for much longer in immunocompromised patients. Transmission is highest in the household setting and other places where people congregate in closed areas. Outbreaks have occurred in cruise ships, nursing homes, college dormitories, homeless shelters, etc. However, many individuals do not report a specific contact.

Clinical Presentation
Adults

Up to 33% of cases can be asymptomatic. Symptomatic disease ranges from mild to moderate to severe/critical illness. Initial reports from China suggested that 80% of those infected had mild disease and about 20% had severe/critical illness with an overall case fatality rate of 2–3%.

Symptoms include fever of 38°C or greater, cough, myalgia/malaise, headache, sore throat, loss of sense of taste and smell, and mild upper respiratory tract symptoms like sneezing and nasal congestion. Pneumonia is the most serious manifestation and is defined by fever, cough, dyspnoea and bilateral lung infiltrates on chest X-ray. Typically, pneumonia develops 7–10 days after onset of symptoms.

Overall case fatality rate is reported to be 0.15–1% of all cases including those that are asymptomatic. The case fatality rate increases dramatically with age with 80% of all deaths being reported in those >65 years of age.

Complications of severe infection include respiratory failure, cardiac and cardiovascular complications (cardiac arrythmias, myocardial injury, heart failure and shock), venous thromboembolism and encephalopathy, especially in critically ill persons.

Those with mild symptoms recover quickly, usually within 2 weeks, but those with severe disease can take weeks or months to recover. Persistence of symptoms 3 months or beyond after first becoming ill is defined as long Covid syndrome. The most common persistent symptoms linked with long Covid are being described as fatigue, cough, not being able to think clearly (described as brain fog), dyspnoea, chest pain/tightness and nausea/vomiting. Among those with long Covid, 15% can experience symptoms for up to a year.

Children

Asymptomatic SARS-CoV-2 infection is common in children. Up to 60% of infected children show no symptoms. Symptoms when they occur are usually mild and, as in adults, consist of fever, cough, shortness of breath, myalgia, sore throat, headache and rhinorrhoea. A small number (2–5%) have moderately severe disease with pneumonia, which may require intensive care treatment.

Multisystem inflammatory syndrome in children (MIS-C) is a rare but serious complication of Covid-19. The clinical features may be similar to those of Kawasaki disease and toxic shock syndrome. They include persistent fever, hypotension, gastrointestinal symptoms, rash and myocarditis. It is thought to occur as a result of immune dysregulation resulting in abnormal immune response to the virus. The exact mechanism by which SARS-CoV-2 triggers this abnormal immune response is not clear.

Most children recover uneventfully but long Covid has been described especially in older children and teenagers.

At-Risk Groups

Immunosuppressed patients of all ages, elderly persons and those with other co-morbidities (e.g. obesity, diabetes mellitus, hypertension, cardiac and chronic kidney and lung disease). In pregnancy, SARS-CoV-2 infection poses a greater risk of pneumonia and fetal death or preterm labour.

The most severe and fatal infections of SARS CoV-2 were in older people >65 years of age. Risk of severe infection and mortality increases by every 5–10 years' increase in age. Data from the USA showed that compared to 18–29 years, the mortality rate was 3.5 times higher in ages 30–39 years and 360 times higher in those aged >85 years. Pre-existing chronic illness and obesity were additional factors for severe SARS-CoV-2 infections.

Management

Oral antiviral agent Paxlovid (a combination of two protease inhibitor drugs, nirmatrelvir and ritonavir) is available for treatment of acute Covid-19 infections in outpatient settings to reduce the risk of Covid-19–associated hospitalisation and death. It is recommended that treatment is started as soon as possible and not later than 5 days after onset of symptoms. The groups to consider for treatment are those at increased risk of complication (see the at-risk groups section) and anyone else without vaccination. There are clear guidelines for its use and the reader should refer to their local and national guidelines.

Treatment for hospitalised patients is likely to be multidisciplinary and dependent upon the presenting illness and complications, which may or may not require intensive care support, and is outside the scope of this chapter.

Long Covid also requires a multidisciplinary approach, depending upon the presenting features. Patients need comprehensive physical, cognitive and psychological assessment to address their long-term needs.

Vaccination strategy has been the mainstay of management for the control of the Covid-19 pandemic. Due to the concerted efforts of scientists, the WHO and governments, the first vaccines were licensed for use in late 2020 and since then the WHO estimates that 70% of the world's population has received at least one dose.

Several vaccines are available, using different vaccine technologies (see Chapter 55). Some of the currently licensed vaccines for use in the West are:

- Pfizer and Moderna – mRNA vaccines
- AstraZeneca; Janssen/Johnson & Johnson – adenoviral vector vaccines
- Sanofi – recombinant viral spike protein vaccine vaccine.

Depending upon the vaccine, the primary course consists of either one or two doses. Boosters are recommended. Currently in the UK, the booster programme consists of 6 monthly spring and autumn boosters for >75 years and for those with risk factors. Everyone else is offered a yearly autumn booster at the same time as the influenza vaccine. It is not clear at present how long in the future such boosters will be required.

Many countries such as China, India and Russia have also manufactured vaccines which have been used in their own countries and also exported to others.

Diagnosis

Depending upon the season, influenza, parainfluenza, RSV, adenovirus and other respiratory viral infections should be considered in the differential diagnosis of infection with SARS-CoV-2 in both adults and children.

Definite diagnosis is by detection of SARS-CoV-2 RNA in the respiratory secretions (nasopharyngeal swab, endotracheal secretions or bronchoalveolar lavage). Several nucleic acid amplification tests (NAATs) including PCR are commercially available. Specimens need to be sent to the laboratory for these tests.

In addition, a diagnosis can be achieved by use of SARS-CoV-2 antigen tests (based on lateral flow technology; see Chapter 51) which are in use in outpatient settings and for home testing.

SARS-CoV-2 serology is useful for seroprevalence studies and for research into vaccine efficacy, etc. It is not useful for the diagnosis of acute Covid-19 infection.

Infection Control

In social/public settings, maintaining a safe distance of at least 2 metres, frequent handwashing, adequate ventilation (opening windows), avoiding overcrowding and wearing face masks indoors all mitigate the spread of the virus.

In healthcare settings, the spread of coronaviruses can be reduced by strict handwashing after patient contact. Use of gloves, aprons and goggles will reduce the risk of transmission. Isolation in single rooms or cohort nursing reduces the risk to other patients.

Patients should be nursed in side rooms, preferably negative pressure rooms, with gloves, aprons and a respirator mask conforming to at least European standard EN149:2001 FFP3 while doing aerosol-generating procedures.

Useful Websites

www.who.int

www.cdc.gov

UK Health Security Agency: www.gov.uk

Chapter

13

Human Herpesviruses Types 6, 7 and 8

The Viruses

Human herpesviruses types 6, 7 and 8 (HHV-6, -7 and -8) all are double-stranded DNA viruses and belong to the family Herpesviridae.

- HHV-6 (betaherpesvirus)
- HHV-7 (betaherpesvirus)
- HHV-8 (gammaherpesvirus)

Epidemiology

Route of Spread

- HHV-6 – aerosol transmission and saliva from mothers to babies and breast milk.
- HHV-7 – aerosol transmission and saliva from mothers to babies and breast milk.
- HHV-8 – there is some evidence of sexual spread via semen and possibly vertically from mother to child. HHV-8 has been transmitted to transplant recipients from donor organs.

Prevalence

- HHV-6 infection is ubiquitous and occurs worldwide. Infection often occurs after 4 months of age, as maternally acquired immunity wanes.
- HHV-7 infection is ubiquitous and occurs worldwide. Most children (95%) acquire the infection by 5 years of age.
- There is considerable worldwide variation in HHV-8 seroprevalence. Infection rates in northern European, Southeast Asia and Caribbean countries are between 2% and 4%. In the Mediterranean they are around 10%, and in sub-Saharan African countries they are 40%. Significant variation can be observed across different countries and regions. Although seroprevalence has been consistently shown to increase with age, countries with high infection rates usually have higher seroprevalence in younger age groups and infection is frequent in childhood, indicating a likely mother-to-child transmission by saliva. In countries with low seroprevalence, HHV-8 is much higher in persons with AIDS and Kaposi's sarcoma.

At-Risk Groups

Immunocompromised patients are at increased risk of more severe infection and clinical disease.

Clinical

Symptoms

HHV-6

- HHV-6 causes sixth disease or roseola infantum, usually in infants between 4 months and 2 years of age. It is also known as exanthema subitum (sudden rash). Children usually have a sudden spiking high fever (39–40°C), followed by a mild maculopapular rash. Rarely, children present with more severe complications, such as encephalitis, lymphadenopathy, myocarditis and myelosuppression. The prevalence of the virus increases with age; rates of infection are highest among infants between 6 and 12 months of age due to the loss of maternal antibodies that protect children from infection.

- The fever can cause convulsions. Rare infection in adolescents and adults has been associated with seizures, glandular fever–like illness and hepatitis, particularly in immunocompromised patients. These are usually reactivated infections of latent virus in association with cytomegalovirus (CMV) reactivation. There are two genetically distinct variants of HHV-6 (HHV-6A and HHV-6B). HHV-6A has not been associated with disease; HHV-6B is associated with the symptoms already listed.

- The virus periodically reactivates from its latent state, with HHV-6 DNA being detectable in 20–25% of healthy adults. In the immunocompetent setting, these reactivations are often asymptomatic, but in immunosuppressed individuals there can be serious complications. HHV-6B reactivation causes severe disease in transplant recipients and can cause several clinical manifestations, such as encephalitis, bone marrow suppression and pneumonitis, as well as graft rejection, often in association with other betaherpesviruses. In people with HIV/AIDS, HHV-6 reactivations cause disseminated infections leading to end organ disease and death.

HHV-7

- More than 95% of adults have been infected and are immune to HHV-7, and over 75% of those were infected before the age of 6. Primary infection with HHV-7 in children usually occurs between the ages of 2 and 5, occurring after primary infection with HHV-6.

- HHV-7 causes similar symptoms to HHV-6 but is less pathogenic. HHV-7, as well as other viruses, can cause the skin condition exanthema subitum, although HHV-7 causes the disease less frequently than HHV-6B. HHV-7 infection is associated with a number of other symptoms, including acute febrile respiratory disease, fever, rash, vomiting, diarrhoea, febrile seizures and low lymphocyte counts, but is usually asymptomatic.

HHV-8

- Infection with HHV-8 is thought to be lifelong, but a healthy immune system will usually prevent clinical symptoms.

- HHV-8 causes Kaposi's sarcoma, a cancer more commonly occurring in AIDS patients, as well as primary effusion lymphoma, which is a large B-cell lymphoma, HHV-8–associated multicentric Castleman's disease and inflammatory cytokine syndrome. It is one of seven currently known human cancer viruses, or oncoviruses.

Laboratory Diagnosis

These viruses are rarely diagnosed in clinical microbiology and virology laboratories except in immunocompromised patients and very young children with meningitis or encephalitis. Molecular assays are available in some laboratories for testing cerebrospinal fluid samples. Other specialist tests may be available in reference laboratories.

Management

Treatment

There are no antiviral drugs approved specifically for treating HHV-6, -7 and -8 infection, although antiviral drugs used to treat CMV (valganciclovir, ganciclovir, cidofovir and foscarnet) have shown some success.

Prophylaxis

There are no vaccines or antiviral drugs available for prophylactic use. Reduction of immunosuppression will often suppress the clinical expression of HHV-8.

Infection Control

Universal precautions are recommended for patients infected with HHV-6, -7 and -8. Additional infection control precautions will vary with the clinical presentation.

Human Metapneumovirus

The Virus

Human metapneumovirus (hMPV) is an RNA virus belonging to genus *Metapneumovirus*, in the family Pneumoviridae.

Epidemiology

Route of Spread

Transmission occurs by direct or close contact with contaminated secretions disseminated via the respiratory route as droplets or large aerosol particles.

Prevalence

The virus is ubiquitous and widespread in its geographical distribution. In 2018 it was estimated that there were 14.2 million acute lower respiratory tract infections in children <5 years of age which were human metapneumovirus. In the west hMPV infections occur in late winter and early spring and most children are infected by the age of 5 years.

Incubation Period

About a week (between 5 and 9 days).

Infectious Period

The relationship between viral shedding and clinical symptoms is not known precisely, but patients are infectious while symptomatic.

At-Risk Groups

Immunosuppressed patients. Lung transplant patients get severe hMPV disease and may develop chronic lung allograft dysfunction.

Clinical

Human metapneumovirus causes mild self-limiting respiratory tract infection in adults and children. Symptoms include cough, fever, rhinitis and wheezing. Severe lower respiratory tract illness and pneumonia may occur especially in the immunocompromised. Seroprevalence studies suggest that most children are infected by the age of 5 years. hMPV can be detected in 5–15% of infants <1 year with acute respiratory illness. The most common cause of hospitalisation in children is bronchiolitis and pneumonia.

77

Laboratory Diagnosis

hMPV infection is difficult to distinguish from other respiratory virus infection, therefore laboratory diagnosis is recommended especially in the immunocompromised. Virus-specific PCR on respiratory secretions (throat swab, nasopharyngeal aspirate or bronchioalveolar lavage) is the mainstay of diagnosis.

Infection Control

Respiratory precautions are recommended (see Chapter 56).

15

Human T-Cell Lymphotropic Viruses

The Viruses

The human T-cell lymphotropic viruses (HTLV) are a group of retroviruses that belong to the family Retroviridae and the genus *Deltaretrovirus*. Like HIV they possess a reverse transcriptase enzyme which converts the viral RNA into DNA in the first step of the replication cycle. This proviral DNA is capable of integrating into the cellular DNA. The viruses cause adult T-cell leukaemia/lymphoma (ATL) and a demyelinating disease called HTLV-1- associated myelopathy/tropical spastic paraparesis. The HTLVs belong to a larger group of primate T-lymphotropic viruses. Members of this family that infect humans are called HTLVs, and the ones that infect Old World monkeys are called simian T-lymphotropic viruses (STLVs). Four types of human HTLVs (HTLV-1, HTLV-2, HTLV-3 and HTLV-4) and four types of simian STLVs (STLV-1, STLV-2, STLV-3 and STLV-4) have been identified.

Epidemiology

HTLV-1 was first isolated accidentally in 1979 from a human T-cell line during experiments to stimulate cells so they could be maintained in cell culture for a longer period of time. The virus was quickly identified as the cause of ATL which had been described in 1977, and because of a clustering of cases in southern Japan it was suspected to have an infectious aetiology. It was the first human retrovirus to be isolated (predating the isolation of HIV). A few years later the second human retrovirus HTLV-2 was also isolated in a human T-cell line.

HTLV-1 and HTLV-2 are both involved in actively spreading epidemics, affecting millions of people worldwide.

HTLV-1 is the more clinically significant of the two. Although most infected persons remain asymptomatic, many of those infected with HTLV-1 eventually develop a rapidly fatal leukaemia, while others develop a debilitative myelopathy. Others will experience uveitis, infectious dermatitis or inflammatory disorders.

HTLV-2 is associated with milder neurological disorders and chronic pulmonary infections.

No specific illnesses have yet been associated with HTLV-3 and HTLV-4.

Route of Spread

HTLV-1 and HTLV-2 can be transmitted sexually, by blood-to-blood contact (e.g. by blood transfusion or sharing needles) and via breastfeeding.

Prevalence

HTLV-1

An estimated 5–10 million people globally are infected with HTLV-1; most infections are asymptomatic. The vast burden of infection is in Japan (southern), Caribbean, Central and South America, and Africa. The prevalence of antibody in Japanese blood donors is about 1%, but is higher in southern Japan and in older age groups. The higher prevalence in the older age group is due to the high rate of transmission when they were born and the low rate in the young now is due to reduction in transmission rates due to interventions (see the section on prevention). In the USA and Europe there is very low (<0.1%) prevalence, infection being mostly identified in immigrants from endemic countries.

HTLV-2

HTLV-2 has a restricted distribution, primarily in the Americas and Africa.

In the USA and Europe, infection is more prevalent in persons who inject drugs (PWIDs).

Incubation Period

As most of infection is asymptomatic it is difficult to define the time of infection from exposure but it is believed to be about 1–2 months for both HTLV-1 and -2.

Infectious Period

Both HTLV-1 and -2 cause chronic infection; therefore infectivity is lifelong.

At-Risk Groups

As indicated by transmission routes:

- children born to infected mothers, especially if breast fed;
- sexual partners of infected individuals, especially female partners of infected males;
- those who receive infected blood products (containing cellular components); and
- PWIDs, especially those sharing equipment.

Clinical

HTLV-1

Most people with HTLV-1 infection are asymptomatic and do not develop severe complications. However, several serious diseases are caused by or strongly associated with the virus. The lifetime risk of developing ATL in people with proven HTLV-1 infection is estimated to be about 5%. ATL has a much higher prevalence in Japan or people of Japanese descent. ATL presents as four clinical subtypes: acute, lymphomatous, chronic and smouldering, with the more aggressive subtypes (acute and lymphomatous) representing the majority of cases. Clinical presentation depends on the subtype. People may present with lymphadenopathy, hepatosplenomegaly or hypercalcaemia through involvement of the skin, lung, bones and other organs.

HTLV-1 also causes HTLV-1-associated myelopathy (HAM) or tropical spastic paraparesis (TSP). TSP is a chronic inflammatory disease of the central nervous system, characterised by progressive spastic weakness of the lower limbs, lower back pain, and bowel and bladder dysfunction. Clinical symptoms can include muscle weakness, hyper-reflexia and clonus in the lower limbs, along with extensor plantar response and a spastic gait. The infection is more common in adults and females. The latent period from acquiring infection to development of HAM/TSP is usually months to years. It is believed that HAM/TSP usually follows those who acquire infection through the sexual route, therefore female predominance is probably due to the fact of high rates of sexual transmission in females.

Estimates of the lifetime risk of this condition in HTLV-1-infected people are 0.18–1.8%.

Other diseases caused by HTLV-1 infection include HTLV-1-associated uveitis, infective dermatitis, bronchiectasis, bronchitis and bronchiolitis, seborrheic dermatitis, Sjögren's syndrome, rheumatoid arthritis, fibromyalgia and ulcerative colitis. There is little evidence that HTLV-1 infections cause other forms of cancer.

HTLV-2

HTLV-2 usually causes no signs or symptoms. Although it has not been definitively linked with any specific syndromes, there have been suggestions that some infected people may later develop neurological problems such as mild cognitive and motor impairment.

Laboratory Diagnosis

Serology is the mainstay of diagnosis. Since there is cross-reactivity between HTLV-1 and -2 viruses, combined HTLV-1 and -2 serological assays are used as screening tests. Positive reaction must be confirmed with more specific Western Blot tests which have the advantage of distinguishing between the two infections. Recent infection can be missed due the length of time between being infected by the virus and seroconversion. This period has been reported to be as long as 65 days. Delayed seroconversion lasting several years has also been reported. Infants born to seropositive mothers have been reported to seroconvert within 1–3 years of age.

Nucleic acid amplification testing for HTLV-1 can detect the virus genome in the blood and is used to confirm infection.

Currently, no single biological marker or clinical feature accurately predicts the development of or quantifies the risk of diseases associated with HTLV-1, although the levels of HTLV-1 proviral load have been suggested as a possible indicator.

Management

Treatment

No antiviral treatment is currently recommended for people with asymptomatic HTLV-1 infection.

Prophylaxis

There is no effective vaccination or other prophylaxis and prevention is the mainstay (see the next section on infection control).

Infection Control

Preventative measures are:

- Reducing vertical transmission by avoidance of breastfeeding. This intervention has virtually eliminated vertical transmission in Japan.
- Screening of all blood/organ donors is highly effective.
- Safe sex using the barrier method.
- Avoidance of sharing drug-injecting equipment.

Chapter

16

Influenza Viruses

The Viruses

Influenza A and B are RNA viruses and belong to the family Orthomyxoviridae. There are four types of influenza viruses, namely influenza virus A, B, C and D. Influenza A virus infects humans, birds and many other animals, influenza B and C infect only humans, while influenza D has been recently identified and infects mainly cattle and pigs.

The RNA genome is split into eight segments for influenza A and B viruses whereas influenza C and D possess only seven RNA segments; each segment encodes for a different viral protein. Influenza A, B and C viruses can be distinguished on the basis of antigenic differences between their nucleocapsid and matrix proteins.

The other important proteins are the two surface proteins, namely haemagglutinin (HA) which binds to the sialic acid residue on the cell surface to allow virus to gain entry, and neuraminidase (NA) which is responsible for cleavage and release of the virus from cells. These two proteins are also used in the classification of influenza A viruses into subtypes and nomenclature of strains (e.g. H2N3 and H5N1).

Epidemiology

For influenza A viruses, 16 HA and 9 NA subtypes have been isolated from birds and a further 2, HA17–18 and NA10–11 have been isolated recently from bats, so in all there are 18 HA subtypes and 11 NA subtypes described for influenza A virus. However, in humans only three HA subtypes (H1, H2, H3) and two NA subtypes (N1, N2) have persisted consistently.

Humans

Influenza viruses are RNA viruses which mutate regularly (especially influenza A virus). Viruses causing outbreaks one year are rarely the same ones causing outbreaks the next year. This is why the composition of influenza virus vaccines is different each year. This gradual change in RNA composition is called *antigenic drift*. It is thought that some new pandemics of influenza A arise because of *antigenic shift* which usually occurs when two different strains of influenza A virus infect the same cell (especially in pigs, which can be infected with human strains). The two infecting viruses are able to exchange RNA segments in a process called reassortment, resulting in new progeny viruses. If these new viruses are pathogenic for humans, because they are new strains previously unknown to humans, a new worldwide pandemic could result.

Both influenza A and B cause seasonal epidemics in winters. The World Health Organization (WHO) estimates that there are 3–5 million cases of severe illness and approximately 300,000–600,000 deaths each year due to influenza virus infection.

There have been several influenza A pandemics in the last 100 years, the most significant being the influenza A H1N1 pandemic in 1918 which infected about 500 million people worldwide (one-third of the world's population at that time) and resulted in about 50 million deaths. Further pandemics occurred in 1957 due to H2N2, 1968 (H3N2) and 2007 (H1N1), but none of them have been as devastating as the 1918 influenza A pandemic.

Avian Influenza

Some influenza A strains infect other animals such as birds and pigs. Avian influenza A virus has been found to infect wild birds, particularly waterfowl and shore birds, with domestic poultry (chickens) being particularly vulnerable. The infecting influenza A subtypes that have been identified in birds are H7N9, H9N2, H5N1 and H5N6. H5N1 has been found in birds throughout the year now and not just in winters, resulting in housing requirements to keep poultry indoors to avoid exposure to infected wild birds. However, infection can be introduced to poultry through fomites, such as soiled infected boots, thus making infection of poultry with avian influenza virus a major public health issue.

Avian influenza viruses can be further subdivided on their pathogenicity in birds as high pathogenic avian influenza A viruses (HPIAV) which present as severe infections in birds leading to fatal infections and low pathogenic avian influenza A viruses which typically cause no symptoms or very mild symptoms in birds.

Infections can spread from these animals to humans. Haemagglutinin type 5 (H5) and haemagglutinin type 7 (H7) strains transmit most commonly from birds to humans and both H5N1 and H7N9 are HPIAV and have been associated with human disease. Usually, these infections are associated with single cases or small clusters of cases in humans. However, there is always the fear that these avian viruses will mutate, becoming much more infectious to humans and causing a worldwide pandemic.

Route of Spread

Influenza viruses are spread by the respiratory route by both droplet and aerosol spread. Infection can also be spread via hands by touching contaminated surfaces.

Prevalence

Prevalence is worldwide. Influenza viruses are constantly mutating. Influenza B viruses are more stable and do not change their antigenic make-up regularly. By contrast, influenza A viruses are constantly mutating, with different strains appearing each year.

The prevalence of human immunity and the incidence of infection varies from year to year, depending on the influenza virus strain circulating in the community. Therefore, annual influenza vaccination with the circulating strains is required. Most people are not immune to the current circulating strain, unless they have received vaccination that includes the circulating strain. Infection usually occurs between October and March.

Incubation Period

1–5 days (average of 2–3 days).

Infectious Period

Viral shedding occurs just before onset of symptoms with little or no detectable virus being present 5–10 days after onset. Patients are therefore infectious for about 24 hours prior to symptom onset and for about 5 days after. Infectiousness, though, is highest while they have respiratory symptoms (especially when coughing). Viral shedding and infectiousness can last for much longer in those who are immunosuppressed.

At-Risk Groups

Immunocompromised patients, elderly persons (>65 years old), patients with chronic heart and lung and kidney disease, high BMI and diabetes. Pregnant women are also at risk of influenza complications.

Clinical

Symptoms

Influenza A and B have similar clinical presentations. However, gastric symptoms such as abdominal pain may be a prominent feature of influenza B infection, therefore it is sometimes also referred to as 'gastric flu'.

Primary influenza illness presents with fever of 38°C or greater, headache, malaise and muscle aches which are primarily due to an interferon-mediated host immune response. These are often accompanied by coryza and respiratory and gastrointestinal symptoms.

Complications of influenza requiring hospital admission are characterised by signs and symptoms of lower respiratory tract infection, that is, hypoxia, dyspnoea, lung infiltrates, exacerbation of underlying respiratory condition and involvement of the nervous system (encephalitis) and myocarditis in severe cases.

Primary influenza pneumonia may occur in the immunocompromised, but the most serious complication of influenza is secondary bacterial lung infection (e.g. with pneumococcus, streptococcus or staphylococcus). This often results in severe or fatal infection, especially in at-risk groups.

Avian influenza virus infection in humans can present as any other severe case of influenza disease. High mortality has been described in previous cases/clusters. Not all cases are severe, and asymptomatic cases have also been picked up as result of screening of poultry workers. It can also present as conjunctivitis.

Differential Diagnosis

Any respiratory infection can be confused with influenza, although severe cases, with significant malaise, fever, chills and myalgia are usually correctly diagnosed as influenza.

Laboratory Diagnosis

See Table 16.1.

Table 16.1 Laboratory diagnosis of influenza virus infection

Specimen	Test	Interpretation of test results
Nose and throat swab in virus transport medium	NAAT* as PCR (sensitive and rapid)	If positive, indicates current infection
	Rapid antigen detection test	If positive, indicates current infection
Nasopharyngeal aspirate (in very young children) or bronchoalveolar lavage (if primary influenza pneumonia suspected)	NAAT as PCR (sensitive and rapid)	If positive, indicates current infection
	Rapid antigen detection test	If positive, indicates current infection

Note: * NAAT – nucleic acid amplification test; of which PCR is most commonly used.

Management

Treatment*

There are many neuraminidase inhibitor (NAI) drugs (oseltamivir, zanamivir and peramivir) which are specific for treating influenza A and B. Baloxavir marboxil which is an endonuclease inhibitor has a different mechanism of action.

Oseltamivir treatment, started as soon as possible, but not later than 48 hours after onset of symptoms and 36 hours in children, reduces the morbidity and duration of illness. Zanamavir should be used as the first-line drug if H1N1 is in circulation as there is a higher risk of developing drug resistance with oseltamivir. However, WHO surveillance of influenza viruses collected in 2016–17 showed that >99% viruses were susceptible to the NAIs in use.

Inhaled or I/V zanamivir or I/V peramivir may also be used as indicated. Treatment should not be withheld from patients at risk of influenza complications despite a presentation later than 48 hours.

Treatment should be started on the basis of clinical diagnosis in the 'influenza season'. Out of the peak influenza season, laboratory confirmation of disease should be sought as most of the cases are likely to be due to respiratory viruses other than influenza.

Prophylaxis*

Pre-exposure Prophylaxis

Annual influenza vaccination of at-risk groups is recommended. In addition, healthcare workers and those working in other emergency services should also be offered vaccination. A live attenuated intranasal vaccine is licensed for use in children. As the circulating influenza strains change constantly, the strains included in the current vaccine are selected on the basis of surveillance of the strains most recently in circulation.

* Note: See latest national guidance and drug data sheets for drug doses and for suitable patients to treat.

Post-exposure Prophylaxis

In those who are not vaccinated, influenza vaccine should be offered along with chemoprophylaxis with a neuraminidase inhibitor, either oseltamivir or zanamivir.

Suspected contacts of avian influenza should be actively followed up for 10 days post exposure and should be offered oseltamivir prophylaxis.

Infection Control

Influenza is spread by the airborne route, both via droplet and aerosol spread and can be transmitted via the hands. Environmental contamination is also known to occur and may be a contributory factor in the spread. It causes outbreaks in hospitals and in the community. In hospitals, infected patients should be put into single rooms (with the door closed) or cohorted until they are asymptomatic. Staff should wear aprons, gloves and face masks and should wash their hands with soap and water before and after patient contact. Staff with influenza-like symptoms should not work with patients, especially those with a higher risk of severe symptoms.

If a patient is suspected of having avian influenza (anyone who develops symptoms within 10 days of contact with avian influenza), should be kept in isolation in a negative pressure room with full barrier precautions, including a FFP 2 face mask. A respirator should be worn while performing aerosol-generating procedures. Healthcare staff and others in contact with these patients should be offered seasonal influenza vaccine and prophylactic oseltamivir and monitored for signs of infection. Special tests are required (usually PCR) for testing for avian influenza virus infection.

Useful Websites

Avian influenza: guidance, data and analysis: www.gov.uk/government/collections/avian-influenza-guidance-data-and-analysis

NICE topics: influenza – seasonal: https://cks.nice.org.uk/topics/influenza-seasonal

Measles Virus

The Virus

Measles virus is an RNA virus belonging to the genus *Morbillivirus* in the family Paramyxoviridae.

Epidemiology

Route of Spread

Measles is highly infectious with a high secondary infection rate in contacts, especially household contacts. The infection is spread by the respiratory droplet route. Infection results in lifelong immunity.

Prevalence

Measles has a worldwide distribution. In 2020, there were 150,000 cases worldwide with over 100,000 in Africa. Incidence of measles is influenced by the percentage of the population (especially young children) receiving vaccine. Even in countries where vaccination has been introduced, vaccination rates may remain low due to parents choosing not to have their children vaccinated. In April 2020, the World Health Organization (WHO) indicated that many countries had started suspending their measles vaccination programmes due to the impact of the Covid-19 pandemic and there were several large outbreaks in countries across Europe where measles, mumps and rubella (MMR) vaccine uptake has been low. After the MMR vaccine controversy began, the MMR vaccination compliance dropped sharply in the UK, from 92% in 1996 to 84% in 2002. In some parts of London, it was as low as 61% in 2003, far below the rate needed to avoid an epidemic of measles. By 2006 coverage for MMR in the UK at 24 months was 85%, lower than the c.94% coverage for other vaccines. After vaccination rates dropped, the incidence of measles and mumps increased greatly in the UK. The UK initially achieved WHO measles elimination status in 2017, based on data from 2014 to 2016. However, in 2018, there was a marked increase in the number of confirmed measles cases, with 991 confirmed cases in England and Wales, compared with 284 cases in 2017. Furthermore, the same strain of measles virus (called B3 Dublin) was detected for more than 12 months across 2017 and 2018. Based on this, the WHO determined that the UK could no longer be considered as 'eliminated' and that transmission of measles had been re-established. While coverage of the first dose in the UK has reached the WHO target of 95% for children aged 5 in 2022, coverage of the second dose is at 87.4%. As measles is highly infectious, even small declines in uptake can have an impact, and anyone who has

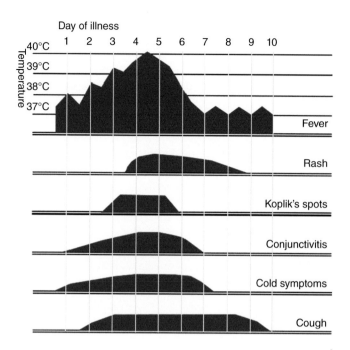

Day of illness

Temperature

Fever

Rash

Koplik's spots

Conjunctivitis

Cold symptoms

Cough

Figure 17.1 Measles symptoms (WHO *Manual for the laboratory diagnosis of measles and rubella infection.* Geneva: WHO Documents Production Services, 2007, UKHSA)

not received two doses of MMR vaccine is at risk, particularly those travelling to countries affected by the ongoing, large outbreaks.

Incubation Period

10–14 days.

Infectious Period

Prodromal period (4 days before the rash appears) to 4 full days after the rash appears.

At-Risk Groups

All susceptible individuals, but especially those who are immunocompromised, pregnant, neonates or malnourished.

Clinical

Symptoms

The typical measles rash is preceded by a prodromal illness of 2–4 days, which includes fever (often greater than 40°C), cough, runny nose and inflamed eyes. Small white spots known as Koplik's spots may form inside the mouth 2 or 3 days after the start of symptoms. Persons are highly infectious in the prodromal stage. A red, flat (maculopapular) rash, which usually starts on the face and then spreads to the rest of the body usually begins 3–4 days after the start of symptoms. The rash and fever fade after 4–5 days (see Figure 17.1).

Complications

Secondary Bacterial Infection

This can cause otitis media, laryngotracheitis and bronchopneumonia. These are common in children in resource-poor countries and occur in part due to measles-induced immunosuppression.

Encephalitis

- *Primary measles encephalitis*: Encephalitis occurring during acute measles infection affects 1–3 per 1,000 patients. The brain becomes infected during the rash phase of the infection. The primary mechanism of infection is unclear, but onset at the early phase suggests a primary viral invasion of neurological cells followed by chemokine induction and lymphocytic infiltration. Measles virus RNA can be found in the cerebrospinal fluid (CSF). Treatment is largely supportive. The mortality rate is 10–15% and a further 25% of patients endure permanent neurological damage.
- *Acute post-infectious encephalitis*: Caused by immune-mediated brain inflammation following shortly after measles infection. Approximately 1 in 1,000 children are affected following a measles infection and 1–2 per 1 million following live measles vaccination. It occurs 2–28 days after infection. Symptoms include headache, irritability, loss of consciousness and fever. Measles virus RNA can be found in the CSF and measles virus IgM and IgG can be detected in serum and detection in the CSF indicates an intrathecal antiviral immune response. MRI examination and finding white blood cells in the CSF can aid diagnosis. It has a high mortality rate.
- *Measles inclusion body encephalitis*: Most commonly occurs in immunodeficient children. The average age of those affected is 6 and onset is within 1 year of measles infection or vaccination. Patients often have an altered mental status, motor deficits and seizures. Measles virus is persistently present and the typical measles rash does not appear or is minimal because of impaired T-cell function. Initially, CSF analysis is usually normal and the amount of measles-specific antibodies in the CSF usually rises as the disease progresses. Measles viral RNA can be detected in brain cells following a biopsy. Mortality is 75%.
- *Subacute sclerosing panencephalitis (SSPE)*: Affects 1 in 25,000 persons with measles infection, but the incidence is higher in children infected at a younger age; those infected with measles under 1 year have a risk of about 1 in 5,000. SSPE is more common in children and symptoms develop 6–15 years after measles infection. Initial symptoms include behavioural changes and cognitive decline. Within weeks or months, these symptoms become more obvious and motor dysfunction symptoms develop. Seizures may occur, often myoclonic in nature, and 50% of patients experience ocular disturbances such as necrotising retinitis. Patients decline into a coma. Death is universal and usually occurs within 3 years. The diagnosis is confirmed by detecting high titres of measles virus antibody in the CSF.

Immunocompromised Patients

These patients do not have a typical rash or may have an atypical measles rash. Measles pneumonitis (giant cell pneumonitis) is seen in immunocompromised and malnourished patients with measles and may occur without a typical measles rash. Measles

Table 17.1 Measles laboratory diagnosis

Clinical indication	Specimen	Test	Significance	Essential information for the laboratory
Acute measles infection	Venous blood or saliva	Measles virus IgM	Positive result* indicates recent infection	Date of onset and symptoms
	Respiratory swab/urine	Measles virus RNA NAAT	Positive result indicates current infection	Date of onset and symptoms
Past measles infection	Venous blood	Measles virus IgG	Positive result (in the absence of measles virus IgM) indicates past infection and immunity	If relevant, history and date of contact with suspected case of measles
Post-vaccination immunity check	Venous blood	Test not indicated as there is no consensus regarding the level of antibody that is consistent with immunity		
SSPE	CSF, brain biopsy (if done)	Measles RNA NAAT	Positive result confirms diagnosis	Detailed clinical history of acute measles and vaccination

Note: * Viral IgM test results need to be interpreted with caution and may be non-specific, especially in specimens giving weak reactions.

pneumonitis has a high mortality rate and can be diagnosed by nucleic acid amplification test (NAAT) on respiratory secretions. Measles inclusion body encephalitis is most commonly seen in immunodeficient children.

Laboratory Diagnosis

See Table 17.1.
See Figure 17.2.

Management

Treatment

There is no licensed antiviral treatment for measles.

Prophylaxis

Pre-exposure

Live attenuated measles vaccine as triple vaccine in MMR is recommended for all young children (see latest schedule advice). The first dose is not given until the second year of life to prevent the maternal, passively acquired antibody from interfering with the vaccine take. High levels of vaccine coverage (approximately 90%) are required for

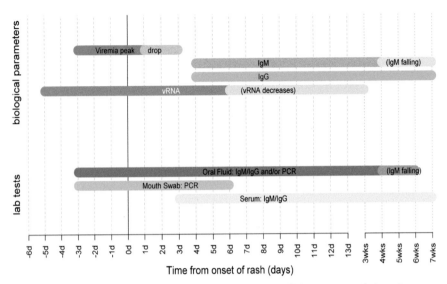

Figure 17.2 Dynamics of biological/viral indicators and timings of laboratory tests during primary measles infection (*National measles guidelines: November 2019*, Public Health England, UKHSA)

interruption of spread. There is no evidence that MMR vaccine is associated with autism and it is regarded as a safe and effective vaccine.

Post-exposure

Intravenous immunoglobulin (IVIG), human normal immunoglobulin (HNIG) or MMR vaccine can be given to susceptible contacts after exposure to a case of measles as post-exposure prophylaxis.

- IVIG is recommended for immunocompromised persons; effectiveness of IVIG is likely to be higher when administered as early as possible following exposure (ideally within 72 hours) although it can be given up to 6 days following exposure.
- HNIG is recommended for susceptible pregnant women.
- HNIG and vaccine are recommended for susceptible infants.

Always refer to the latest guidance on government websites, listed at the end of this chapter, for current advice. The most vulnerable individuals (immunosuppressed persons, pregnant women and infants) are the highest priority to be considered for prophylactic treatment. Recommendations for prophylaxis in pregnant women are based on a combination of age, history and/or antibody testing. The main aim of measles post-exposure prophylaxis for pregnant women is attenuation of disease and therefore HNIG can be used. This will be issued up to 6 days after exposure. Urgent measles virus IgG testing is available in all regional public health laboratories, as well as many National Health Service laboratories. Most testing can be done the same day or out of hours.

Infection Control

Measles is one of the most highly contagious infections with attack rates of >80% in household contacts. As it is spread by the respiratory route, respiratory precautions

(Chapter 56) should be instituted for those at risk. Contact tracing should be prioritised for the most vulnerable individuals (immunosuppressed persons, pregnant women and infants). Susceptible healthcare workers who work with at-risk patients should be excluded from work during the incubation period if exposed to measles. All infected healthcare workers should be excluded from work during the infectious period.

Useful Websites

Public Health England: National measles guidelines, February 2024: https://assets .publishing.service.gov.uk/government/uploads/system/uploads/attachment_data/file/ 849538/PHE_Measles_Guidelines.pdf

Chapter

18

Mumps Virus

The Virus
The mumps virus is a single-stranded RNA virus and belongs to the family Paramyxoviridae.

Epidemiology

Route of Spread
Infection is spread by aerosol or hand and fomite contact with infected salivary or respiratory secretions.

Prevalence
Mumps is an endemic childhood infection worldwide. Cases occur all year round although in temperate climates they tend to peak in colder months. Mumps is highly infectious and outbreaks occur in institutionalised settings like schools and universities provided there are sufficient numbers of susceptible individuals to allow the infection to spread.

Incubation Period
10–21 days, average of about 2 weeks.

Infectious Period
Virus is shed in the saliva and respiratory secretions. Maximum infectivity is at 48 hours prior to appearance of parotitis but patients are infectious from about a week before to after the appearance of parotitis. The virus can be shed in the urine for much longer than this.

At-Risk Groups
All those who are susceptible, particularly post-pubertal males as 20–30% may develop acute mumps orchitis.

Clinical

Acute Parotitis
Up to 50% of acute cases of mumps infection in children may be subclinical (e.g. asymptomatic). When symptoms develop they comprise uni- or bilateral parotid gland

(parotitis) swelling; other salivary glands may also be involved. There is usually a 24-hour prodrome of fever and malaise preceding the parotitis.

Complications

The following complications may occur with or without clinical parotitis.

Orchitis develops in 20–30% of young adult or adolescent males. It follows 4–5 days after parotitis (if present) and may involve pain and swelling in one or both testes, which is often accompanied by headache and fever. The resulting severe testicular pain may raise testicular torsion as a differential diagnosis, especially if mumps orchitis is not preceded by parotitis (clinical mumps). However, the symptoms of mumps orchitis subside in 3–4 days. Infertility is a rare occurrence but testicular atrophy may follow in about 30%.

Similarly, inflammation of ovaries (oophoritis) may occur in post-pubertal women but is much less common (5%). Rarely, mumps pancreatitis and arthritis may occur.

Central Nervous System Complications

Meningitis is the most common complication and may occur in up to 15% of mumps cases. It is normally self-limiting but may spread to the brain to cause the more serious meningoencephalitis. Sensorineural deafness in a small number of cases may result as a consequence of this infection. Central nervous system infection can be difficult to diagnose clinically, especially in the absence of parotitis.

Laboratory Diagnosis

See Table 18.1.

Table 18.1 Laboratory diagnosis of mumps

Clinical indication	Specimen	Test	Significance	Essential information
Acute mumps	Venous blood-clotted	Mumps IgM	Positive result indicates recent infection. Test may take up to a week to become positive so may be negative in first week of infection.	Clinical symptoms, date of onset, relevant epidemiology, e.g. history of contact, outbreak, etc.
Acute mumps	Parotid or salivary swab, urine	Mumps NAAT**/ PCR	Positive result indicates current infection	As above
Mumps meningitis/ encephalitis	Cerebrospinal fluid	Mumps NAAT/ PCR	Positive result indicates current infection	As above
Mumps immunity*	Venous blood – clotted	Mumps* IgG	Positive IgG (in the absence of IgM) indicates past infection	History of at-risk contact with date, etc.

Note: * It is not possible to test reliably for post-vaccination immunity to mumps because there is no consensus on the amount of antibody which is consistent with immunity. Post-vaccination mumps immunity tests are therefore not recommended.
** NAAT – nucleic acid amplification test; of which PCR is most commonly used.

Management

Treatment

There is no treatment. Treatment is supportive with painkillers, etc.

Prophylaxis

Mumps is a component of the measles, mumps and rubella (MMR) vaccine (see Chapter 55) and in countries where the MMR vaccine is incorporated in childhood vaccination programmes, mumps infection has declined. Unfortunately, in the 1980s the mumps component was withdrawn from the vaccine due to vaccine-induced mumps meningitis; this resulted in a large cohort of mumps-susceptible young adults resulting in several large mumps outbreaks in university students in the UK, some of which were controlled by offering mass vaccination to university students. The mumps component of the vaccine was subsequently substituted with a more suitable mumps virus vaccine strain.

Infection Control

This is achieved by instituting respiratory droplet precautions (Chapter 56) over the infectious period.

Chapter

19

Noroviruses

The Viruses

Noroviruses are a genetically diverse group of non-enveloped single-stranded, positive-sense RNA viruses belonging to the family Caliciviridae and the genus *Norovirus* has one species, *Norwalk virus*. Noroviruses are classified into at least seven different genogroups (GI, GII, GIII, GIV, GV, GVI and GVII), which can be further divided into different genetic clusters or genotypes.

Individual noroviruses are often named after the place where they were first identified and the majority of those isolated in cases of acute gastroenteritis belong to two genogroups. Genogroup I (GI) includes Norwalk virus, Southampton virus and Desert Shield virus and genogroup II (GII) includes Bristol virus, Toronto virus, Lordsdale virus, Hawaii virus, Mexico virus and Snow Mountain virus.

Most noroviruses that infect humans belong to genogroups GI and GII. Noroviruses from genogroup II, genotype 4 (GII.4) account for the majority of adult outbreaks of gastroenteritis and often cause worldwide outbreaks.

Epidemiology

Route of Spread

Noroviruses most frequently spread from person to person by the ingestion or inhalation of aerosolised vomit and faeces. Patients frequently have no prior warning that they are about to vomit, which results in environmental contamination. Vomiting transmits infection very effectively and noroviruses are very contagious; fewer than 20 virus particles can cause an infection. Noroviruses can also be transmitted via contaminated food and water. Shellfish (e.g. bivalve molluscs such as cockles and oysters) and salad ingredients are the foods most often implicated in norovirus outbreaks. Eating shellfish that have not been sufficiently heated (<75°C) creates a high risk for norovirus infection when the shellfish have been harvested from sewage-contaminated waters. Most bacteria can be removed from contaminated shellfish by being exposed to clean running water for several days, but this does not work for noroviruses, which adhere to the shellfish flesh. Salad ingredients grown in soil fertilised by human excrement pose a high risk for transmitting noroviruses. Foods other than shellfish may be contaminated by infected food handlers. Many norovirus outbreaks have been traced to food that was handled by only one infected person.

Prevalence

Norovirus infection is common and 90% of adults have been infected at some time in their lives. After infection, immunity to the same strain of the virus (genotype) protects against reinfection for between 6 months and 2 years and reinfection can occur with the same or different strains. Immunity gained after a norovirus infection does not fully protect against infection with the other genotypes of the virus.

Noroviruses cause about 20% of cases of acute gastroenteritis across the world, with higher prevalence in resource-rich countries. Noroviruses have caused large outbreaks on cruise ships, but preventative action has reduced this incidence in recent years. Outbreaks can affect 25% of cruise passengers with a lower incidence in staff (most of whom will have been exposed in previous outbreaks).

Incubation Period

12–48 hours after contact with contaminated environment or eating contaminated food.

Infectious Period

From onset of symptoms to 48 hours after symptoms stop.

At-Risk Groups

All ages. Infection can be more severe in the very young and the elderly and those with weakened immunity, in whom dehydration and electrolyte imbalance are important.

Clinical

Symptoms

Severe and fatal infection is rare. Noroviruses are associated with projectile vomiting, watery diarrhoea and abdominal pain as a result of the virus infecting the small intestine. Symptoms usually last for 24–72 hours.

Differential Diagnosis

In very young and old persons, sporadic cases and outbreaks of diarrhoea and vomiting can be caused by rotaviruses (especially between December and March). Other enteric viruses such as adenoviruses, sapoviruses and astroviruses can cause sporadic diarrhoea and vomiting, but seldom cause outbreaks. Testing for noroviruses and rotaviruses in cases of gastroenteritis and at the start of outbreaks of diarrhoea and vomiting is useful.

Outbreaks

Noroviruses cause large outbreaks in hospitals, cruise ships and in the community, especially in schools and nursing homes. Outbreaks occur more frequently in the winter, but when new variants emerge, outbreaks in the summer occur. Strict infection control is required, especially in hospitals, in order to bring outbreaks under control (see Chapter 56).

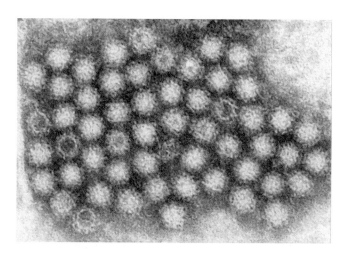

Figure 19.1 Electron micrograph of negatively stained noroviruses (courtesy of CDC; details – Public Health Image Library (PHIL): https://phil.cdc.gov/Details.aspx?pid=10704cdc.gov)

Laboratory Diagnosis

Faeces samples should be taken as soon as possible and <3 days after the onset of symptoms. Nucleic acid amplification testing (RT-PCR) is the preferred laboratory method (but samples can be tested by electron microscopy or enzyme immunoassay, although these are less sensitive methods). An electron micrograph of noroviruses is shown in Figure 19.1.

Management

Treatment

There is no antiviral treatment for norovirus infections. Replacement of fluid in severe cases should be considered.

Prevention

There are currently no licensed vaccines for noroviruses and rapid diagnosis and strict infection control procedures are important in limiting the spread of infection.

Infection Control

- In hospitals, isolation or cohorting of infected patients is very important. Patients are infectious until 48 hours after the last symptoms.
- Thorough handwashing with soap and water is important. Alcohol rubs are less effective than handwashing, as noroviruses lack a lipid viral envelope.
- Exclusion of symptomatic staff until 48 hours after the last symptoms is also important.
- Do not move patients from a ward with symptomatic patients to other wards or care homes.
- Restrict staff movement.

- Thoroughly clean the ward when the outbreak has finished (48 hours after the last symptomatic case) with diluted hypochlorite or hot soapy water before admitting new patients.
- In cruise ships, where norovirus outbreaks can be a big problem, increased passenger awareness/exclusion of symptomatic passengers, prohibition of passengers touching food on buffet tables and prompt decontamination of public areas are the principal tools used to reduce the risk of outbreaks.

Papilloma and Polyoma Viruses

20

The Viruses

Human papillomaviruses and polyomaviruses are non-enveloped DNA viruses. Human papillomaviruses belong to the family Papillomaviridae and polyomaviruses belong to the family Polyomaviridae.

There are hundreds of known species of papillomaviruses infecting many vertebrate species, some of which are oncogenic. Those infecting humans are known as human papillomaviruses (HPV); there are over 170 types divided into 5 genera. They cause skin, laryngeal and genital lesions, some of which are associated with genital cancers.

There are over 100 species of polyomaviruses which infect mammals and birds, 14 of which infect humans. Most of these are common asymptomatic infections in humans, infrequently causing disease. However, BK virus is associated with nephropathy in solid organ transplant recipients, JC virus is associated with progressive multifocal leukoencephalopathy in immunocompromised people and Merkel cell virus with Merkel cell cancer.

Papillomaviruses

Epidemiology
Route of Spread

- Direct contact with infected material, usually introduced through abraded skin (e.g. sharing towels, swimming pools, walking barefoot). Common skin warts are normally transmitted by this route.
- Sexual: The main route of spread for genital warts is sexual and therefore it is a sexually transmitted infection.
- Vertical: Laryngeal papilloma or warts in children are usually due to transmission to the baby at the time of delivery if mother has genital warts.

Prevalence

Infection is prevalent worldwide. Skin infection with HPV (causing warts) is very widespread and most common in childhood and lesions typically appear and regress spontaneously over the course of weeks to months. HPV1–4 cause skin lesions; HPV4 typically causes plantar warts and HPV1 produces lesions on fingers and trunk. Recurring skin warts are common.

HPV infection of the skin in the genital area is the most common sexually transmitted infection worldwide. These infections are associated with genital or anal warts (condylomata acuminata). The strains of HPV that can cause genital warts are usually different from those that cause warts on other parts of the body (e.g. on the hands or feet or inner thighs). A wide variety of HPV types can cause genital warts, but types 6 and 11 together account for about 90% of all cases. Some genital infections (types 6 and 11) in pregnant women can be transmitted to their newborns, causing laryngeal papillomas in the infants. The majority of genital HPV infections never cause any overt symptoms and are cleared by the immune system in a matter of months. HPV is estimated to be the most common sexually transmitted infection in most developed countries; most sexually active men and women will probably acquire genital HPV infection at some point in their lives. Worldwide, 10–15% of women are positive for HPV DNA, with rates varying by age and country. The highest rates of HPV are in younger women (25% in women under 25 years of age). Rates decline in older age groups in Europe and the Americas, but less so in Africa and Asia. HPV disproportionately affects low-income and resource-poor countries.

Types 16 and 18 are responsible for causing most of HPV-caused cancers. About a dozen HPV types (including types 16, 18, 31 and 45) are linked to cancer of the oropharynx, larynx, vulva, vagina, cervix, anus and penis. These cancers are all caused by sexually transmitted infections, with individuals infected with both HPV and HIV at an increased risk of developing cervical or anal cancer. The wider availability of HPV vaccines has dramatically reduced the incidence of HPV-induced genitally transmitted cancers worldwide in recent years.

Incubation Period
- Warts: Genital warts normally appear 3 months after exposure to an infected partner.
- Cancer: There is usually a latency period of several years from the acquisition of infection to development of cervical cancer.

Infectious Period
Lesions, when present, are highly infectious; asymptomatic shedding of the virus from the genital tract may occur. Lesions on the skin, once they disappear, are no longer infectious.

At-Risk Groups
The viruses infect both sexes and all age groups. Warts may recur with waning immunity; therefore, those who are immunosuppressed and the elderly may have frequent recurrences with more severe symptoms and more extensive lesions.

Clinical
HPVs cause infection of the mucus membrane and skin. The virus infects the rapidly replicating epithelial cells and therefore may cause lesions both on the skin and mucus membrane. Different genotypes are associated with different clinical manifestations and anatomical sites of infection although there is an overlap (see Table 20.1).

Skin
Common Warts (Verrucae Vulgaris) HPV Types 1, 2, 4, 7, 22
Warts are caused by a rapid growth of cells on the outer layer of the skin. They are small in size and occur in large numbers anywhere on the body but most commonly on the

Table 20.1 Human papillomaviruses and their associated lesions

Type of lesion		Associated HPV genotype
Non-malignant lesions	Common warts	1, 2, 4, 7, 22
	Verrucas	1, 2, 4, 63
	Flat warts	3, 10, 28
	Genital warts	6, 11, 42, 44
	Laryngeal papilloma	6, 11
Premalignant lesions	Epidermodysplasia verruciformis	2, 3 and others
Malignant lesions	Cervical cancer	16, 18, 31, 33, 35 and others
	Oropharyngeal cancer	16

hands and feet and have a roughened surface. Skin warts are most common in childhood and typically appear and regress spontaneously over the course of weeks to months. Recurring skin warts are common. Patients' complaints are related mostly to the cosmetic appearance. However, because of the pressure on the warts they are painful when they occur on the soles of the feet.

Flat Warts (Verrucae Planae) HPV Types 3, 10, 28

Flat warts are most commonly found on the arms, face and forehead. They are flat and smooth and generally affect children.

Epidermodysplasia Verruciformis: HPV Types 2, 3 and up to 20 Other HPV Types

This condition is characterised by the appearance of multiple flat lesions all over the body which may persist. It is associated with a specific T-cell deficiency and is a premalignant condition.

Mucus Membrane

Genital Warts HPV Types 6, 11, 42, 44

Genital warts (condylomata acuminata) are the most common sexually transmitted infection and commonly occur in association with other sexually transmitted infections on the genitals and anus. More than 40 HPV types can be transmitted by sexual contact and may cause genital warts, although they may also remain asymptomatic. The HPV types that cause genital warts are usually different from those that cause warts on other parts of the body, such as the hands or feet. Ninety per cent of genital warts are due to HPV genotypes 6 and 11. The lesions may appear as papules or papillomatous and the size may vary from small to very large especially when several lesions coalesce into one.

- Men
  - penis mostly around glans and prepuce
  - urethra
  - anus and rectum – especially in those who practise receptive anorectal sex (e.g. men who have sex with men)

- Women
  - vulva
  - vagina

- o cervix – typically flat lesions
- o anus and perinium

Laryngeal Warts HPV Types 6, 11

These occur in the mouth and larynx, especially in small children as a result of vertical transmission at delivery from the mother's genital infection.

Cancers

Several HPV types (including types 16, 18, 31, 33, 35 and 45) are called high-risk types because persistent infection is associated with cancer of the oropharynx, larynx, vulva, penis, anus, vagina and cervix. Two HPV early proteins (E6 and E7) are primary oncoproteins, associated with induction of cancers in HPV infections.

These cancers are all sexually transmitted HPV infections infecting the stratified epithelial tissue. Individuals infected with both HIV and HPV have an increased risk of developing cervical or anal cancer. HPV type 16 is the type most likely to cause cancer and is present in about 46% of all cervical cancers and in many vaginal, vulvar, penile and anal cancers and cancers of the head and neck.

Cervical Cancer HPV 16, 18, 31, 33, 35 and Higher Genotypes

Most cases of cervical cancer result from HPV infection, and about 70% of all HPV-associated cancers are due to types 16 and 18; the rest are due to the other HPV types. Persistent HPV infection increases the risk of developing cervical carcinoma, particularly in women with HIV/AIDS, who are at a 20-fold increased risk of cervical cancer. See also Chapter 46.

Other Cancers

Squamous cell carcinoma of penis, vulva, vagina and some laryngeal carcinomas are also associated with HPV infection. Men who are HIV positive and have sex with men have an 80-fold higher risk of developing anal carcinoma.

Laboratory Diagnosis

Routine laboratory diagnosis is not available and the diagnosis is on the basis of routine cervical screening programmes, clinical history and appearance of the lesions on examination, with follow-up nucleic acid amplification tests (NAAT) to confirm. HPV testing is part of the cervical screening programme. In 2019 the primary screening test was changed from cytology to high-risk HPV testing, due to its increased sensitivity for cervical cell changes and high negative predictive value. There is no blood test for HPV. During cervical screening, a small sample of cells is taken from the cervix and tested for high-risk HPVs. If these types of HPV are found, the sample is then checked for any changes in the cells of the cervix. The test is offered to women in England aged 25–49 every 3 years and those aged 50–64 every 5 years. Some sexual health clinics may offer anal screening to men with a higher risk of developing anal cancer, such as men who have sex with men. There are a number of tests approved for use in the UK which can detect the commonest high-risk HPVs.

Management

Treatment

Warts

There is no specific antiviral treatment as the lesions are usually self-limiting and normally recede in 6–12 months. Warts or verrucae can be frozen, so they fall off. Other treatments include covering them up (occlusion) and chemical burning with salicylic acid. Patients may need referral to a skin specialist. Genital warts should be treated in a sexual health clinic.

Cervical Cancer

Cervical cancer requires management by gynaecological oncologists.

Prophylaxis

There are currently three different HPV vaccine products. Cervarix® contains virus-like particles (VLPs) for two HPV types (16 and 18 – bivalent vaccine), Gardasil® contains VLPs for four HPV types (6, 11, 16 and 18 – quadrivalent vaccine) and Gardasil®9 contains VLPs for nine HPV types (6, 11, 16, 18, 31, 33, 45, 52 and 58 – nine valent vaccine). The Cervarix® HPV vaccine helps protect against cancers caused by HPV, including cervical cancer, some mouth and throat (head and neck) cancers and some cancers of the anal and genital areas. The Gardasil® HPV vaccine also helps protect against genital warts.

Girls and boys aged 12–13 years in the UK are offered the HPV vaccine as part of the National Health Service vaccination programme. The bivalent vaccine Cervarix® was the HPV vaccine offered initially in 2008 but subsequently from 2012 the quadrivalent vaccine Gardasil® has been offered. In February 2014, the UK Joint Committee on Vaccination and Immunisation concluded that a two-dose schedule in adolescents could be recommended up to (and including) 14 years of age for both Cervarix® and Gardasil®. Since 2023, the UK recommendation has been for a one-dose Gardasil®9 regime for the vaccination of adolescents. Since different countries may have varying vaccination schedules, which may change over time, it is important to check the latest national and local guidelines.

More than a decade after the introduction of the national HPV immunisation programme, evidence of the impact of vaccination has shown reductions in HPV type 16/18 infection, genital warts, precancerous lesions and cervical cancer among vaccinated cohorts.

Infection Control

Prevention includes using barrier methods during sexual intercourse. Cover the warts especially while swimming, do not share towels or walk barefoot on wet floor in public areas (e.g. swimming pools).

Polyomaviruses

Polyomaviruses belong to the family Polyomaviridae. There are two viruses that cause infection in humans (human polyoma virus 1 (BK virus) and human polyomavirus 2 (JC virus).

Human Polyomavirus 1 (BK Virus)

BK virus was named after the initials of the patient from whom it was first isolated. BK virus rarely causes disease, but severe symptoms can occur in kidney transplant recipients. Primary infection is usually asymptomatic, but any symptoms tend to be mild (respiratory infection and fever). The virus then disseminates to the kidneys and urinary tract where it persists for life. After primary infection, the virus establishes latency in the renal uroepithelium and particularly in tubular epithelial cells. In some immunosuppressed solid organ transplant recipients, the virus reactivates and begins to replicate, triggering a cascade of events starting with tubular cell lysis and consequent viruria. The BK virus then multiplies in the interstitium and crosses into the peritubular capillaries, causing viraemia and may also invade the allograft, leading to the tubulointerstitial lesions that characterise BK virus nephropathy. Approximately 20–60% of renal transplant recipients present with viruria; one-third of patients with viruria will develop BK viraemia. BK virus nephropathy develops in 2–10% of recipients. The most consistent risk factor identified for the development of BK virus nephropathy is the overall level of immunosuppression. Approximately 80% of the population contains a latent form of the virus, which remains latent until some form of immunosuppression awakens it. This is usually seen in kidney or multi-organ transplant recipients in whom symptoms are much more severe. Clinical manifestations include renal nephropathy (detected by a progressive rise in serum creatinine). A total of 1–10% of renal transplant patients progress to BK virus–associated nephropathy and up to 80% of these patients lose their kidneys. The onset of nephritis can occur from several days to 5 years after transplantation. BK reactivation is also associated with urethral stenosis and interstitial nephritis. In bone marrow transplant recipients BK reactivation is associated with haemorrhagic cystitis. Infection can be diagnosed by detection of the virus in urine and blood by NAAT (usually PCR). Regular monitoring by BK virus testing of urine and blood by NAAT may help identify infection early and evaluate the success of treatment strategies. Quantitative PCR (see Chapter 51) is particularly helpful as a high or rising viral load especially in blood is predictive of clinical illness. A BK DNA viral load >185,000 copies/ml at the time of the first positive BK reactivation diagnosis is a predictor for BKV-associated nephropathy.

Prevention

BK virus viruria screening is recommended in renal transplant recipients in the first 2 years after transplantation in order to detect the early stages of BK virus infection (when patients are still viruric or viraemic) and to facilitate intervention before the development of overt nephropathy. This timely intervention is crucial, as when BK virus nephropathy is established, treatment becomes more complex and immunosuppression reduction is often not sufficient to stabilise renal function.

Treatment

Treatment comprises reducing immunosuppression where possible or employing different immunosuppressive drugs (e.g. ciclosporin). However, immunosuppression reduction alone is often not sufficient to stabilise renal function. The main objective of immunosuppression reduction is to reduce viral replication without triggering rejection. Antiviral agents that have been associated with anecdotal success include intravenous immune globulin, cidofovir and brincidofovir. Brincidofovir is a lipid conjugate of the acyclic nucleotide phosphonate cidofovir, but unlike cidofovir, it is not concentrated in the proximal tubules of the kidney and less likely to produce renal toxicity. It has been proven effective against polyomavirus. Leflunomide in combination with a low-dose calcineurin inhibitor and prednisone has been shown to facilitate virus clearance and to stabilise graft function without increasing the risk of rejection.

Human Polyomavirus 2 (JC Virus)

JC virus was also named after the initials of the patient it was first isolated from. Antibody to the virus is highly prevalent in the general population, but so far it is not clear what primary illness the virus causes. Its clinical importance is in patients who are immunosuppressed due to T-cell dysfunction (e.g. patients with AIDS or immunosuppressed) in whom the virus reactivates to cause progressive multifocal leucoencephalopathy (PML), which is a progressive degenerative brain disease caused by demyelination and loss of oligodendrocytes. PML usually begins insidiously with changes in intellect, reduced motor function or sensory loss. It rapidly progresses to give rise to multifocal neurological signs and invariably leads to death within a year. Prior to effective antiretroviral therapy, PML developed in 2–4% of AIDS patients. There is no effective treatment for PML. Laboratory confirmation of clinical diagnosis is by finding JC virus in the cerebrospinal fluid or brain biopsy by PCR.

Simian Virus 40 (SV40)

This is a monkey virus which replicates in their kidneys without causing disease and does not cause human disease. However, in the 1950s, it was inadvertently introduced into humans with some contaminated batches of killed polio vaccine grown in monkey kidney cells. All such individuals have been followed up with no evidence of any associated SV40 disease.

Parainfluenza Viruses

The Viruses

Parainfluenza viruses (PIV) are single-stranded RNA enveloped viruses and members of the Paramyxoviridae family which also includes mumps and measles. There are four major serotypes, PIV-1–4. PIV-1 and PIV-3 belong to the genus *Respirovirus* and PIV-2 and PIV-4 belong to the genus *Rubulavirus*.

Epidemiology

Route of Spread

PIV are spread by the respiratory route primarily via inhalation of large droplets or fomites. PIV initially infect the epithelial cells of the nose and oropharynx and then spread distally to the airways.

Prevalence

PIV have a worldwide distribution and are commonly isolated from children <5 years of age. The age at infection varies with serotypes; most children have been infected with PIV-1 by 1 year of age, whereas the other serotypes tend to affect slightly older children at 2–4 years of age. In population-based studies PIV accounted for 7% of hospitalisations due to pneumonia in children under 2 years of age. Serological surveys show that by adulthood >90% of adults have had PIV infection.

PIV do not show seasonal variation in tropical countries, but in temperate climates certain serotypes predominate in spring or autumn/winter. For example, PIV-3 tends to predominate in spring/summer whereas PIV-4 predominates in autumn/winter.

Reinfections with PIV are common but tend to be milder than the initial infection.

Incubation Period

2–6 days (most infections occur within 1–3 days after exposure).

Infectious Period

Patients are infectious while they have respiratory symptoms (especially when coughing).

At-Risk Groups

Immunocompromised patients, especially those with haematological malignancies, bone marrow and solid organ transplant recipients, HIV/AIDS and those with severe T-cell deficiencies. These viruses cause severe and fatal infections in bone marrow transplant recipients and cause outbreaks in bone marrow transplant units. In addition, for adults, older age and cardiac and pulmonary comorbidities are additional risk factors for severe PIV infection.

Clinical

Infection limited to the nasopharynx is associated with mild upper respiratory disease. Spread to the lower respiratory tract is associated with the viral load in the nasopharynx. As with other respiratory viruses, host immune response plays an important role in the symptomatology of PIV infections.

Children

In children, most infections occur in the upper respiratory tract and otitis media is a common complication. About 15% of infections present as lower respiratory tract infections. Croup is generally associated with PIV-1 and PIV-2 infections, whereas PIV-3 is more commonly associated with lower respiratory tract infections. PIV cause 60–75% of cases of croup and 10–20% of all viral bronchiolitis in children.

In the immunocompromised, PIV are detected in 10–15% of all respiratory virus infections and clinical presentation ranges from upper respiratory infection to severe pneumonia especially in the bone marrow transplant recipients.

Adults

Symptoms range from asymptomatic infection to mild upper respiratory tract infection (URTI) to severe and fatal pneumonia depending upon risk factors. Clinical features associated with URTI are similar to other respiratory viruses and include fever, rhinorrhoea, cough and sore throat and most cases are self-limiting. Lower respiratory tract infection presents as pneumonia and acute bronchitis with associated symptoms.

PIV infection is also associated with exacerbations of asthma and chronic obstructive pulmonary disease. As in children immunocompromised adults, especially bone marrow transplant recipients, are at increased risk of pneumonia. PIV infections have been associated with lung allograft dysfunction and rejection.

Differential Diagnosis

It is impossible to diagnose PIV infections clinically and to distinguish infection from many other respiratory viruses and bacteria.

Laboratory Diagnosis

See Table 21.1.

Management

Treatment

Infection is self-limiting in immunocompetent children and adults and requires symptomatic relief. In the immunocompromised, supportive treatment and reduction in

Table 21.1 Laboratory diagnosis of parainfluenza virus infection

Specimen	Test	Interpretation of positive result
Nose and throat swab in virus transport medium	NAAT* (sensitive and rapid)	If positive, indicates current infection
	Point of care test (POCT), i.e. immunofluorescence test (rapid but not very sensitive)	If positive, indicates current infection
Nasopharyngeal aspirate (in very young children) or bronchoalveolar lavage (in immunocompromised patients and those in ITUs)	PCR (sensitive and rapid)	If positive, indicates current infection
	POCT, i.e. immunofluorescence test (rapid but not very sensitive)	If positive, indicates current infection

Note: * NAAT – nucleic acid amplification test; of which PCR is most commonly used.

immunosuppression, where possible, is advised. Evidence to support the use of the antiviral drug ribavirin is variable with no evidence of proven efficacy, but aerosolised or intravenous ribavirin has been used to treat infected bone marrow transplant and lung transplant recipients.

Infection Control

PIV are spread by the airborne route and can cause outbreaks in hospitals and the community. Infection control is paramount in transplant setting (especially bone marrow transplant units) as a PIV outbreak has serious consequences. In hospitals, infected patients should be put into single rooms (in a negative pressure room or with the door closed) or cohorted until they are asymptomatic. Staff should wear aprons, gloves and eye and face masks (if involved in procedures likely to generate respiratory aerosols) and should wash their hands with soap and water before and after patient contact.

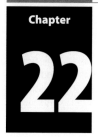

Parvovirus B19

The Virus

Parvovirus B19 is a small DNA virus and belongs to the genus *Erythroparvovirus* in the family Parvoviridae. It was first discovered in 1975. It is the only known human parvovirus. Many other mammalian species including dogs have parvoviruses, but they do not cause infection in humans.

The virus replicates in the erythroid precursor cells which it infects by attachment to one of the blood group antigens (P antigen) expressed at the surface of the cells and which act as the receptor for the virus.

Epidemiology

Route of Spread

The virus replicates initially in the respiratory mucosa and is spread by droplet (rather than aerosol) transmission by the respiratory route. Attack rate is about 50% in susceptible household contacts but much lower in the community setting.

There is a short period of viraemia before the rash appears; therefore, occasional transmissions by blood transfusion have been recorded where a donor has donated in the prodromal period.

Prevalence

Parvovirus B19 has a worldwide prevalence. It is a childhood infection with the prevalence of antibody rising with age with about 50% of young adults showing evidence of previous infection.

Incubation Period

About 12–18 days.

Infectious Period

The highest infectivity period is in the prodromal phase which is 2 days before the rash appears, but patients are not infectious after the rash appears.

At-Risk Groups

Pregnant women, immunocompromised patients and those with haemolytic anaemia.

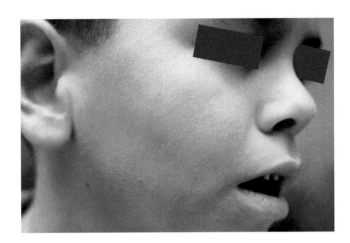

Figure 22.1 A boy with skin rash of erythema infectiosum, or fifth disease, caused by the human parvovirus B19 (courtesy of CDC; details – Public Health Image Library (PHIL): https://phil.cdc.gov/Details.aspx?pid=4509)

Clinical

Erythema Infectiosum

Erythema infectiosum (EI) is also called fifth disease. About 50% of infections, especially in childhood, are asymptomatic. Symptomatic infection is characterised by a biphasic illness of fever, malaise, upper respiratory symptoms for a few days followed by a fine maculopapular rash which is immune-mediated. Typically, the rash is on the cheeks (malar eminences) hence the name of slapped cheek syndrome as the child gives the appearance of having been slapped on both cheeks (see Figure 22.1). A generalised rash on the limbs and body may occur but is usually very transient although a persistent rash for up to 2–3 weeks has been described. Joint pains (arthralgia) occurs in up to 30–50% of adults with parvovirus infection and may be the only presenting feature. Arthralgia is less common in children and associated with EI in about 10% of cases. It may persist for several weeks; generally the large joints are involved but small joints may be involved. True rheumatoid factor–positive arthritis may occasionally occur as a result of infection.

Complications

Transient infection of the erythroid precursor cells leads only to a transient fall in red cells which does not clinically manifest itself as anaemia in healthy immunocompetent children or adults. However, in the following at-risk groups complications occur due to manifestations of severe anaemia of aplastic nature.

Infections in Pregnancy

Fetal transmission may occur in up to 30% of cases, but congenital malformation or birth defects are not associated with it. Fetal loss occurs in about 7–10% of infected women if infected prior to 20 weeks' gestation. The most severe fetal complication is hydrops foetalis, which occurs in 2–3% of infected women. The condition is due to fetal oedema and ascites as a result of severe fetal anaemia and is managed by giving the fetus intrauterine blood transfusion until the condition resolves in a few weeks. It is important to note that about 30% of pregnant women infected with human parvovirus B19 have asymptomatic infection and yet can still infect their unborn babies.

After 20 weeks of gestation, although fetal infection may occur it is not accompanied by untoward fetal outcome.

Evidence also suggests that asymptomatic infection in pregnancy has a higher risk of transmission to the fetus as compared to symptomatic infection as the former suggests a poor host immune response and failure to clear the virus effectively.

Infection in the Immunocompromised

Infection in the immunocompromised may result in chronic parvovirus infection due to the failure of the immune system to clear the virus. This can lead to hypoplasia or aplasia of erythroid cells and precursors leading to the patient developing chronic intractable aplastic anaemia. The blood picture shows significant reduction of reticulocytes. Besides anaemia, leukopenia and thrombocytopenia has also been reported. Other complications such as hepatitis, myocarditis, encephalitis and pneumonitis associated with parvovirus B19 infection have also been reported in the immunocompromised.

Infection in Patients with Haemolytic Anaemia

Transient aplastic crisis develops due to red blood cell death and a sharp fall in red blood cells and haemoglobin. Patients with haematological abnormalities and those with sickle cell disease, thalassemia and hereditary spherocytosis are at risk. Eighty per cent of patients with sickle cell disease who get infected develop transient aplastic crisis. The patient is normally viraemic at the time of the aplastic crisis. Once the immune response is mounted, the patient recovers from the aplastic crisis with a reticulocytic response. Typically, these patients do not develop a rash. Patients generally present with pallor, weakness and lethargy secondary to anaemia.

Myocarditis

Parvovirus B19 has been frequently demonstrated in the cardiac muscle by PCR; however, a direct causal link with myocarditis has not been established.

Laboratory Diagnosis

See Table 22.1.

Management

Treatment

There is no specific treatment in immunocompetent patients; the treatment is supportive.

- *Immunocompromised and in aplastic crisis.* Blood transfusions to improve and maintain the haemoglobin level. Use of intravenous immunoglobulin has been shown to be effective in resolving infection.
- *Hydrops foetalis.* Pregnancy should be monitored by regular ultrasound scans and intrauterine blood transfusions should be given to manage fetal anaemia in cases of hydrops foetalis. The hydrops resolves itself once the fetus is able to limit the infection. There is no evidence of long-term damage to the fetus and such pregnancies successfully go to term with a normal outcome.

Table 22.1 Laboratory diagnosis of human parvovirus B19 infection

Clinical indication	Specimen	Test	Significance	Essential information for the laboratory
Diagnosis of acute parvovirus infection	Serum	Parvovirus IgM	Positive result denotes recent infection	Clinical symptoms, date of onset, any history of any risk factor, e.g. pregnancy, immuno-compromised or aplastic crisis.
Diagnosis of acute infection in immunocompromised and in patients with aplastic crisis	Serum	Parvovirus DNA PCR	Positive result indicates recent or chronic infection. Specific IgM may be negative in immuno-compromised patients due to poor immune response.	Clinical details and symptoms with risk factors if any, date of onset.
Diagnosis of fetal infection	Cord blood by cordocentesis	Parvovirus DNA PCR and IgM if fetus is more than 20 weeks.	Positive IgM and/or PCR indicates fetal infection	Gestational age of the fetus, presence of hydrops.
Check immune status	Serum	Parvovirus IgG by enzyme immunoassay	A positive IgG in the absence of parvovirus specific IgM indicates past infection.	History of and date of recent contact if any, risk factors for infection.

- *Pregnancy*. Pregnant women with acute parvovirus infection should be referred to an obstetrician so that the pregnancy can be followed and managed appropriately if hydrops foetalis develops.

Prophylaxis

There is no specific prophylaxis or vaccine.

Pregnant women who are in contact with a known case of parvovirus B19 infection should be tested for parvovirus IgG to establish immunity. Those found to be susceptible should have a repeat test 4 weeks after contact to ensure that they have not had a subclinical infection (50% of adults have subclinical infection).

Infection Control

Patients do not need to be isolated once the rash appears. Patients with haemolytic anaemia in aplastic crisis do not normally develop a rash and have a prolonged period and a high level of infectivity.

Advice to avoid exposure to infection should be given to patients at risk of parvovirus complications. Patients with infection should also be advised to avoid contact with pregnant women and those who are immunocompromised or suffer from haemolytic anaemia. If in contact, patients at risk of complications from parvovirus infection should be screened for immunity and observed if susceptible and managed appropriately if signs of infection develop.

Healthcare workers who have had a significant exposure to parvovirus B19 infection either at work or at home and work with the at-risk group of patients should be excluded from work from 7 days to 3 weeks after exposure to cover the incubation period.

Chapter 23

Poxviruses

The Viruses

These viruses are double-stranded DNA viruses belonging to the family Poxviridae. They are the largest in size of all known viruses. There are 83 species in the Poxviridae family. Four genera of poxviruses infect humans:

- *Orthopoxvirus* – smallpox virus, vaccinia virus, cowpox virus, monkeypox virus
- *Parapoxvirus* – including orf virus, pseudocowpox virus, bovine papular stomatitis virus
- *Yatapoxvirus* – tanapox virus, yaba monkey tumour virus
- *Molluscipoxvirus* – molluscum contagiosum virus.

Introduction

Poxvirus infections, with the exception of molluscum contagiosum and monkeypox, are rare in the UK. Smallpox was eradicated from the world in 1977. The most commonly diagnosed infections in the UK are molluscum contagiosum, monkeypox (usually sexually transmitted), cowpox (most often acquired from cats), orf (transmitted by sheep) and milker's nodule (acquired from cows). All these viruses cause characteristic pustular skin lesions that develop into large scabs, which can leave permanent pockmarks. These skin lesions and their distribution are different, facilitating clinical diagnosis. However, clinical diagnosis is not foolproof, with monkeypox, smallpox and chickenpox (caused by a herpes virus) being mistaken for each other before smallpox eradication in Africa. Laboratory diagnosis used to be made by electron microscopy and via culture in embryonated eggs. Although diagnosis can still be made by electron microscopy, molecular diagnosis is most commonly used.

Smallpox

Smallpox is transmitted from human to human through the respiratory route, after close contact with an infected person. Smallpox was highly contagious, but generally spread more slowly and less widely than some other viral diseases. Although the virus used to be transmitted to and between monkeys, there is currently no animal reservoir of the virus because smallpox has been eradicated from the world after a concerted international vaccination campaign co-ordinated by the World Health Organization. The last case occurred in Africa in 1977 and the virus is held in two high-security units in the USA and Russia.

Smallpox has an incubation period of 10–12 days. Patients are infectious after the rash has appeared. Once the rash has formed scabs, patients are not infectious. Although virus can be found in scabs, they are not a significant source of infection.

There are two forms of smallpox: variola major, which has a mortality of 20–30%, and variola minor, with a case fatality rate of 1%. The most characteristic feature of smallpox is the rash, which evolves over several days from macule to vesicle to pustule. Finally, a scab forms, which falls off, leaving a pockmark. The rash first appears on the face, then on the arms, and later on the lower limbs. It is usually more profuse on the face and limbs than on the trunk.

The first symptoms are a sudden onset of fever, headache and backache. The fever often falls on the second or third day, as the rash appears and rises again as it becomes pustular. Immunosuppression, pregnancy and malnutrition are associated with more severe infection.

Chickenpox would be the major differential diagnosis if the disease were ever to emerge again. The chickenpox rash is similar, but is more prevalent on the body (trunk) than on the face and limbs. Smallpox lesions tend to be larger. There are several other pox viruses (e.g. cowpox and monkeypox) which cause vesicular lesions on the skin.

There are no really effective antiviral drugs available to treat smallpox.

Suspected smallpox cases should be treated in strict isolation in negative pressure isolation facilities, preferably in designated specialist units.

Smallpox Vaccine

Smallpox was eliminated from the world by use of the smallpox vaccine. Current smallpox vaccines have a much-improved side-effect profile compared to previous vaccines. The modified vaccinia Ankara (MVA-BN) vaccine, used in the UK, is a third-generation smallpox vaccine containing a defective virus, attenuated through multiple passages in chicken embryo fibroblast cells. The MVA-BN vaccine has been authorised for active immunisation against monkeypox as well as smallpox in adults in the UK and USA. Vaccination in the UK is restricted to those personnel who would be involved in the emergency response to smallpox and for close contacts of monkeypox cases or those at greatest risk of acquiring monkeypox through sexual exposure. Staff caring for patients with smallpox or monkeypox must be vaccinated with MVA-BN smallpox vaccine. The vaccine is given using a bifurcated needle that is dipped into the vaccine solution. The needle is used to prick the skin (usually the upper arm) several times in a few seconds. If successful, a red and itchy bump develops at the vaccine site in 3 or 4 days.

Cowpox

The first description of cowpox was recorded by Jenner in 1798. 'Vaccination' is derived from the Latin adjective *vaccinus*, meaning 'of or from the cow'. Cowpox used to be commonly transmitted to farmworkers, often milkmaids, from cows. The virus is not now commonly found in cattle. The reservoir hosts for the virus are woodland rodents, particularly bank voles, field voles and wood mice. Domestic cats contract the virus from these rodents and can then pass on the infection to humans. Symptoms in cats include lesions on the face, neck, forelimbs and paws, and, less commonly, upper respiratory tract infections.

The incubation period in humans is 9–10 days. The virus is most prevalent in late summer and autumn. Symptoms of infection with cowpox virus in humans are localised, pustular lesions generally found on the hands and face and limited to the site of contact with the infected cat. The skin lesions eventually crust over; when the crust falls off, patients are no longer infectious. Patients can sometimes have more systemic symptoms including headache and malaise as well as localised skin redness, swelling and local lymph node involvement. The illness usually lasts from 6 to 12 weeks. Occasional deaths from cowpox have been recorded and infection can be more severe in atopic patients and immunocompromised patients, who often have a more generalised and widespread infection, which can be fatal. There is no antiviral treatment. Occasionally infection can be misdiagnosed as orf or milker's nodule.

Monkeypox

Monkeypox (now referred to as mpox) is a rare disease that is caused by infection with the monkeypox virus, which is related to, but distinct from, the viruses that cause smallpox and cowpox. The name monkeypox originates from the initial discovery of the virus in monkeys in a Danish laboratory in 1958.

Monkeypox used to occur most commonly in West and Central Africa and is still endemic there. Infection in Africa is thought to be acquired by eating bushmeat and contact with infected animals. The West African clade occurs in countries from Sierra Leone to South Sudan and the Central African clade occurs mainly in the Democratic Republic of Congo. Rats, mice, squirrels and rabbits can also be infected by monkeypox virus. Recently, infection outside Africa has become more common and has spread widely across the world, largely as a result of sexual transmission (especially in men who have sex with men). Between 2018 and 2022, the UK experienced a small number of imported cases, all from West Africa. From April 2022, the UK identified a rapid increase in monkeypox cases, which led to a prolonged outbreak. By September 2022, over 3,500 cases had been confirmed, mainly in London, and the vast majority in males. The outbreak appeared to be associated with cases in similar populations worldwide including Canada, Portugal, Belgium and Germany. Monkeypox occurs when a person comes into close contact with lesions, body fluids, respiratory droplets from an animal or human with the infection or contact with material contaminated with the virus (e.g. bedding). The virus enters the body through broken skin, the respiratory tract or the mucous membranes. The incubation period is 10–12 days, after which patients experience fever, headache, backache, malaise, lymphadenopathy and muscle ache. The vesicular rash appears about 3–5 days later, becoming pustular and then scabbing over. Traditionally, monkeypox rash has been found on the face, limbs and trunk of the body. However, in the current outbreak, it has been common for lesions to occur on the genitalia and perineal area. The illness usually lasts for 2–4 weeks. Most patients experience a mild, self-limiting illness, with spontaneous and complete recovery seen within 3 weeks of onset although bacterial superinfection can result in severe disease, which can sometimes result in death. The risk of severe disease is higher in children, pregnant women and immunosuppressed individuals. In Africa, mortality rates for the West African cases are 1–3% and up to 10% for the Central African cases; in developed countries, the mortality rate is about 0.05%. There are currently no antivirals in use to treat monkeypox, but clinical trials are under way to evaluate the efficacy of brincidofovir and tecovirimat; smallpox vaccination will protect against monkeypox infection. In the recent UK outbreak, vaccine was used prophylactically in persons and healthcare staff at increased risk of infection and post-exposure (see website listed at end of chapter for details). Infection control measures include avoiding skin contact with people who have a rash that looks like monkeypox and avoiding handling clothes, sheets, blankets or other materials that have been in contact with an infected person.

Molluscum Contagiosum

Molluscum contagiosum is the most common poxvirus infection in humans worldwide. Infection is most common in children. It causes small (2–6 mm) wart-like lesions on the skin, often in clusters on exposed areas of skin (hands, arms, face, neck, chest, abdomen and eyelid margins). They are raised dome-shaped areas of skin with a central dimple. They eventually form a crust and then heal up. Patients rarely have any other symptoms. Molluscum contagiosum is infectious and is usually spread among young children by direct contact. The virus is spread either by direct contact, including sexual activity, or via contaminated objects such as towels and toys. The condition can also be spread to other areas of the body by the person themselves. More severe and widespread infection can occur in immunocompromised persons and those with atopic dermatitis, and who live in crowded living conditions. It is possible to get reinfected. Diagnosis is typically based on the appearance of the lesions. Although infectious, no exclusion from school, work or swimming pools is necessary, although sharing of towels and sponges should be avoided for those infected. There is no antiviral treatment but squeezing individual lesions will result in the molluscum body, full of infectious virus, to be forced out of the central dimple in the lesion; this will result in the lesion resolving. This is easier after a bath. Freezing (cryotherapy) and burning (laser therapy) can also be used. Piercing the lesions with a sharp object dipped in podophylin or cimetidine is sometimes used for treatment, but this can leave scars.

Orf and Milker's Nodule

These diseases have an identical clinical presentation and are acquired by close contact with sheep and goats (orf) and cows (milker's nodule). They are caused by a parapox virus which has a different morphological appearance to orthopox viruses, from which it can be distinguished easily (see Figure 23.1).

They produce large (1–2 cm) vesicular lesions which become pustular and then scab over. They are often surrounded by a red erythematous area which can be quite tender to touch. Patients with a severe form of disease can have symptomatic symptoms such as headache, malaise and fever as well as swollen lymph nodes. There is no treatment and infection cannot be passed to other humans. Although the lesions may often appear severe, patients can be reassured that symptoms will resolve in 2–3 weeks.

Laboratory Diagnosis

Several laboratory methods can be used to diagnose pox and parapox virus infections. Nucleic acid amplification tests (NAATs) can distinguish between different viruses and some are so specific that they can differentiate different strains of the same virus. Electron microscopy (EM) can easily distinguish between pox and parapox viruses by morphology but only experienced electron microscopists could accurately distinguish between smallpox, vaccinia and molluscum contagiosum viruses (Figure 23.1); EM can also easily differentiate herpes viruses, which have a very different morphology, from pox viruses.

See Table 23.1.

Table 23.1 Laboratory diagnosis of poxvirus infections

Specimens	Test	Interpretation of positive result
Vesicle fluid, vesicle swab or scab	NAAT	Specific virus infection*
	Electron microscopy	Pox virus or parapox virus infection

Note: * Varicella-zoster virus (VZV) and herpes simplex virus (HSV) PCR tests should also be conducted as part of the differential diagnosis if the type and distribution of vesicular lesions are similar to those produced by VZV and HSV.

(a)   (b)   (c)

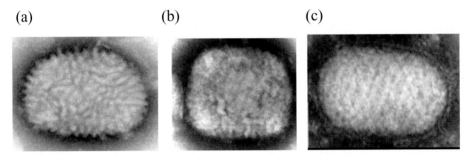

Figure 23.1 Electron micrographs of pox and parapox viruses (courtesy of CDC)
a Vaccinia virus.
b Monkeypox virus.
c Orf virus.

Infection Control

Pox viruses spread by physical contact (especially with monkeypox) or via fomites. When in healthcare settings, patients should be in single rooms with the door closed, using universal precautions. The skin lesions are infectious if touched and when the skin scabs fall off; they can remain infectious for many weeks. Therefore, infected persons should ideally be in isolation for the duration of illness, which typically lasts 2–4 weeks and should not be in contact with other humans. Their bedding and other items which could be contaminated with the virus should be laundered or disinfected and items that have been worn or handled and surfaces that have been touched by a lesion should be decontaminated.

Useful Website

Smallpox and monkeypox, *The Green Book on Immunisation*, chapter 29 (Public Health England): www.gov.uk/government/publications/smallpox-and-vaccinia-the-green-book-chapter-29

Chapter

24

Rabies Virus

The Virus

Rabies virus is a single-stranded RNA virus and belongs to the genus *Lyssavirus* in the family Rhabdoviridae.

Epidemiology

Route of Spread

Rabies is a zoonotic disease and is transmitted from animals (particularly dogs, foxes, wolves, jackals, monkeys and bats) to man. Dogs are responsible for 99% of human cases in rabies-endemic areas. Infection can be transmitted from a bite or scratch via a puncture wound through the skin or through a lick on an open wound or sore. Human-to-human spread does not occur but has exceptionally been reported in the rare circumstance of tissue/organ transplantation from an infected patient.

Prevalence

According to the World Health Organization (WHO), rabies is responsible for about 59,000 human deaths globally every year. Rabies occurs in every region of the world, but there are some countries that have eradicated the infection from terrestrial animals although related lyssaviruses may exist in bats. Rabies can be reintroduced into countries that have eradicated it, so it is always wise to check if it is present in countries that are being visited so one can be aware of the risk and the need for prophylactic rabies vaccine.

Incubation Period

The incubation period in man is usually 1–3 months, but it can be as short as 10 days and as long as 2 years, following exposure. The incubation period in the dog is usually from 14 to 60 days, but it may be much longer.

Infectious Period

Animals are infectious via infected saliva.

At-Risk Groups

People are at risk when they have not received prophylactic vaccine and they are bitten or scratched by an infected animal or licked on an open wound in a country where rabies is prevalent. Risk of infection depends on the severity and location of the wound and timeliness of post-exposure prophylaxis. Risk is highest the closer the bite is to the head. It is estimated that the probability of developing rabies after a bite to the head/neck is 55% as compared to about 10% after bites to the lower limb/trunk.

Clinical

Symptoms

The virus first multiplies in the tissue around the site of inoculation. For the first 2–4 days patients usually develop malaise, fever, headache, sore throat and lack of appetite. Pain and tingling around the site of inoculation in the infected limb is usually the first indication that the virus has entered the nervous system and it is due to virus replication in the corresponding dorsal root ganglia. The virus then spreads via the peripheral nerves to the spinal cord and eventually to the brain where it gives rise to acute encephalitis. Symptoms therefore usually travel up the limb or spread around the face or neck, depending on the site of infection. Jerky movements and increased muscle tone may well follow. Dilation of the eye pupils and excessive secretion of tears and saliva often occurs next. The patient may next become anxious and frightened when examined or disturbed and the patient's temperature rises to 38–40°C. Localised paralysis may follow, resulting in difficulty in swallowing, resulting in the patient being terrified of drinking. The fear of drinking water (hydrophobia) is very suggestive of rabies. Patients may be very excited (in the furious form of rabies) or apathetic (in the paralytic or dumb form). With very few exceptions, patients die within a week of the onset of symptoms. Tetanus can cause similar convulsions.

Laboratory Diagnosis

Several laboratory methods and clinical specimens can be used to diagnose rabies; all the tests should be performed in a high-security specialist laboratory. In life, a hairline biopsy is usually tested for presence of rabies virus by PCR or immunofluorescence in a reference laboratory. After death, additional specimens such as a brain biopsy can be tested for rabies virus by PCR or immunofluorescence. 'Negri bodies' (rabies virus inclusions in the neuronal cells) are typically seen on brain histology (see Figure 24.1).

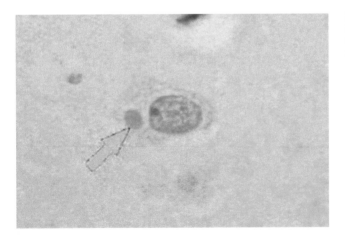

Figure 24.1 Negri body (arrowed) in an infected neuron (image courtesy of CDC)

Management

Treatment

Once symptoms have become established, there is no effective treatment other than supportive care.

Prophylaxis

Prophylaxis is by inactivated rabies vaccine which is given by the intramuscular route. However, the intradermal route is equally effective, and as it uses a smaller vaccine dose this route may be preferred in resource-poor countries as it saves on vaccine doses.

Pre-exposure prophylaxis is with three doses of rabies vaccine. Post-exposure prophylaxis is either by five doses of rabies vaccine, over a period of a month, or, if the risk of rabies exposure is likely, by means of vaccine and human anti-rabies immunoglobulin (injected around the site of inoculation and any remaining given intramuscularly). It is very important to seek urgent medical advice in case of a bite or a lick or scratch from a suspect animal abroad, especially if it was behaving aggressively. Even in people who have had previous rabies vaccine, it is strongly advised to have post-exposure vaccine where a significant risk of exposure has occurred. Administration of prompt post-exposure prophylaxis is highly effective in preventing rabies. In the UK, the UK Health Security Agency (UKHSA) Virus Reference Laboratory provides expert advice on the need for giving rabies vaccine and immunoglobulin after an exposure and it issues vaccine and immunoglobulin after the patient and exposure information has been provided via the forms included in the websites shown in the Useful Websites section.

Infection Control

Rabies does not spread from human to human, but gloves and apron should be worn when treating patients with suspected rabies. Healthcare workers caring for an infected patient should be offered rabies vaccination.

As dogs are responsible for almost 99% of all rabies cases in endemic areas, the WHO has launched a global framework to eliminate rabies transmitted by dogs by 2030 via a programme of mass vaccination of dogs to interrupt the transmission cycle to humans.

Useful Websites

UKHSA: Guidelines on managing rabies post-exposure, January 2023: https://assets .publishing.service.gov.uk/government/uploads/system/uploads/attachment_data/file/ 1130673/UKHSA-guidelines-on-rabies-post-exposure-treatment-January-2023.pdf

UKHSA: Annexe 3: Summary of risk assessment and treatment: https://assets .publishing.service.gov.uk/government/uploads/system/uploads/attachment_data/file/ 1127795/UKHSA-guidelines-on-rabies-post-exposure-treatment-January-2023-annexe-3.pdf

Rabies, *The Green Book on Immunisation*, chapter 27 (Public Health England): www .gov.uk/government/publications/rabies-the-green-book-chapter-27

25

Respiratory Syncytial Virus

The Virus

Respiratory syncytial virus (RSV) is a single-stranded RNA virus belonging to the family Pneumoviridae. Its name is derived from the large cells (syncytia) that form when infected cells fuse.

Epidemiology

Route of Spread

RSV is spread by direct contact with respiratory secretions in air droplets through the nose and eyes. The virus infects the epithelial cells of the upper and lower airways, causing inflammation, cell damage and airway obstruction.

Prevalence

RSV has a worldwide distribution and is the most common cause of respiratory illness in infants requiring hospital admission. Reinfection is common in later life: it is an important infection in all age groups. Worldwide, RSV is the leading cause of bronchiolitis and pneumonia in infants and children under the age of 5. The risk of serious infection is highest during the first 6 months of life. In young children, 70% are infected and 30% have clinical illness in their first year of life. All children are infected by 3 years of age, some having had more than one infection and 2% of infants have severe lower respiratory tract symptoms. Immunity is short lasting (just a few weeks or months). In families with pre-school-aged children, 50% of family members will be infected. There are higher attack rates in nurseries and schools. Infection rates are higher during the cold winter months (November to February in the UK), causing bronchiolitis in infants, common colds in adults, and more serious respiratory illnesses such as pneumonia in the elderly and immunocompromised. Healthy young adults rarely develop severe illness with RSV requiring hospitalisation. However, it is a significant cause of morbidity and mortality in certain adult populations, including the elderly and those with underlying heart or lung conditions and who are immunosuppressed. Approximately 5–10% of nursing home residents will experience RSV infection each year, with significant rates of pneumonia and death.

Incubation Period

3–6 days.

Infectious Period

- Children are infectious for 9 days on average, but this can be much longer.
- Adults are infectious for about 2–3 days.
- Immunocompromised patients can be infectious for several weeks.

At-Risk Groups

Immunocompromised patients (e.g. those with severe combined immunodeficiency syndrome, haematopoietic stem cell transplant recipients, those on chemotherapy and HIV infected patients).

Clinical

Symptoms

RSV infection produces a wide variety of signs and symptoms that range from asymptomatic to mild upper respiratory tract infections to severe and potentially life-threatening lower respiratory tract infections requiring hospitalisation.

- In young children with symptoms, approximately 15–50% develop more serious lower respiratory tracts infections, such as bronchiolitis, viral pneumonia or croup. Bronchiolitis is characterised by inflammation and obstruction of the small airways in the lungs. Several viruses can cause bronchiolitis, but RSV is responsible for about 70% of cases. It usually presents with 2–4 days of runny nose and congestion followed by worsening cough, noisy breathing, tachypnoea and wheezing.
- Infection in adults often produces only mild to moderate symptoms indistinguishable from the common cold but may also be asymptomatic. Symptoms are generally confined to the upper respiratory tract (runny nose, sore throat, fever and malaise). Only about 25% of infected adults have significant lower respiratory tract symptoms.
- Elderly adults have a similar presentation to younger adults but tend to have more severe symptoms and an increased risk of lower respiratory tract involvement. Elderly adults are more likely to experience pneumonia, respiratory distress and death.
- Immunocompromised persons are at a significantly increased risk of severe infection with RSV and are more likely to progress from upper to lower respiratory tract involvement and have prolonged shedding. The severity of symptoms is related to the amount and type of immune suppression. Patients who have received hematopoietic stem cell transplants, intensive chemotherapy or lung transplants are particularly susceptible. Bone marrow transplant patients appear to be at highest risk, especially prior to marrow engraftment, when RSV infection carries an 80% risk of pneumonia and death.

Differential Diagnosis

Influenza, parainfluenza, adenovirus, Covid-19 and other respiratory viral infections. RSV infections in nursing homes for the elderly can mimic influenza.

Laboratory Diagnosis

Several laboratory methods and clinical specimens can be used in diagnosing RSV infection. Laboratory diagnosis may not always be indicated but is important in patients

Table 25.1 Laboratory diagnosis of RSV infection

Specimens	Test	Comments
Nasopharyngeal aspirate and bronchoalveolar lavage	NAAT*	Very sensitive Result in a few hours
	Immunofluorescence	Less sensitive than NAAT. Sensitivity dependent on receiving a good quality specimen. More sensitive in young children (more viral shedding) but less sensitive in older children and adults. Result in 1–2 hours.
Nose and throat swab	NAAT	Very sensitive Result in a few hours
Nasal aspirate or wash Nasopharyngeal swab	Rapid 'bedside' antigen tests (including EIA** and chromatographic immunoassays)	Rapid (<1 hour) but less sensitive than PCR. More sensitive in young children (more viral shedding) but less sensitive in older children and adults.
	NAAT	Very sensitive Results in a few hours

Note: * NAAT – nucleic acid amplification test; of which PCR is most commonly used.
** EIA – enzyme immunoassay.

with severe disease and to facilitate infection control. Serology is not helpful. See Table 25.1.

Management

Treatment

Ribavirin is licensed for administration by inhalation for the treatment of severe bronchiolitis caused by RSV in children less than 2 years of age, especially when they have other serious diseases. However, there is no evidence that ribavirin produces clinically relevant benefit in RSV bronchiolitis. As ribavirin is potentially teratogenic, pregnant healthcare workers should avoid exposure to the aerosolised drug particles.

Intravenous ribavirin is sometimes given under expert medical supervision to immunocompromised children with life-threatening RSV infection but it is currently not licensed for this use.

Prophylaxis

Passive immunisation is available in the UK by giving Synagis® (palivizumab) which is a humanised monoclonal antibody produced using recombinant DNA techniques in mouse myeloma host cells. It provides passive immunity against RSV. The recommended dose of palivizumab is 15 mg/kg of body weight, given once a month. Where possible, the first dose should be administered at the start of the RSV season (calendar week 40). Subsequent doses should be administered monthly throughout the RSV season up to a maximum of five doses. The objective of the passive immunisation is to protect at-risk infants for whom RSV infection is likely to cause serious illness or death. These include:*

- all children less than 24 months of age with severe combined immunodeficiency syndrome;
- those at high risk due to bronchopulmonary dysplasia:
  - pre-term infants who have moderate or severe BPD;
  - infants with respiratory diseases who are not necessarily preterm but who remain in oxygen at the start of the RSV season;
- those at high risk due to congenital heart disease.

Note: * Refer to the latest version of the Green Book for the latest guidance (see weblink in the Useful Website section).

Infection Control

The spread of RSV can be reduced by strict handwashing after patient contact. The use of gloves, aprons, face masks and goggles will reduce the risk of transmission. Isolation in single rooms or cohort nursing reduces the risk to other patients. During the RSV season, many paediatric centres screen for RSV before admission so they can cohort nurse the infected babies separately from those who are not infected.

Useful Website

Respiratory syncytial virus, *The Green Book on Immunisation*, chapter 27a (Public Health England): https://assets.publishing.service.gov.uk/media/5a80e88ae5274a2e87 dbc7ff/Green_Book_Chapter_27a_v2_0W.PDF

26
Chapter

Rhinoviruses

The Viruses

Rhinoviruses are single-stranded RNA viruses and belong to the family Picornaviridae.

Epidemiology

Route of Spread

Rhinoviruses are spread readily by direct contact with respiratory secretions, fomites and large droplets through the nose and eyes. Nosocomial infections are common. The name rhinovirus derives from the fact that these viruses infect the nasal passages and these viruses are one of several causes of the 'common cold'. There are over 100 serotypes of rhinoviruses.

Prevalence

Rhinoviruses have a worldwide distribution. They occur in epidemics in autumn, winter and spring, with peaks of infection at those times of the year. Infection occurs in people of all ages, but the incidence is higher in children than adults. Children experience 4–8 infections per year as compared to adults experiencing 2–3 infections per year.

Incubation Period

1–3 days.

Infectious Period

Infected individuals are usually infectious for about 5 days, when they are sneezing and have a nasal discharge.

At-Risk Groups

Immunocompromised patients (severe combined immunodeficiency, bone marrow transplant, chemotherapy, HIV) are at greatly increased risk of developing pneumonia. Patients with underlying asthma and other chronic respiratory conditions are at risk of exacerbation of the disease.

Table 26.1 Laboratory diagnosis of rhinovirus infections

Specimens	Test	Comments
Nasopharyngeal aspirates and bronchoalveolar lavages	NAAT*	Very sensitive. Can have results in a few hours.
Nose and throat swab	NAAT	Very sensitive. Can have results in a few hours.

Note: * NAAT – nucleic acid amplification test; of which PCR is most commonly used.

Clinical

Symptoms

Almost all rhinovirus infections in young children are associated with clinical illness, whereas 50% of infections in older children and adults may be asymptomatic. Infections with various serotypes begin in early childhood and continue throughout life, usually resulting in typical 'common cold' symptoms. The infection has no prodrome; sneezing and nasal discharge are usually the first symptoms to become apparent. The nasal passages, paranasal sinuses, oropharynx, Eustachian tubes, middle ear, larynx and large airways can all be involved. Symptoms include sneezing, nasal obstruction, sore throat, facial pressure, hoarseness, cough, headache, malaise and fever. Symptoms usually last for about 5 days. Complications such as acute bacterial otitis media and acute bacterial sinusitis occur, but in a minority of those infected.

Differential Diagnosis

Influenza, parainfluenza, RSV, adenovirus and other respiratory viral infections.

Laboratory Diagnosis

Diagnosis is usually clinical and laboratory investigations are normally not indicated. If required several laboratory methods and clinical specimens can be used to diagnose infection (Table 26.1). Serology is not helpful.

Management

Treatment

There are no specific antiviral treatments available, although compounds with anti-rhinovirus activity have been identified in the laboratory. Symptomatic treatments for headache, nasal congestion, cough and sore throat are appropriate.

Prophylaxis

There are no viral vaccines available for preventing rhinovirus infections.

Infection Control

The spread of rhinoviruses can be reduced by strict handwashing after patient contact. Use of gloves, aprons and goggles will reduce the risk of transmission. Isolation in single rooms or cohort nursing reduces the risk to other patients.

Chapter 27

Rotaviruses

The Viruses

Rotaviruses are double-stranded RNA viruses with segmented genomes belonging to the family Sedoreoviridae. They are called rotaviruses because by electron microscopy, the virus particles resemble a wheel (see Figure 27.1). There are nine species of the genus (A, B, C, D, F, G, H, I and J); Rotavirus A, the most common species, causes more than 90% of rotavirus infections in humans. Rotavirus strains are classified based on the outer layer proteins VP7 (G type) and VP4 (P type). Although there are at least 15 G types and 28 P types, only 10 G and 11 P types have been identified in humans.

Epidemiology

Route of Spread

Rotaviruses are transmitted mainly by the faecal-oral route, via contact with contaminated hands, surfaces and objects. Viral diarrhoea is highly contagious. It has been estimated that fewer than 100 virus particles are required to transmit infection to another person. Rotaviruses are stable in the environment and have been found in sewage and estuary samples. They can survive for up to 20 days in these environments; despite this they are not associated with food-borne gastroenteritis outbreaks.

Prevalence

Rotaviruses are the most common cause of diarrhoeal disease in infants and young children worldwide, with 90% of children in the UK being infected at least once by the age of 5. Each year, rotaviruses cause millions of cases of diarrhoea in developing countries, over a million of which result in hospitalisation, with many deaths. Immunity develops with each infection and therefore subsequent infections are less severe or asymptomatic. Infections in young adults are rarely reported, although they are not uncommon in individuals in contact with children who have rotavirus gastroenteritis. Rotavirus diarrhoea outbreaks are common among hospitalised infants, young children attending nurseries and elderly people in nursing homes, with infections peaking in the winter months, in the UK, between January and March.

Incubation Period

The incubation period of rotavirus infection is between 1 and 2 days.

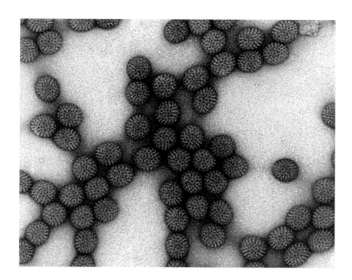

Figure 27.1 Rotavirus electron micrograph (courtesy of CDC)

Infectious Period

Persons are most infectious when symptomatic with diarrhoea and vomiting.

At-Risk Groups

The most severe symptoms occur in children 6 months to 2 years of age, the elderly and those with immunodeficiency, who have prolonged symptoms and virus excretion.

Clinical

Symptoms

Rotaviruses infect and damage the cells that line the small intestine and cause gastroenteritis. Rotavirus gastroenteritis symptoms usually last from 3 to 8 days. Rotavirus enteritis is associated with nausea, vomiting, watery diarrhoea and low-grade fever. Symptoms often start with vomiting followed by 4–8 days of profuse watery diarrhoea. Dehydration is more common in rotavirus infections than in gastroenteritis caused by bacteria and is the most common cause of death, especially in resource-poor countries.

Differential Diagnosis

Other viruses such as noroviruses, astroviruses, sapoviruses and adenoviruses, as well as bacteria, can cause sporadic cases of diarrhoea and vomiting, but these are under-diagnosed because most cases of gastroenteritis presenting to the health service do not include laboratory confirmation of the causal organism. Rotaviruses are seldom associated with outbreaks of diarrhoea and vomiting but outbreaks can occur in very young and elderly persons.

Laboratory Diagnosis

See Table 27.1.

Table 27.1 Laboratory diagnosis of rotavirus infections

Specimen	Test	Interpretation of results
Faeces	NAAT* (RT-PCR)	If positive, indicates current infection**
	EIA***	If positive, indicates current infection
	Dipstick/rapid test device	If positive, indicates current infection
	Electron microscopy	If positive, indicates current infection

Note: * NAAT – nucleic acid amplification test; of which PCR is most commonly used.
** The increased sensitivity of the RT-PCR for rotavirus detection means that asymptomatic infection, characterised by low viral loads, can be detected and results must be interpreted with caution.
*** EIA – enzyme immunoassay.

Management

Treatment

There is no antiviral treatment available. Rehydration is appropriate in severe cases, especially in very young children.

Prophylaxis

In 1998, a rotavirus vaccine was licensed for use in the USA. Clinical trials found it to be over 80% effective at preventing severe diarrhoea caused by rotavirus A and no significant serious adverse effects were reported. However, in 1999, after it was discovered that the vaccine may have contributed to an increased risk for intussusception (a severe type of bowel obstruction) in 1 in every 12,000 vaccinated infants, the vaccine was withdrawn from the market.

In 2006, two new vaccines against rotavirus A infection were shown to be safe and effective in children and in 2009, the World Health Organization recommended that rotavirus vaccine be included in all national immunisation programmes. Rotavirus vaccines have reduced rotavirus hospitalisations by 49–92% in those countries using rotavirus vaccine in their national immunisation programmes. Rotarix® is the vaccine offered as part of the UK national childhood immunisation programme. It is a live attenuated vaccine administered orally. It has been shown to protect against gastroenteritis due to rotavirus serotypes G1P, G2P, G3P, G4P and G9P; some efficacy against uncommon rotavirus genotypes G8P and G12P has also been demonstrated. The vaccine is over 85% effective in protecting against severe rotavirus gastroenteritis in the first 2 years of life. The first dose is given at approximately 8 weeks of age, with the second dose at least 4 weeks after the first dose. Although the vaccine is a live attenuated virus, with the exception of severe combined immunodeficiency, the benefit from vaccination may exceed any risk in other forms of immunosuppression; therefore, there are very few infants who cannot receive rotavirus vaccine.

Infection Control

Rotaviruses are spread principally by the faecal-oral route and can cause outbreaks in hospitals and in the community. In hospitals, infected patients should be put into single rooms (with the door closed) or cohorted until they are asymptomatic. Staff should wear aprons and gloves and should wash their hands with soap and water before and after patient contact. In household and community settings, although good hygiene measures can help prevent spread of the disease, the stability of rotaviruses and the low infectious dose (10–100 virus particles) makes standard sanitary measures to halt transmission of the virus relatively ineffective.

Useful Website

Rotavirus, *The Green Book on Immunisation*, chapter 27b (Public Health England): https://assets.publishing.service.gov.uk/media/5a80848aed915d74e622eea8/ Green_Book_Chapter_27b_v3_0.pdf

Chapter

28

Rubella Virus

The Virus

Rubella virus is a single-stranded RNA virus which is the only member of the genus *Rubivirus* within the family Togaviridae. The outer envelope protein E1 is the viral haemagglutinin protein responsible for binding to the cell receptors to initiate infection.

Epidemiology

Prevalence

Rubella has a worldwide prevalence. Before the introduction of vaccination, it circulated in epidemic form with an epidemic cycle every 6–8 years. In countries with effective childhood rubella vaccination programmes, this pattern has been interrupted as has been the number of reports of endemic cases. In countries without vaccination programmes, it remains an infection of childhood. About 15–20% of young adults remain susceptible, putting them (especially pregnant women) at risk of acute infection as the virus is endemic and continues to circulate in the community.

Route of Spread

Infection is spread via respiratory secretion droplets. The virus is highly infectious with attack rates of 50–80% in susceptible individuals in communities during outbreaks.

Incubation Period

The rash usually develops 16–18 days after exposure but the incubation period may range from 14 to 21 days. Infection is first initiated in the respiratory epithelium and then spreads and replicates in the regional lymph node. This is then followed by viraemia and dissemination of virus to multiple sites.

Infectious Period

Maximum viral shedding from respiratory tract of infected individuals occurs from 5 days before to 7 days after the appearance of the rash.

At-Risk Groups

Pregnant women, especially those in the first trimester of pregnancy.

Clinical

Postnatal Rubella

Approximately 25–50% of infections in adults are asymptomatic; infections in childhood are more likely to be asymptomatic. Symptoms are usually mild and consist of fever and a maculopapular rash which may be transient. Arthralgia (joint pains) or frank arthritis may occur in up to 30% of adolescents and young adults with rubella but are less common in children. Usually, big joints are involved and pain may be fleeting in nature. Development of post-auricular shotty lymph nodes is almost pathognomic of rubella.

Congenital Rubella

Sir Norman Gregg, an Australian ophthalmologist, was the first to describe congenital rubella syndrome, which consists of the classical triad of bilateral cataract, microcephaly and sensorineural deafness. Other features are hepatosplenomegaly, thrombocytopaenia and a purpuric rash.

The risk of fetal malformation is highest (80%) after maternal rubella in the first trimester, especially in the first 6 weeks of pregnancy. The risk of fetal malformation decreases from the second trimester onwards and maternal infection after 20 weeks of gestation, although leading to fetal infection, has little risk of fetal abnormality, that is, congenital malformation. However, a minority of infants may develop sensorineural deafness later on, so long-term follow-up is advisable.

Complications

Postnatal acute rubella is a self-limiting illness; in adults rare complications are rubella hepatitis and encephalitis.

Acute infection, especially in the first trimester of pregnancy, leads to fetal infection and congenital infection.

Laboratory Diagnosis

See Table 28.1.

Management

Treatment

- *Postnatal rubella*: There is no treatment and acute rubella is a self-limiting illness, complications are rare and management is supportive.
- Rubella infection in the first trimester of pregnancy has a high risk of fetal infection and malformation. Risk should be discussed and an informed decision made regarding the option for termination of pregnancy.
- *Congenital rubella*: Prognosis depends upon the fetal age at acquisition of congenital infection. The neonate should be followed as late sequelae of congenital infection, especially deafness (not apparent at birth), may develop. There is no specific treatment and treatment will depend upon the management of the presenting condition, for example sensorineural deafness, cataracts, etc.

Table 28.1 Laboratory diagnosis of rubella infection

Clinical indication	Specimen	Test	Significance	Essential information for the laboratory
Diagnosis of acute rubella infection in children and adults	5–10 ml of clotted venous blood	Rubella IgM Rubella IgG avidity	Positive IgM result denotes recent infection. Spurious positive IgM result may occasionally occur therefore result should be confirmed by rubella IgG avidity test. Mature (high avidity IgG) antibody indicates that infection has occurred more than 3 months ago.	Clinical symptoms, date of onset, history of contact, if pregnant then period of gestation.
Diagnosis of congenital infection in neonates	As above	Rubella IgM	Presence of rubella IgM in newborn is indicative of congenital infection as IgM does not cross the placental barrier.	History of suspected or confirmed maternal rubella infection. Clinical signs and symptoms.
Diagnosis of fetal infection	Fetal blood by cordocentesis (taking of fetal cord blood under ultrasound guidance)	Rubella IgM Rubella PCR	Positive result indicates fetal infection. Positive IgM must be confirmed.	History of suspected or confirmed maternal rubella infection.
Check for past infection or immunity	5–10 ml of clotted venous blood	Rubella IgG	Positive result indicates immunity due to past infection or vaccination	History of vaccination

Prophylaxis

Post-exposure

Pregnant women with suspected rubella contact should have a blood test for rubella IgG antibody to determine their immune status. Those who are found to be susceptible should have a second blood test 4 weeks after the suspected contact to ensure that they have not acquired infection and should be offered measles, mumps and rubella (MMR) vaccine after delivery.

Pre-exposure

Rubella immunisation programmes are well established in many countries, especially in the West. Most countries follow a universal childhood vaccination programme.

In the UK, universal vaccination as combined MMR vaccine is offered at 12–15 months, followed by a second dose before school entry at 3–5 years. Unvaccinated older children and adults should be offered two doses of MMR 1 month apart.

Any woman found to be susceptible in pregnancy should be offered vaccination in the post-partum period as rubella vaccination is contraindicated in pregnancy. Inadvertent administration of rubella vaccine in pregnancy is not an indication for therapeutic intervention as there has been no association to date of rubella vaccine virus causing fetal malformation.

Infection Control

Respiratory precautions (Chapter 56) should be applied. Rubella virus can be shed for a long period in the urine of congenitally infected babies. Handwashing and wearing of gloves when dealing with infected secretions should be practised. Infected healthcare workers should be excluded from work during the infectious period.

Rubella immunisation remains the mainstay of infection control. Healthcare workers and women working with small children who do not have documented vaccination history should be screened and immunised.

Chapter 29

Varicella-Zoster Virus

The Virus

Varicella-zoster virus (VZV) is a double-stranded DNA virus and a member of the Herpesviridae family of viruses.

Epidemiology

Route of Spread

VZV is transmitted by the airborne route from respiratory secretions and from vesicles on the skin. After entry through the respiratory route there is an initial period of viraemia which seeds the virus in the reticulo-endothelial system. This is followed by a second episode of viraemia resulting in dissemination of the virus throughout the body and manifestations of the typical chickenpox vesicular rash on the skin surface. The virus then travels down the sensory nerves to the dorsal route ganglia adjacent to the spine, circularises its DNA and becomes latent. At some future time the virus may reactivate, usually in one ganglion, with the virus travelling back down the sensory nerve(s) to the area of the skin served by the nerve (s) and producing clusters of vesicles (shingles/zoster). Persons with shingles can transmit VZV infection to non-immune persons, who will experience chickenpox.

Prevalence

VZV infection occurs worldwide and the prevalence of infection varies considerably. While >90% of people in industrialised countries have had chickenpox by the age of 20 years (although about 20% will have had such a mild infection that they may be unaware of this), in the tropics, only 50% of people have had chickenpox by the age of 20 years.

Incubation Period

10–23 days (mean 14 days).

Infectious Period

From 1 day before the onset of symptoms until 5 days after the rash or all the skin lesions are fully crusted.

At-Risk Groups

- Immunocompromised persons
- Pregnant women

- Unborn children in the first 20 weeks of pregnancy and 1 week before or after delivery

Clinical

Symptoms

Chickenpox (varicella) infection produces a generalised vesicular skin rash. The lesions normally first appear on the upper part of the body before becoming generalised. The rash involves the whole body (including scalp) but the lesions are most dense on the central part of the body (the trunk) as compared to the limbs. Vesicles may be so few as to be missed in some persons. Lesions of chickenpox continue to appear over the first 48 hours of onset and lesions at various stages of development can be seen in clusters (cropping). It is usually a fairly mild infection in children, but severe infection can occur, particularly in immunocompromised children. Adults (especially pregnant women in the third trimester) are at much higher risk of severe or fatal chickenpox, particularly if they develop varicella pneumonitis which is much more common in smokers rather than non-smokers. Rarely, encephalitis may occur as a complication. Symptoms are more severe in immunocompromised adults and haemorrhagic chickenpox (almost always fatal) with multi-organ involvement can occur in transplant recipients.

Shingles (zoster) results when VZV reactivates from a dorsal root ganglion; the virus then travels down a sensory nerve to the skin supplied by that nerve (dermatome). It usually produces a group of fluid-filled blisters (vesicles) on the skin. Sometimes vesicles do not appear on the skin, but patients experience pain in the affected dermatome (zoster sine herpete). Shingles is often associated with pain (post-herpetic neuralgia), particularly in older persons and prompt antiviral treatment given less than 48 hours after the onset of the symptoms is indicated in these patients.

Infection in Pregnancy

Pregnant women are more likely to have severe symptoms than other adults (especially pneumonia). Chickenpox in the first 20 weeks of pregnancy can result in severe infection in the fetus (congenital varicella syndrome) in 1–2% of cases. Occasional cases of fetal damage, comprising chorioretinitis, microcephaly and skin scarring following maternal varicella between 20 and 28 weeks' gestation, have been reported. If the mother has chickenpox in the second and third trimesters of pregnancy, zoster can develop in an otherwise healthy infant in the first year of life. Babies with congenital varicella syndrome are born with skin scarring, microphthalmia, chorioretinitis, cataracts, hypoplasia of the limbs and neurological abnormalities (microcephaly, cortical atrophy, mental retardation or dysfunction of bowel and bladder sphincters). These defects do not occur at the time of the initial fetal infection; they are caused by subsequent herpes zoster reactivation in utero. Prenatal diagnosis of congenital varicella syndrome can be achieved by ultrasound (by detecting evidence of limb deformity, microcephaly, hydrocephalus, soft tissue calcification and fetal growth restriction). In order to maximise detection of defects, ultrasound scans should be done at least 5 weeks after chickenpox infection in the mother.

If maternal infection occurs in the last 7 days before delivery or within 7 days of delivery, there is a significant risk of severe or fatal chickenpox in the neonate. A planned

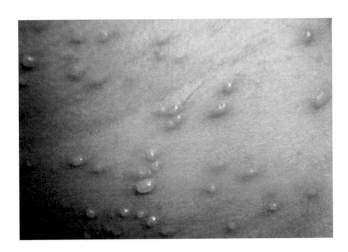

Figure 29.1 Typical chickenpox rash (copyright Dr Tim Wreghitt)

delivery should normally be avoided for at least 7 days after the onset of the maternal rash to allow for the passive transfer of antibodies from mother to child, provided that continuing the pregnancy does not pose any additional risks to the mother or baby. Neonates should be given prophylactic varicella-zoster immune globulin (VZIG) and/ or aciclovir.

Expert advice should be sought from a specialist if a pregnant woman presents with chickenpox or she has had recent contact with a person with chickenpox or shingles.

Differential Diagnosis

Vesicular skin lesions caused by VZV can be mistaken as herpes simplex virus (HSV) infection (or monkeypox). Chickenpox usually causes widespread lesions, especially on the body, with vesicles at various stages of development in one cluster (Figure 29.1). Shingles vesicles are usually confined to an area of skin (dermatome) on one side of the body served by a sensory nerve (although immunosuppressed patients can have much more extensive lesions). HSV lesions are usually all at the same stage of development in the same cluster. Reactivated HSV lesions and clusters of zoster vesicles can look very similar. It may be important to ensure, by laboratory tests, whether persons are infected with VZV or HSV (to ensure appropriate infection control procedures are instituted and the correct dose of antiviral drugs are given, if treatment is required).

Laboratory Diagnosis

Several laboratory methods and clinical specimens can be used to diagnose VZV infection (see Table 29.1).

All herpes viruses have the same morphology and cannot be differentiated by electron microscopy (see Figure 29.2).

Management

Treatment

Several drugs are available for treating VZV infections (Table 29.2).

Table 29.1 Laboratory diagnosis of VZV infection

Clinical indication	Specimens	Test	Interpretation of positive result
Chickenpox	Vesicle fluid or vesicle swab	PCR	Indicates VZV infection
		Electron microscopy	Indicates a herpes virus infection (all herpes viruses look alike in the EM, so cannot distinguish between VZV and HSV, but can differentiate from other viruses (e.g. pox viruses). No longer used for routine diagnosis.
	Clotted blood taken at least 7 days after onset	VZV IgM	Indicates recent VZV infection
Shingles	Vesicle fluid or vesicle swab	PCR	Indicates VZV infection
		Electron microscopy	Indicates a herpesvirus infection (VZV or HSV). No longer used for routine diagnosis.
	Clotted blood	VZV IgM	Indicates recent VZV infection (but may be negative in cases of shingles).
	Paired clotted blood samples (first taken in first 5 days of illness)	VZV IgG	A significant seroconversion rise in VZV IgG titre indicates recent shingles.
Encephalitis/ meningitis	CSF	PCR	Indicates VZV central nervous system infection
Has the patient had VZV infection before?	Clotted blood	VZV IgG	Indicates previous VZV infection if sufficient VZV IgG is found.*

Note: * Refer to current guidelines for correlation between VZV IgG units and correlation to immunity in different patient groups.

Prophylaxis*

Chickenpox infection in immunosuppressed persons, pregnant women and neonates can result in severe and life-threatening disease. Post-exposure prophylaxis is recommended to attenuate disease and reduce the risk of complications such as pneumonitis, rather than to prevent infection in these at-risk individuals. Oral aciclovir (or valaciclovir) is the first choice of post-exposure prophylaxis for susceptible immunosuppressed individuals, all susceptible pregnant women at any stage of pregnancy and infants at high risk.

They should be given from day 7 to day 14 after exposure. The day of exposure is defined as the date of onset of the rash if the index is a household contact.

Post-exposure prophylaxis is recommended for individuals who fulfil all of the following three criteria:

Table 29.2 Antiviral drugs for treating chickenpox and shingles*

Clinical indication	Drug
Chickenpox	Oral aciclovir
Severe chickenpox (encephalitis or pneumonitis)	IV aciclovir
Severe chickenpox in immunocompromised patients	IV aciclovir
Shingles	Oral aciclovir Oral valaciclovir Oral famciclovir
Severe shingles in immunocompromised patients	IV aciclovir

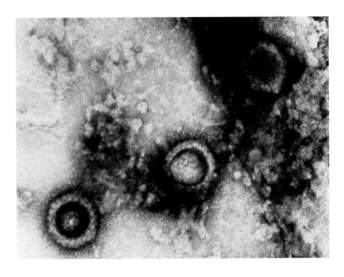

Figure 29.2 Electron micrograph of herpes viruses (courtesy of CDC; details – Public Health Image Library (PHIL): https://phil.cdc.gov/Details.aspx?pid=6493)

- significant exposure to chickenpox or shingles during the infectious period;
- at increased risk of severe chickenpox such as immunosuppressed individuals, neonates and pregnant women; and
- no or insufficient antibodies to VZV.

In immunocompetent individuals, the infectious period should be taken as being from 24 hours prior to rash onset to 5 days after rash. For immunosuppressed individuals, the infectious period should be taken from 24 hours prior to rash onset until all lesions have crusted over. For individuals who are unable to take oral antivirals, and for susceptible neonates exposed within 1 week of delivery (in utero or post-delivery), VZIG should be given.

* Note: Always refer to nationally agreed protocols and drug data sheets for latest recommended treatment and prophylaxis regimes.

Vaccine

Varicella vaccines for the prevention of chickenpox are lyophilised preparations containing live, attenuated virus derived from the Oka strain of VZV. Transmission of vaccine virus from immunocompetent vaccinees to susceptible close contacts has occasionally been documented but the risk is very low. The two-dose vaccination schedule provides about 98% protection in children and about 75% protection in adolescents and adults.

Both a live attenuated and a recombinant subunit vaccine to prevent shingles is available and recommended for elderly at increased risk of shingles.

Infection Control

Patients with chickenpox and zoster should be nursed in isolation and expert infection control and patient management advice should be sought if a pregnant woman or immunocompromised person or healthcare worker in contact with these patients develops chickenpox or shingles or is in contact with a case of chickenpox or shingles. Non-immune staff in clinical contact with cases of chickenpox or shingles should be removed from clinical contact work from days 8–16 after contact.

Useful Websites

Varicella: the Green Book, Chapter 34: www.gov.uk/government/publications/varicella-the-green-book-chapter-34

UK Health Security Agency (UKHSA) guidelines on post exposure

prophylaxis (PEP) for varicella or shingles (January 2023): https://assets.publishing .service.gov.uk/government/uploads/system/uploads/attachment_data/file/1134812/UKHSA-guidelines-on-VZ-post-exposure-prophylaxis-january-2023.pdf

Royal College of Obstetricians and Gynaecologists, Chickenpox in Pregnancy (Green-top Guideline No. 13): https://www.rcog.org.uk/guidance/browse-all-guidance/green-top-guidelines/chickenpox-in-pregnancy-green-top-guideline-no-13/

| Section 2 | **Other Related Agents** |

Chapter

30

Chlamydia

Chlamydia are obligate intracellular gram negative bacteria. They have a dimorphic growth cycle of elementary bodies (EB) which are electron-dense infectious structures and reticulate bodies (RB) which are non-infectious intra-cellular forms. EBs attach to the cell to initiate cell infection. Once inside the cells they differentiate into reticulate bodies. RBs divide by binary fission and subsequently differentiate back to EBs to be released from the cell to initiate further infection.

Chlamydia belong to the family Chlamydiaceae which has one genus, *Chlamydia*, and the following species:

- *C. trachomatis* is further subdivided into serovars:
  o serovars A, B, Ba and C which cause trachoma (tropical eye infection);
  o serovars D–K which cause genital infection; and
  o lymphogranuloma venereum (LGV) serovars 1, 2 and 3 which cause genital infection with inguinal lymphadenopathy in the tropics.

- *C. psittaci* is a natural infection in birds, both psittacine (parrots, budgerigars, etc.) and other birds (e.g. pigeons). Human infection is acquired as a zoonosis from birds.
- *C. pneumoniae* is a human pathogen.
- *C. abortus* primarily infects sheep and causes abortion in pregnant ewes (hence the name). Human infection is accidental from sheep.
- *C. caviae* causes infection in guinea pigs. It does not cause human infection.

For *C. psittaci*, *C. pneumoniae* and *C. abortus*, see Chapter 33 on atypical pneumonia. See Table 30.1.

Epidemiology

Chlamydia is prevalent worldwide. Trachoma is a disease of underdeveloped and developing countries and the most important cause of blindness in these parts. Genital *C. trachomatis* infection is the most common bacterial sexually transmitted infection (STI) in the UK with 8–10% of all 15–25 year-olds being infected at any given time in 2020/21. LGV is limited purely to those who have partners from tropical countries as their sexual contacts.

C. psittaci and *C. pneumoniae* are prevalent worldwide; about 60–80% people worldwide acquire *C. pneumoniae* infection, the incidence being 1–2% a year.

LGV and trachoma are limited to tropical countries.

Table 30.1 Infections due to *Chlamydia* species

Agent	Clinical infection	Route of spread
C. trachomatis A, B, Ba, C	Trachoma	Infected fomites, flies
C. trachomatis D–K	Genital chlamydia, adult inclusion conjunctivitis, ophthalmia neonatorum	Sexual Mother to baby
LGV 1, 2, 3	Genital ulcers and enlarged inguinal lymph nodes	Sexual
C. psittaci	Febrile illness, atypical pneumonia, rarely endocarditis	Respiratory
C. pneumoniae	Upper respiratory tract infection or atypical pneumonia	Respiratory
C. abortus	Febrile illness, miscarriage in pregnancy	Respiratory

Clinical

C. trachomatis

Trachoma: Trachoma is an infection of childhood in the tropics. It is spread as a result of poor hygiene through infected fomites or close personal contact. Flies are an important route of spread for trachoma as they can carry the bacteria from person to person. Active trachoma presents as follicular conjunctivitis. Reactivation and reinfections occur resulting in severe fibrosis of eyelids and inward turning of eyelid (entropion) due to contracture; this in turn results in the eyelashes constantly rubbing against the cornea (trichiasis) and leads to blindness in adult life.

Genital chlamydia infection: Those who have unprotected casual sexual intercourse with multiple partners are the most at risk.

Male genital infection is mostly asymptomatic. Clinical infection presents as urethritis. Chlamydia infection is the commonest cause of non-specific urethritis in males. Infection may spread to the upper genital tract and cause epididymo-orchitis and prostatitis and may cause male infertility. Inclusion conjunctivitis and proctitis occur in case of eye and rectal infection.

Female genital infection: As in males >50% of infection is asymptomatic. Clinically, cervicitis with cervical discharge is the most common presentation, urethritis being relatively uncommon in females. If untreated, ascending infection leads to salpingitis (infection of fallopian tubes) and pelvic inflammatory disease (PID), leading to complications such as ectopic pregnancy and infertility. Fitz-Hugh–Curtis syndrome is the name given to chlamydia perihepatitis and is a rare complication of intra-abdominal extension of PID. Infertility may occur due to blockage of fallopian tubes as a result of salpingitis or infection of ovaries (oophoritis).

Extra genital infection: Inclusion conjunctivitis, proctitis and oral/throat infection occur in both men and women as result of oro-genital or anal sex.

Ophthalmia neonatorum: This is neonatal conjunctivitis which typically presents between 5 and 15 days of age due to acquisition of infection from the mother at the time of birth. Approximately a third of the babies will have nasopharyngeal carriage of

Table 30.2 *C. trachomatis* diagnosis

Clinical presentation	Specimen type for NAAT test	Serology
Trachoma, inclusion conjunctivitis and ophthalmia neonatorum	Conjunctival swab	Not indicated
Female genital tract infection	Self-taken vulvo-vaginal swabs, cervical swab or FVU. Other swabs as indicated by clinical presentation.	Only useful for diagnosis of PID, otherwise not indicated
Male genital tract infection	FVU. Other swabs as indicated by clinical presentation.	Not indicated

chlamydia, therefore it is essential to treat the infection with systemic antibiotics. Untreated infection may give rise to chlamydial pneumonia which presents around 6 weeks of age or later.

LGV: This causes genital ulcers and inguinal lymphadenopathy. Inguinal buboes may be a feature.

***C. psittaci*:** This presents clinically as atypical pneumonia (Chapter 33). Infection may be asymptomatic or present as a febrile influenza-like syndrome with general malaise, sore throat, headache and photophobia. Rare complications are endocarditis, myocarditis, arthritis or meningoencephalitis. The infection is acquired from birds and should be suspected on epidemiological grounds. Pigeon, bird fanciers and those who keep birds as pets or work in bird pet shops are most at risk.

***C. pneumoniae*:** This is a human chlamydial infection and a common cause of community-acquired pneumonia. Outbreaks in young, institutionalised adults (e.g. military recruits) occur. Infection may also present as pharyngitis, sinusitis and bronchitis.

***C. abortus*:** This is an infection of sheep which causes abortion in ewes. Farmers and those coming into contact with sheep, especially at lambing time, are at risk of infection as the bacteria are present in high concentration in the sheep placenta. Infection in pregnant women may lead to miscarriage therefore it is advisable for pregnant women to avoid contact with pregnant ewes at lambing time.

Laboratory Diagnosis

Laboratory diagnosis of *C. trachomatis* is by demonstration of chlamydia in swabs taken from the relevant sites and first-void urine (FVU) (Table 30.2) by nucleic acid amplification techniques (NAATs). The chlamydia NAAT tests are usually able to detect all *C. trachomatis* serovars including those that cause trachoma and LGV. However, false negative results occurred in certain commercial NAATs in 2006 in relation to emergence of a new strain (the Swedish strain) which had a mutation in the target region used in these tests. Epidemiological surveillance for emerging strains is therefore important.

C. psittaci and *C. pneumoniae* infection are diagnosed serologically by demonstration of rising antibody titres in paired acute and convalescent serum samples. As the bacteria are intracellular, they cannot be cultured on the traditional bacterial medium in the laboratory. Direct detection by NAAT tests on respiratory secretions is diagnostic.

Management

Treatment

Chlamydia (genital and respiratory) infections respond to treatment with antibiotics. Tetracyclines are the first-line drugs for treatment. Erythromycin should be used in pregnancy and in children as tetracyclines are contraindicated in them.

Azithromycin is equally effective against chlamydia. It is available as a single-dose treatment for *C. trachomatis* hence results in better patient compliance.

The UK National Chlamydia Screening Programme for genital chlamydia infection aims to identify the pool of infected 15–25 year-old young adults. The aim is to reduce the burden of genital infection and thus the associated complications of PID and infertility by targeting this population through opportunistic screening, identifying the infected and offering them and their partners treatment.

Infection Control

Good personal hygiene, avoidance of unprotected sexual intercourse with casual partners by use of barrier method of protection. *C. psittaci* and *abortus* infections are zoonoses and human-to-human spread does not occur. However, since these infections can be more severe in pregnant women and their unborn children, pregnant women should not come into contact with sheep and goats that are giving birth or that have recently done so. *C. pneuminiae* is a common respiratory infection in the community and so it is difficult to control.

Toxoplasma gondii

The Organism

Toxoplasma gondii is an obligate intracellular protozoan parasite which can infect almost all warm-blooded animals; felids (including domestic cats) are the only known definitive host in which the parasite undergoes sexual reproduction.

Life Cycle

The sexual component of the life cycle occurs only in felids (e.g. domestic or wild cats). The asexual component of the life cycle can occur in almost all warm-blooded mammals (including humans, cats, pigs, cows, goats, sheep and birds). When a cat is infected with *Toxoplasma gondii* by eating a mouse carrying the organism in tissue cysts, this enables the organism to undergo sexual reproduction in the cat's gastrointestinal tract, with the resulting thick-walled oocysts being shed in the cat faeces; they are very hardy and can survive in the environment in an infectious form for several months. Oocysts take 1–5 days to sporulate in the environment and become infective (so changing cat litter regularly is beneficial). Almost all mammals can be infected either by ingesting cat faeces or by eating tissue cysts (e.g. in meat). Tissue cysts lie dormant in their mammalian hosts (usually in muscle and brain), only reactivating when the host is immunosuppressed, causing symptomatic infection. The infection can be passed around mammals by eating tissue cysts.

Epidemiology

Route of Spread

Toxoplasma gondii is transmitted to humans by four principal routes (although it can also be transmitted very rarely via blood transfusions):

- the ingestion of cat faeces containing oocysts;
- the ingestion of uncooked or undercooked meat containing tissue cysts;
- mother to child (in utero); and
- from donated organs to solid organ transplant recipients
  (especially heart transplants).

Prevalence

Toxoplasma gondii is a worldwide infection in humans which infects approximately 10% of people in the UK by the age of 50. In the elderly, evidence of previous infection is higher. The prevalence is also higher in people living in countries (e.g. France) where undercooked meat is more frequently consumed. Infection rates differ significantly from country to country; it has been estimated that 30–50% of the worldwide population overall have been infected. It is more prevalent in countries with a warm wet climate.

Incubation Period
4–21 days (mean 10 days).

Infectious Period
Humans cannot acquire *Toxoplasma gondii* infection from other humans.

At-Risk Groups
Immunosuppressed persons (e.g. transplant recipients, HIV-positive persons) and pregnant women, as unborn babies can acquire infection from mothers who have active infection during pregnancy.

Clinical

Symptoms
Most *Toxoplasma gondii* infections in humans are asymptomatic. Those persons who do have symptoms from primary infection experience pyrexia, lymphadenopathy, myalgia and malaise. The frequency of lymphadenopathy varies with age and sex; it is more prevalent in boys under the age of 15 and more prevalent in women than men. The most common sites for lymphadenopathy are neck (65%), axillae (24%) and groin (11%). In most persons (60%) lymphadenopathy lasts less than 2 months, but it can last for longer than 6 months in 6% of cases. Therefore, Toxoplasma infection should be excluded in patients presenting with persistent lymphadenopathy.

Immunocompromised persons (see Chapter 45) can experience severe and life-threatening infection (encephalitis, pneumonia, myocarditis and retinitis) both as primary and reactivated infection. Approximately 1% of *Toxoplasma gondii* antibody-positive solid organ transplant recipients will experience symptomatic reactivated *Toxoplasma gondii* infection in the first few months after transplantation.

Babies can be infected in utero following maternal infection (see Chapter 39) and this can cause damage to the baby at any stage of pregnancy. There is a 40% risk of maternal-fetal transmission if a woman is infected while pregnant, but not all infected babies will develop congenital infection. If the mother has *Toxoplasma gondii* infection in the first trimester of pregnancy, 25% of babies will have congenital infection. Not all infected babies will have congenital damage, so it is very important to consider the difference between infection and disease. The infection rates for the second and third trimesters are approximately 54% and 60–70% respectively. Infection of the placenta is a prerequisite for congenital transmission. The severity of symptoms in the baby depends on the trimester in which infection occurred. Infection acquired in the first trimester of pregnancy leads to congenital damage in 75% of infected fetuses; infection later in pregnancy is less likely to cause fetal damage with virtually no damage associated with

Table 31.1 Laboratory diagnosis of *Toxoplasma gondii* infection*

Sample	Laboratory test	Result interpretation
Clotted blood (serum)	*Toxoplasma gondii* IgG	If positive, indicates infection at some time
	Toxoplasma gondii IgM	If positive, indicates recent infection. This needs confirmation in a reference laboratory in pregnant women, neonatal and immunocompromised persons.
	Toxoplasma gondii dye test	The gold standard test. Only done in a reference laboratory, which will do other confirmatory tests and interpret the results.
EDTA blood	*Toxoplasma gondii* DNA PCR	If positive, indicates active infection

Note: * Toxoplasma PCR on fetal blood sample obtained at cordocentesis is required to confirm or exclude fetal infection.

infections acquired in the third trimester. Congenital symptoms include hydrocephalus, meningoencephalitis, intracranial calcifications, chorioretinitis, hepatosplenomegaly, jaundice, petechial rash, anaemia and thrombocytopenia. Retinal chorioretinitis is the most frequent sign in babies with congenital damage (in 76% of cases). Some, who may be asymptomatic at birth, may present with retinal lesions (often unilateral) later in life (often in their teens).

Differential Diagnosis

Epstein–Barr virus, cytomegalovirus, adenovirus and several bacterial infections can present with similar symptoms, although those with Epstein–Barr virus infection are more likely to have a sore throat and persons with *Toxoplasma gondii* infection are more likely to present with lymphadenopathy (particularly cervical lymphadenopathy) (see Chapter 37). Lymphoma can present with similar symptoms.

Laboratory Diagnosis
See Table 31.1.

Management

Treatment

Infections can be treated with antimicrobials. Pyrimethamine, sulfadiazine, clindamycin, clarithromycin and azithromycin may be used individually or in combination to treat persons with severe *Toxoplasma gondii* infection. Treatment of Toxoplasma infection in pregnant women reduces the risk of in-utero transmission to the foetus and may limit foetal damage. Specialist advice should always be sought when interpreting laboratory results and in deciding appropriate antimicrobial treatment, especially in pregnant women, neonates and immunocompromised persons.

Prophylaxis

Some patients (notably those with HIV infection or those who have recently received transplanted organs or bone marrow) may require antimicrobial prophylaxis to prevent donor-acquired infection or symptomatic reactivation.

Infection Control

There are no infection control issues with *Toxoplasma gondii* infection. It does not spread from person to person. Infection prevention advice such as not eating uncooked or undercooked meat, wearing gloves and an apron when gardening and changing cat litter and strict handwashing after such activities, should be given to all persons at increased risk of severe infection.

Useful Website

Antiprotozoal drugs | Treatment summaries | BNF | NICE: https://bnf.nice.org.uk/treatment-summaries/antiprotozoal-drugs/#toxoplasmosis

Transmissible Spongiform Encephalopathies (CJD and vCJD)

Transmissible spongiform encephalopathies (TSE) are a group of agents that give rise to spongiform degeneration in the brain. These agents do not possess any nucleic acid (DNA or RNA) and are very resistant to inactivation. They consist of only a glycoprotein core and the term 'prion' or 'prion protein' (PrP) has been coined to describe them.

They infect both humans and animals and have recently been shown to cross the species barrier (e.g. vCJD which crossed into humans from cattle).

Epidemiology

The first agent to be described was scrapie. Scrapie has been known to cause infection in sheep in the UK for more than 100 years. In the late 1980s there was an outbreak of a bovine form of scrapie namely bovine spongiform encephalopathy (BSE) which had previously not been described. This led to the destruction of hundreds of thousands of cattle in the UK and a public health crisis in the confidence of beef for human consumption.

Creutzfeldt-Jakob disease (CJD) is the human form of prion disease and has been known to occur throughout the world since 1920. Kuru is the name given to infection that was limited to parts of Papua New Guinea only. In the 1990s a new form of CJD was described for the first time in the UK as a result of BSE transmission. This was named as variant CJD (vCJD) to distinguish it from the already existing CJD.

Human prion disease can be acquired through either the inherited or the infectious route. To understand this and to understand how an agent consisting of protein only can be 'infectious' it is important to understand the pathogenesis of prion disease.

Pathogenesis of Prion Disease

A cellular form of PrP exists naturally in cells. This cellular 33–37 kDa protein is a referred to as PrP^c (c for cellular). Mutations in the cellular protein (PrP^c) lead to changes in its conformational (folding pattern) structure and make it resistant to protease enzyme. This mutated protein is 27–30 kDa in size and referred to as PrP^{Sc} (Sc for scrapie) or PrP^{Res} (Res for resistant).

As this PrP^{Sc} is resistant to protease enzyme it is not destroyed and accumulates in the brain. Even though the exact mechanism is not clear this accumulation initiates the process of spongiform brain degeneration (encephalopathy). Folded PrP^{Sc} or 'scrapie fibrils' can be demonstrated by electron microscopy in the infected brain tissue.

There is considerable experimental evidence to show that when this PrP^{Sc} is injected in a normal brain it can induce the normal cellular PrP^c to change to the resistant PrP^{Sc} by contact thus explaining the infectious aetiology of prion disease.

Route of Spread

TSE in humans can be acquired as an inherited (due to the inheritance of defective genes causing the PrP^c mutation) or infectious form.

The main route of infectious spread is through consumption of infected meat or exposure of cuts and abrasions to infected material.

Iatrogenic spread of CJD through use of pituitary growth hormone, dura mater and corneal grafts and through contaminated neurosurgical instruments has been well documented. vCJD has also been shown to be transmitted via lymphocytes in blood transfusion and other lymphatic-rich tissues (e.g. tonsils).

In animals, the vertical route of transmission (e.g. from the mother to the newborn) has been shown for both BSE and scrapie.

Prevalence

Scrapie is known to exist in many other countries besides the UK; Australia is considered as a scrapie-free country. Although the BSE outbreak occurred in the UK, sporadic cases in cattle were identified in France, Germany and other European countries.

Sporadic CJD has an incidence of 1/million population and probably occurs because of chance mutation of the PrP^c to PrP^{Sc}. Familial forms are due to inheritance of the defective gene, have higher incidence than sporadic CJD and are limited to family clusters or certain races.

Incubation Period

The incubation period is prolonged and varies from months to years depending upon the species and clinical presentation of the prion disease.

Infectious Period

Infectivity lasts throughout the period of infection and is highest in the neural tissue especially the central nervous system. vCJD is also present in high concentration in the tonsils and appendix as it has tropism for lymphoid tissues/cells. It is likely that both animals and humans are infectious in the incubation period (e.g. before any symptoms appear).

At-Risk Groups

Some forms of CJD have been shown to occur in family clusters. For vCJD, consumption of infected beef, especially prior to safety measures being instituted, and blood transfusions from potentially infected donors were also risk factors.

Clinical

Animal Prion Disease

Scrapie

As the name implies, scrapie presents as intense itching which results in the sheep scraping themselves against objects. This is normally accompanied with ataxia.

BSE

In cattle, BSE presented as ataxia, excessive response to sensory stimuli and aggressive behaviour, which gave it the popular name of 'mad cow disease'. The BSE outbreak was likely to have been started by feeding of scrapie-infected bonemeal to cattle. There was some debate though that sporadic low-level BSE already existed and the outbreak was due to BSE-infected bonemeal getting into the feed chain due to changes in the process of bonemeal extraction. The outbreak was brought under control by the slaughter of hundreds of thousands of potentially infected cattle and by banning bonemeal as cattle feed.

Human Prion Disease

All human prion diseases have common neurological features such as neuronal loss, proliferation of glial cells, absence of inflammatory response and presence of protease-resistant PrP.

Creutzfeld-Jakob Disease (CJD)

Sporadic CJD has an incidence of 1 case/million and is slowly progressive disease with a long incubation period (decades) and occurs after 50 years of age. Disease onset starts with tremors, insomnia and depression progressing to ataxia and dementia. It is invariably fatal, death normally occurring within a few months to years after onset. Diagnosis is clinical and at autopsy the brain biopsy shows spongiform degeneration.

Kuru is another form of CJD and was limited to the Fore tribe of Papua New Guinea who practised ritualistic cannibalism. It was mainly seen in the women and children as the brains of the dead elders were consumed mostly by them. The disease was eradicated in the 1950s subsequent to the banning of cannibalism in the country.

Iatrogenic CJD is similar to sporadic CJD but acquired as a result of some medical intervention (see Route of spread section).

Variant CJD (vCJD) was first reported in UK in 1995/6 and was directly linked to BSE and consumption of infected beef. The prion of vCJD and BSE has been shown to have the same structure. vCJD has a longer clinical course than CJD and affects a younger age group with an average age of around 25 years. The number of case reports since the start have been small (between 200 and 300); the majority (about 75%) of cases have occurred in the UK with a smattering of cases across the world including the USA and Europe. All cases were related to food consumption and most have been traced back to the UK. There were case reports of vCJD transmission via blood transfusion; this led to the policy in the UK of leucodepletion (since vCJD has a predilection for lymphoid cells) for safe blood transfusion.

Gerstmann–Straussler–Scheinker disease (GSS) and *fatal familial insomnia (FFI)* are familial forms of the disease.

See Table 32.1.

Laboratory Diagnosis

There are no specific laboratory tests except for histology on brain biopsy. However, tests to detect PrP^{Sc} in blood, tonsillar tissue and cerebrospinal fluid are being developed. One prototype blood-based vCJD assay looks promising for screening of blood.

Table 32.1 List of animal and human TSEs

Animal TSEs	Route of transmission
Sheep, goats (scrapie)	Grazing on infected pastures Vertical from mother to newborn
Cattle (BSE)	Feeding infected bonemeal Vertical from mother to newborn
Domesticated elk, deer, minks, domestic cats (wasting transmissible encephalopathy)	Feeding of contaminated food

Human TSEs	Route of transmission
Sporadic CJD	Probably due to chance mutation of the cellular prion protein. Occurs in older individuals.
Iatrogenic CJD	Infection acquired as a result of medical intervention
Kuru	Ritualistic cannibalism, children and women affected
vCJD	Consumption of contaminated beef, blood transfusion
GSS and FFI	Autosomal inherited

Diagnosis is clinical. Histology on brain biopsy is the only definitive diagnosis and shows spongiform degeneration of brain with astrocytosis and an absence of inflammatory response. Amyloid-like plaques in the brain are a feature of most of the TSEs; the folded PrP^{Sc} protein or 'scrapie fibrils' can be seen by electron microscopy in these plaques.

Management
No effective treatment or prophylaxis exists and all the TSEs are invariably fatal.

Infection Control
The BSE epidemic was controlled by banning bonemeal as cattle feed and by slaughtering infected herds (e.g. all herds with any infected cows) to prevent introduction of infected beef to the food chain.

There are strict guidelines to prevent the iatrogenic spread of CJD and vCJD. These include:
- single-use neurosurgical instruments on high-risk patients;
- removal of leucocytes from blood to be transfused (reducing risk of vCJD); and
- sourcing plasma from countries free of vCJD.

Useful Website
GOV.UK guidance on minimising transmission risk of CJD and vCJD in healthcare setting: www.gov.uk/government/publications/guidance-from-the-acdp-tse-risk-management-subgroup-formerly-tse-working-group

Chapter

33

Atypical Pneumonia

Epidemiology

Atypical pneumonia is caused by bacteria, rather than viruses, but it is included in this book because laboratory tests for evidence of infection with these organisms are often carried out in virology laboratories. They are called 'atypical' because they produce a type of pneumonia not caused by one of the pathogens most commonly associated with the disease (e.g. *Streptococcus pneumoniae* causing lobar pneumonia). Persons with atypical pneumonia are more likely to present with 'atypical' generalised symptoms (e.g. fever, headache, sweating and myalgia) and bronchopneumonia. Atypical pneumonia organisms tend to produce less severe and more protracted symptoms than other bacterial pneumonias; however, they can cause severe or fatal infection.

Atypical pneumonia is caused mainly by five different bacteria:

- *Mycoplasma pneumoniae*
- *Chlamydia psittaci*
- *Chlamydia pneumoniae*
- *Coxiella burnetii*
- *Legionella pneumophila*.

Prompt diagnosis of infection is important because these organisms can cause severe or fatal infection and they all respond to appropriate antibiotic treatment (e.g. macrolides), but do not respond to antibiotics such as sulfonamide and beta-lactams (e.g. penicillins).

Mycoplasma pneumoniae

Mycoplasma pneumoniae causes respiratory symptoms including mild to severe pneumonia. Primary infection usually occurs in school-age children but immunity only lasts for a few years, so individuals can be infected several times during their life. *Mycoplasma pneumoniae* is associated with prolonged carriage, and is associated with outbreaks in military camps, schools and hospitals.

The illness starts with a persistent non-productive cough, sore throat, malaise and fever, which develop over several days, with headache and chills. Over 95% of infected persons have a persistent cough and 25% have a maculopapular rash, which starts on the trunk and then moves to the limbs but not face. Children under 5 years of age normally have upper respiratory tract symptoms; pneumonia is relatively uncommon. Children aged 5–15 years are more likely to develop bronchopneumonia. Adults usually have asymptomatic infection or mild symptoms, but bronchopneumonia develops in 3–10%. Other symptoms such as haemolytic anaemia and neurological complications (e.g. encephalitis, meningitis, polyradiculitis and Guillain–Barré syndrome) can occur about

2 weeks after the onset of symptoms and can be life-threatening. Stevens–Johnson syndrome (erythema multiforme) can also develop 10–14 days after the onset of symptoms. Myalgia and polyarthropathy occur in approximately 14% of cases.

The infection can be effectively treated with macrolide antibiotics such as clarithromycin, azithromycin or doxycycline.

Chlamydia psittaci

Chlamydia psittaci infection is transmitted from birds to humans (causing psittacosis) but does not transmit from human to human. Contact with birds is the greatest risk factor for psittacosis, and more than 70% of cases have a traceable exposure. Infections are usually associated with psittacine birds (parrots, cockatiels and parakeets) but many other avian species, notably pigeons, as well as canaries, chickens, turkeys and ducks, have been linked with human infection. The incubation period is 5–14 days.

Infection is most common in persons aged 40–70 years. Symptoms usually develop rapidly, with high fever and chills; they may evolve slowly. Symptoms include severe headache, arthralgia and painful myalgia. Most infected persons have a dry, non-productive cough. Other symptoms, seen less frequently, include myocarditis, pericarditis, endocarditis, encephalitis, arthritis and hepatitis. Severe infection is associated with confusion and abnormal liver function tests and can be fatal, especially in elderly persons. Most cases are not diagnosed, but a history of bird contact should be sought in all patients with atypical pneumonia. Birds carry the infection in their gut and are often asymptomatic; infection in humans results from breathing in dried bird faeces.

Psittacosis can be treated with macrolides (e.g. doxycycline or tetracycline).

Humans can acquire a severe respiratory infection with a closely related organism (*Chlamydia abortus*), which is a cause of abortion and fetal loss in sheep, cattle and goats. Infected and aborting ewes excrete the organism in large amounts from placentas, uterine discharges and faeces. Human infection can result from breathing in these infected materials. Infection can be asymptomatic, but symptoms, when they occur, include an influenza-like illness with non-productive cough, headache, chills, fever and joint pains. Infection can be more severe or fatal in pregnant women with most reported cases occurring between 24 and 36 weeks' gestation. Severe infection in pregnancy is characterised by a systemic illness with disseminated intravascular coagulation, renal failure and hepatitis. The main effects of infection in pregnancy are severe – sometimes life-threatening disease in the mother and stillbirth or miscarriage, which occurs 3–8 days after the symptoms start. There is no evidence that *Chlamydia abortus* causes congenital damage. Pregnant women are advised not to help to lamb or milk ewes, avoid contact with aborted or newborn lambs or with the afterbirth and not to handle clothing or boots which have come into contact with ewes or lambs. There is a vaccine available for sheep, but not for humans. *Chlamydia abortus* infections can be treated with macrolides (e.g. doxycycline or tetracycline).

Chlamydia pneumoniae

Chlamydia pneumoniae infection is transmitted from humans to humans, with no animal reservoir. It produces symptoms similar to those caused by *Chlamydia psittaci*, but usually less severe, which usually begin 3–4 weeks after exposure. It usually causes infection in school-aged children and young adults, but reinfections occur throughout life. *Chlamydia pneumoniae* infection causes acute wheezing, which may become chronic, leading to asthma. Chlamydia pneumoniae infections can be treated with macrolides (e.g. doxycycline or tetracycline).

Coxiella burnetii

Coxiella burnetii infection (also known as Q fever – the Q stands for 'query' and was first used at a time when the causative agent was unknown) is a worldwide zoonotic infection transmitted from sheep, cattle and goats to humans, often by them breathing in dried faeces or products of conception, but it can also be transmitted from humans to humans. The organism is very resistant and can survive in the environment for many weeks. It can be blown in the wind and has been associated with large outbreaks, which need to be investigated so that the source of infection can be identified and eliminated. The incubation period is 9–30 days. Infection is asymptomatic in about 50% of persons but symptomatic infection often presents as an influenza-like illness, with abrupt onset of fever, malaise, severe headache, muscle pain, joint pain, loss of appetite, dry cough, pleuritic pain, chills, confusion, nausea, vomiting and diarrhoea. Infection can also cause hepatitis, often in the absence of jaundice but with abnormal liver enzyme values. The most serious complication is endocarditis, which is associated with chronic infection, which can occur months or decades following the infection. It is usually fatal if untreated; however, with appropriate antibiotic treatment, the mortality rate is less than 10%. Specialist serological tests, performed in reference laboratories, can be used to test serial serum samples from patients, to predict the likelihood of chronic infection developing. There are distinct antibody responses to two different antigenic phases (phase I and phase II) of *Coxiella burnetii* infection. IgG antibody to *Coxiella burnetii* phase II antigens is higher in acute infection, and the response to phase I antigens is higher in chronic infection.

Coxiella burnetii infections can be treated with antibiotics including doxycycline, tetracycline, chloramphenicol, ciprofloxacin, ofloxacin and hydroxychloroquine. Chronic *Coxiella burnetii* infection often requires up to 4 years of treatment; specialist treatment advice is required. Infection in pregnancy is difficult to treat because doxycycline and ciprofloxacin are contraindicated in this context.

Legionella pneumophila

Legionnaires' disease is caused by infection with any species of Legionella (usually *Legionella pneumophila*). The disease is named after the outbreak where it was first identified, in 1976, at an American Legion convention in Philadelphia. Over 90% of cases of Legionnaires' disease are caused by *Legionella pneumophila* (this is an overestimate, since other species are rarely tested for); other types include *Legionella longbeachae*, *Legionella feeleii*, *Legionella micdadei* and *Legionella anisa*. *Legionella pneumophila* is found naturally in fresh water, where it normally causes no problems but it can contaminate hot water tanks, hot tubs and cooling towers of large air conditioners; it usually causes infection in humans only when present in these environments in high concentrations. Infection does not spread directly between people, and most people who are exposed do not become infected. Risk factors for symptomatic infection include older age, a history of smoking, chronic lung disease and immunosuppression. Infection is acquired by humans from breathing air contaminated with *Legionella pneumophila* in

Table 33.1 Diagnosis of atypical pneumonia infections

Sample	Laboratory test	Result interpretation
Lower respiratory tract secretions (e.g. sputum, bronchoalveolar lavage)	NAAT* (e.g. PCR) for individual organisms Growth on specialist culture media (e.g. charcoal yeast extract agar only for *Legionella pneumophila*)	If positive, indicates infection with that organism If positive, indicates infection with that organism
Urine	Legionella antigen test	If positive, indicates infection with *Legionella pneumophila* type 1
Clotted blood (serum)	Specialised tests (such as EIA** and micro-immunofluorescence) can be performed in reference laboratories	If significant amount of antibody (or seroconversion), indicates infection with that organism

Note: * NAAT – nucleic acid amplification test; of which PCR is most commonly used.
** EIA – enzyme immunoassay.

water mist from air conditioning units, spa pools, water features or hot water systems. It causes respiratory symptoms, including cough, shortness of breath, fever, muscle pains and headaches, with lobar pneumonia. Symptoms often begin 2–10 days after exposure and infection can have a mortality rate of up to 40%, especially in immunocompromised and elderly persons. Treatment is by antibiotics including most macrolides, tetracyclines, ketolides and quinolones. When a case is diagnosed, the source of infection should be sought urgently and remedial action taken promptly in order to prevent further cases. Cases should be reported promptly to the appropriate public health body so that clusters of cases can be identified, the source of infection identified and prompt action taken.

Laboratory Diagnosis

See Table 33.1.

If serological tests are employed, antibody can be present at the time of presentation (especially *Mycoplasma pneumoniae*) but may not be detectable until 10 days after the onset of symptoms (up to a month for *Legionella pneumophila*). Paired serum samples, the first taken on presentation and the second taken 10 days after the onset of symptoms, are recommended, if serological diagnosis is being pursued.

Urine taken (for antigen detection) in the first 5 days of *Legionella pneumophila* infection is the best way to diagnose it. However, legionella antigen may not be detected in all cases and therefore other diagnostic methods may need to be considered.

Useful Website

Public Health England guidance on investigating cases, clusters and outbreaks of Legionnaires' disease: https://assets.publishing.service.gov.uk/government/uploads/system/uploads/attachment_data/file/961760/guidance_on_investigating_cases_clusters_and_outbreaks_of_legionnaires_disease.pdf

Chapter

34

Central Nervous System Viral Infections

The brain and spinal cord make up the central nervous system (CNS), for which several viruses have predilection.

Clinical

There are several viruses which can cause meningitis and/or encephalitis. Listed in the next sections are the viruses most commonly associated with these symptoms. However, it must be remembered that any virus causes encephalitis only rarely. For more details on individual viruses, refer to virus-specific pages.

Viral Encephalitis

Herpes Simplex Virus

Herpes simplex virus (HSV) infection is the most common cause of sporadic fatal encephalitis worldwide. The incidence of HSV encephalitis in the West is estimated to be 2.2 per million population per year. Nearly all the cases are due to HSV-1 with <10% due to HSV-2 infection. In neonates, HSV encephalitis may be caused by either HSV-1 or HSV-2. The infection presents as fever, headache, seizures, focal neurologic signs and impaired consciousness. Local HSV skin lesions are often absent. The infection arises in all age groups, with one-third of all cases occurring in children and adolescents. The pathogenesis of HSV encephalitis is not fully understood, and possibly both direct virus and immune-mediated CNS damage are responsible. HSV encephalitis can occur due to reactivation of latent virus as well as primary or reinfections. Prompt antiviral treatment with intravenous aciclovir (10 mg/kg body weight given every 8 hours) is essential, since HSV encephalitis can have a mortality of 70% when untreated. Early antiviral therapy within 24 hours of onset of symptoms can reduce morbidity and mortality. Even when prompt treatment is given, about 10–30% of patients will be left with some sort of neurological deficit. The duration of treatment of HSV encephalitis in immunocompetent patients should be 14–21 days and treatment should only be stopped once a negative polymerase chain reaction (PCR) result is obtained on the cerebrospinal fluid (CSF) as rebound of infection can occur in those in whom treatment is stopped prior to the virus clearing from the CSF.

HSV can also cause meningitis (usually HSV-2), but this rarely requires antiviral treatment.

Varicella-Zoster Virus

Varicella-zoster virus (VZV) can cause meningitis or meningoencephalitis, usually as a result of reactivation of the virus in the brain. As with HSV, few patients have VZV lesions on the skin. Patients usually experience zoster with no external manifestations. One of the most feared but rare complications of chickenpox is encephalitis, which can be fatal, especially in pregnant women and should be treated promptly with high-dose intravenous aciclovir.

In the immunocompromised patients, cytomegalovirus (CMV), Epstein–Barr virus (EBV), human herpesvirus 6 (HHV-6) and JC virus should always be considered and excluded. In HIV/AIDS patients primary infection with HIV should also be excluded as a cause of their CNS symptoms.

Other Viruses

Other viruses causing encephalitis are rabies, arbovirus infections (West Nile encephalitis, St Louis encephalitis, Western equine encephalitis, California encephalitis, Eastern equine encephalitis, Japanese encephalitis), other herpesviruses (CMV, EBV) and other miscellaneous viruses (e.g. enteroviruses, influenza A viruses, mumps virus, adenovirus, measles virus, rotavirus and HHV-6 in children and progressive multifocal leukoencephalopathy caused by JC virus in the immunocompromised patients). Clue to diagnosis often lies in the other symptoms related to the causal virus and epidemiological history including travel history. A confirmed diagnosis can only be made by the demonstration of the infecting agent in the CSF.

Congenital Viral Encephalitis

Neonates can be born with encephalitis as a result of congenital infection. Herpes viruses HSV-1 and -2, VZV and CMV are usually the cause, but rubella virus and *Toxoplasma gondii* can also be responsible.

Post-infectious Encephalitis

Infection with several viruses (e.g. measles virus, rubella virus, mumps virus and VZV) can rarely be associated with post-infectious encephalomyelitis. This syndrome can also be caused by vaccination against these infections but this is much less likely. For example, the risk of post-infectious encephalomyelitis with rubella virus is 1 in 6,000, whereas the risk after receiving rubella vaccine is less than one in a million.

Acute post-infectious encephalitis typically occurs about a week or 10 days after the viral symptoms appear. In measles, this is usually 10 days after the rash disappears. It is accompanied by headache, irritability, loss of consciousness and fever. This is due to demyelination as a result of autoimmune reaction to the virus and therefore the virus cannot be found in the CNS. It is relatively uncommon (e.g. 1 in 1,000 cases of measles) and has a high mortality.

Subacute Sclerosing Panencephalitis

Subacute sclerosing panencephalitis (SSPE) is a rare condition with an incidence of one in a million measles cases but is invariably fatal. Typically, symptoms appear several years (10–15) after the initial acute attack of measles in early childhood. The first signs are deterioration in intellect (poor performance at school) followed by motor dysfunction and seizures. A defect in the measles virus allows it to persist in the brain by 'hiding' from the immune system. Virus can therefore be found in the brain and CSF in SSPE by molecular techniques and confirms the diagnosis.

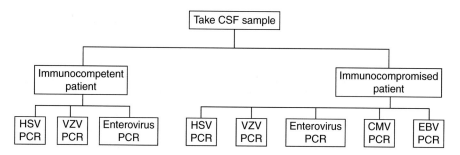

Note: this algorithm assumes that, when clinically indicated, appropriate investigations will also be carried out by culture, antigen detection and PCR to exclude bacterial pathogens, fungal pathogens and parasitic infections.

Figure 34.1 Investigation of viral encephalitis or meningitis

Guillain–Barré Syndrome

This is an acute ascending symmetrical paralytic disease associated with flaccid paralysis, which can be triggered by various viral and bacterial infections (e.g. CMV, EBV, HIV, Japanese encephalitis virus and *Campylobacter jejuni*). Guillain–Barré syndrome is more common in adults than in children. Overall, 80% of those affected by this syndrome recover to lead normal lives, but some are left with permanent disability.

Viral Meningitis

Viral meningitis is usually less severe than bacterial meningitis (such as meningococcal meningitis), which can be fatal and needs prompt treatment. The most common causes of viral meningitis are enteroviruses (especially echoviruses and coxsackie A and B viruses), herpes simplex type 2 virus, VZV and mumps virus.

Viral meningitis typically presents with fever, severe frontal headache and meningism or meningitis. Clinically, the viral cause of meningitis is difficult to establish, but there may be clues in accompanying clinical signs (e.g. parotitis suggesting mumps virus infection or genital herpes lesions suggesting HSV-2 meningitis). VZV meningitis is due to reactivation of the virus and very often precedes the appearance of shingles lesions or lesions may not appear at all. Diagnosis is confirmed by detection of the virus in the CSF by PCR. Symptoms normally resolve in a few days with conservative treatment including those of HSV-2 and VZV meningitis but antiviral treatment with oral aciclovir or valganciclovir is available for HSV-2 and VZV meningitis.

Laboratory Diagnosis

Figure 34.1 and Table 34.1 show the investigation of viral encephalitis and meningitis.

CSF findings show the presence of lymphocytes in cases of encephalitis and meningitis, but early in infection white cells may be absent in the CSF. CSF from patients with encephalitis or meningitis should be tested by molecular techniques such as PCR for virus infections (HSV, VZV, enteroviruses), which should include HHV-6 in neonates and children less than 1 year old and CMV and EBV in immunocompromised patients.

Table 34.1 Laboratory diagnosis of viral encephalitis and meningitis

Virus	CNS symptoms	Best specimen	Other useful specimens to take if CSF is not available
HSV types 1 & 2	Encephalitis	CSF for PCR	–
HSV type 2	Meningitis	CSF for PCR	–
VZV	Encephalitis or meningo- encephalitis	CSF for PCR	Clotted blood taken at least 7 days after onset of symptoms for VZV IgM tests
Enteroviruses • Echoviruses • Coxsackie A viruses • Coxsackie B viruses	Meningitis	CSF for PCR	Faeces and throat swab for PCR
• Enterovirus type 71	Encephalitis	CSF for PCR	As for other enteroviruses
• Poliomyelitis viruses	Poliomyelitis	CSF for PCR	As for other enteroviruses
Mumps	Meningitis or meningo-encephalitis	CSF for PCR	Clotted blood taken at least 3 days after onset of symptoms for mumps virus IgM tests. Throat swab/parotid gland mouth swab in virus transport medium for virus culture or PCR.
Human herpesvirus type 6	Meningitis in neonates and young children, petechial rash	CSF for PCR	EDTA blood for PCR
Other viruses (see text above)	Meningitis/ encephalitis. Other clinical symptoms depending on the infecting virus.	CSF for PCR	Blood samples for serology/PCR and other samples for PCR as indicated
Viruses in immunocompromised persons (see text above)	Meningitis/ encephalitis	CSF for PCR	Blood samples for serology/PCR and other samples for PCR as indicated

Useful Website

Article on acute encephalitis – diagnosis and management: www.ncbi.nlm.nih.gov/pmc/articles/PMC6303463/

Common Cold

The Viruses

The main viruses associated with the 'common cold' are rhinoviruses (over 100 types), coronaviruses, influenza viruses, respiratory syncytial virus and parainfluenza viruses, but any respiratory virus can present with common cold symptoms.

Epidemiology

Route of Spread

The mechanism of transmission of the common cold is different for different viruses. There are three main routes of transmission: direct contact (the virus is transmitted by skin contact from handling an infected object and transmission to the mouth or nose); via inhalation of small particle aerosols (these hang around in the air and can be highly infectious); and/or droplet infection by large particle aerosols (created by coughing and sneezing).

Prevalence

As its name suggests, the common cold occurs throughout the year. It is most prevalent in children, especially in younger children. Preschool or primary school children have about 3–8 colds a year, whereas adults usually have 2–4 per year. Parents, teachers and others in frequent contact with young children have more colds than those with minimal contact. Women have more colds than men, probably reflecting their increased contact with children.

The common cold is more prevalent in winter months (usually caused by rhino-viruses or parainfluenza virus types 1 and 2. Summer colds are more likely to be caused by coronaviruses or parainfluenza virus type 3. Quite why parainfluenza viruses types 1 and 2 cause winter infections and parainfluenza virus type 3 causes summer infections is not clear. It is a myth that colds are more likely to be acquired in cold and wet weather.

Incubation Period

1–5 days depending on the virus.

Infectious Period

Persons are infectious when they are symptomatic, especially if they are coughing and sneezing. They are likely to be most infectious in the first few days of the illness.

Clinical

Symptoms

Sore throat is often the first symptom. Nasal congestion, nasal discharge and sneezing usually follow. Laryngitis sometimes occurs and 30% of people will develop a cough (often after the nasal symptoms have gone). Some will have sore eyes. Low-grade fever is often present. Headache and muscle pain are more frequent in cases of influenza, but mild influenza can present with common cold symptoms.

Sinusitis and lower respiratory tract infections caused by bacterial superinfection are the most common complications in adults. Sinusitis occurs in 0.5–2% of adults and older children. Lower respiratory tract infection occurs more frequently in elderly persons, immunocompromised patients and those with asthma, chronic obstructive airway disease and in smokers. Lower respiratory tract infection may be a result of community-acquired pneumonia (*Mycoplasma pneumoniae*, *Chlamydia psittaci*, *Chlamydia pneumoniae*, *Coxiella burnetii* or *Legionella pneumophila*) (see Chapter 33) which should be investigated because appropriate treatment is usually with different antibiotics to other chest infections, and there may be environmental and public health issues which need to be explored.

Laboratory Diagnosis

If patients present with typical common cold symptoms, laboratory investigation is not recommended. If they are admitted to hospital, swabs and or respiratory secretions for virus investigation should be sent to the laboratory, especially if patients are immunosuppressed. Patients with suspected community-acquired pneumonia should be investigated.

See Table 35.1.

Table 35.1 Laboratory diagnosis of common cold virus infections

Clinical indication	Specimens	Test	Interpretation of positive result
Severe respiratory infection in hospitalised patients	Nose and throat swab in virus transport medium	Direct antigen detection tests	Indicates infection with a particular type of respiratory virus
		PCR	Indicates infection with a particular type of respiratory virus
	Nasopharyngeal aspirate in children <2 years old or bronchoalveolar lavages in patients in intensive care	Direct antigen detection tests especially for respiratory syncytial virus and parainfluenza and influenza viruses	Indicates infection with a particular type of respiratory virus
		PCR	Indicates infection with a particular type of respiratory virus
	Clotted blood	Serology for atypical pneumonia antibody detection	Indicates infection with a particular atypical pneumonia bacteria

Management

Treatment

There is no antiviral treatment for the common cold but analgesics can be used to treat fever, headache and muscle aches. Decongestants are helpful for reducing nasal congestion. Atypical pneumonia bacterial infections should be treated with appropriate antibiotics.

Infection Control

Patients with the common cold admitted to hospital should be isolated in single rooms or cohorted in isolation bays, if possible.

Genital Tract and Sexually Transmitted Infections

True sexually transmitted infections are those that are transmitted only through sexual activity, but there are many in which sexual transmission is one of the routes and others which even though not strictly transmitted via the sexual route may be transmitted through related sexual practices. It is important to remember that many of these patients may not perceive themselves at risk of a sexually transmitted infection and therefore may present outside the Sexually Transmitted Disease medicine setting.

Clinical

Sexually transmitted viral infections can be divided into two groups:

- those that present with localised genital lesions or symptoms; and
- those that are systemic infections but may also be transmitted via the sexual route or during related sexual activity.

This chapter will consider only those pathogens that cause local genital lesions. Refer to the appropriate chapters in the book for those that have a systemic manifestation. See Table 36.1.

Vesicular or Ulcerative Genital Lesions

Herpes simplex virus (HSV) is the commonest cause, but occasionally varicella-zoster virus (VZV) may also cause localised genital lesions which may be clinically difficult to distinguish from herpes. Clinical examination may reveal shingles-like distribution along a sensory nerve in case of VZV infection. The distinction is important to make as a higher dose of aciclovir is required to treat varicella-zoster.

Acute syphilis may present as an ulcerative gummatous lesion.

Non-vesicular or Non-ulcerative Genital Lesions

Papilloma virus, or genital warts, are sexually transmitted, and multiple warts may be present on the genital area. Papilloma virus types 6 and 11 are the commonest cause of warts and are not associated with cervical cancer. Papilloma virus 16, 18 and the other types associated with cervical cancer do not present as warts.

Molluscum contagiosum virus is a poxvirus, which spreads by close personal contact resulting from sexual encounters. Lesions may be present on the genital area only or may form a part of more generalised skin infection. The lesions are typical and discharge a caseous material when squeezed.

Widespread genital warts and molluscum lesions can occur in immunocompromised patients, especially those with HIV infection.

Table 36.1 Sexually transmitted infection with local and systemic manifestations

Clinical presentation	Infecting agents	Route of transmission
Localised genital vesicular or ulcerative lesions	Herpes simplex virus 1 and 2 Varicella-zoster virus	Sexual Local reactivation (zoster) involving sensory nerve supplying genital area
Localised genital ulcerative lesion	Treponema (syphilis)	Sexual
Localised lesions other than vesicular or ulcerative	Papilloma virus (genital warts) Molluscum contagiosum	Sexual Direct contact with infected lesions
Cervical/urethral discharge due to cervicitis or urethritis	*Chlamydia trachomatis* including lymphogranuloma venereum	Sexual
Systemic infections	HIV HTLV-1 and -2 Hepatitis A, B, C, D and E Epstein–Barr virus Cytomegalovirus	Sexual, coincidental ulcerative genital lesions aid in transmission Anal-oral sex Close contact with infected saliva as in kissing

Urethritis and Urethral Discharge

Chlamydia trachomatis is the commonest cause of non-specific discharge and urethritis in males. This may be accompanied with some urinary symptoms, and therefore may be misdiagnosed as urinary tract infection especially in men. Gonococcal infection should be considered in the differential diagnosis and ruled out; many patients have dual infection with both chlamydia and gonococci. Urethral infection and urethritis in females on their own are rare and occur as an accompaniment to cervical infection.

Cervicitis and Vaginal Discharge

Bacterial causes including gonococcal infection should be ruled out. Chlamydia is the commonest cause of cervicitis, but about 50% women have no symptoms; therefore, the infection can only be diagnosed by opportunistic screening.

Lymphogranuloma Venereum

Symptoms are those of *Chlamydia trachomatis*, but in addition large inguinal lymphadenopathy is present and there is normally a history of sexual contact in the tropics or with someone from the tropics.

Prostatitis and Epididymo-Orchitis

Chlamydia trachomatis infection, if untreated, ascends to the upper genital tract to cause prostatitis and epididymitis; this has been associated with male infertility. Mumps virus is the commonest cause of orchitis, which is bilateral in nature, but unilateral orchitis may occur and should be considered in the differential diagnosis of orchitis.

Pelvic Inflammatory Disease

Chlamydia is the most important cause of pelvic inflammatory disease (PID), being responsible for most of the cases. Thirty per cent of women with chlamydia, if untreated, will develop PID resulting in salpingitis and female infertility and/or risk of ectopic pregnancy. A vaginal discharge is often absent.

Fitz-Hugh–Curtis Syndrome

Chronic upper genital tract infection in females may lead to pelvic adhesions and perihepatitis with the adhesions extending to the liver.

Genital Infection in Pregnancy

Genital herpes, chlamydia and papilloma virus (genital warts) infection can be passed on vertically to the fetus at the time of delivery.

Genital herpes simplex lesions, especially if due to primary infection, are a high risk factor for neonatal herpes simplex infection due to vertical transmission at the time of delivery; therefore, caesarean section is recommended if active lesions of primary HSV infection are present.

Laboratory Diagnosis

Serology: Is of limited use.

Type-specific HSV IgG tests have been used to study the prevalence and epidemiology of genital herpes. HSV type 1 and type 2–specific IgG tests can be useful to determine if sexual couples are discordant with respect to their previous HSV type 1 and type 2 infection. Appropriate advice to prevent infection can be given to antibody-negative pregnant female partners.

Chlamydia antibody tests are useful in diagnosis of PID as high levels are diagnostic of PID and endocervical swabs for chlamydia may be negative.

Virus Detection

HSV/VZV: A lesion or ulcer swab should be sent to the laboratory for virus-specific PCR.

Molluscum: Electron microscopic examination of the central caseous-like material in the lesion shows typical pox-like virus.

Genital warts: Clinical diagnosis; laboratory diagnosis is not routinely indicated but PCR can be done on biopsy material if required. Typing can also be done to determine if patients are infected with a potentially cancer-causing papilloma virus genotype.

Chlamydia: Nucleic acid amplification tests (NAATs) on first-void urine (FVU) specimen in males and endocervical or self-taken vulvo-vaginal swab or FVU in females should be sent for diagnosis of lower and upper genital tract chlamydia infection. FVU in females has lower sensitivity than the other specimen types therefore self-taken vulvo-vaginal swabs are the specimen of choice. Swabs from other sites such as rectal or pharyngeal should be sent from men who have sex with men and from others depending upon history of sexual practice.

In addition, appropriate tissue biopsies and venous blood sample should be sent for diagnosis of PID in females.

Management

Good history, examination, diagnosis and treatment of specific condition.

Aciclovir, valaciclovir or famciclovir should be used for treatment of HSV infections. Chlamydia is sensitive to treatment by oxytetracycline, but azithromycin has replaced oxytetracycline as treatment of choice. Erythromycin should be used in pregnant women as the drug of choice.

There is no specific treatment for molluscum contagiosum and it is usually a self-limiting condition.

Genital warts are also self-limiting in nature, but if multiple and large lesions are present these can be removed by cryosurgery with liquid nitrogen.

Prophylaxis and Control of Infection

Contact tracing of sexual contacts, their screening and treatment is the mainstay of control of infection. There is no vaccination for herpes or chlamydia. Vaccines are available against papilloma virus strains responsible for causing cervical cancer and those that cause genital warts. In the UK all 12–13-year-old children are offered papilloma virus vaccine.

Glandular Fever–Type Illness

Clinical

Glandular fever is a broad clinical description given to a cluster of symptoms and signs including lymphadenopathy, sore throat, atypical mononuclear cells in the blood, fever and malaise (often prolonged). Symptoms and signs of infection with Epstein–Barr virus (EBV) and cytomegalovirus (CMV) include jaundice and abnormal liver enzyme test results. EBV infection typically presents as infectious mononucleosis (IM) in young adults. Primary HIV infection may present as glandular fever–like illness and HIV infection should be excluded.

Differential Diagnosis

This broad clinical syndrome is associated with a number of different infections. Table 37.1 indicates the symptoms and signs most usually associated with different infections.

Infectious mononucleosis due to EBV infection is usually, but not always, clinically diagnosed accurately. The blood picture in IM typically shows lymphocytosis of >50% and atypical lymphocytes of >10% in blood smear. Other causes of glandular fever–like illness (e.g. CMV, adenoviruses and *Toxoplasma gondii*) are less easy to diagnose

Table 37.1 Symptoms associated with various infectious causes of glandular fever–like illness

Symptoms/signs	Infectious organism			
	EBV	CMV	Adenovirus	*Toxoplasma gondii*
Sore throat	*****	**	**	*
Lymphadenopathy	**	*	***	*****
Fever	***	***	**	**
Malaise	****	****	*	**
Hepatitis	***	****		
Abnormal liver function test results	****	****		
Night sweats	*	*****		
Relapsing illness	*	****		
Prolonged symptoms	****	****	*	****

Table 37.2 Laboratory diagnosis of glandular fever–like illness

Specimen	EBV	CMV	Adenovirus	Toxoplasma gondii	HIV
Clotted blood (serum)	EBV VCA IgM and IgG and EBNA antibody[1] Paul Bunnel test[6]	CMV IgM[2] CMV IgG avidity[3]	Adenovirus antibody[4]	Toxoplasma gondii IgM[5] Reference laboratory testing required to confirm results	HIV antibody and antigen
EDTA blood	EBV DNA by PCR[7]	CMV DNA by PCR[7]	Adenovirus DNA by PCR[7]	Toxoplasma gondii DNA by PCR[7]	HIV PCR
Throat swab	No	No	Adenovirus DNA by PCR[7]	No	No

Notes: Interpretation of laboratory results:
1. Recent primary EBV infection: EBV IgM positive, EBV IgG positive, EBNA antibody negative.
2. Recent primary CMV infection: CMV IgM positive (beware of weakly reactive results which could be non-specific).
3. Recent primary CMV infection: CMV low avidity IgG.
4. Recent adenovirus infection if titre raised significantly (e.g. CFT titre >64).
5. Recent Toxoplasma gondii infection if positive. Toxoplasma gondii IgM test results can be non-specific and should always be confirmed in a reference laboratory.
6. Recent EBV infection in adults likely if positive. Paul Bunnell and Monospot tests detect heterophile antibody and can give false positive and false negative results and are not suitable for children <16 years old because of false negative results.
7. Positive result indicates current infection in immunocompromised persons.

clinically, but Table 37.1 may be a useful guide to the likely diagnosis in order to better direct laboratory testing. To be absolutely certain, laboratory investigation is required.

Laboratory Diagnosis

A diagnostic approach is shown in Table 37.2.

Chapter

38

Haemorrhagic Fevers

Haemorrhagic Fever Viruses

Haemorrhagic fever viruses are viruses which cause outbreaks of severe or fatal infections with haemorrhagic symptoms, principally in the tropics. These infections are occasionally imported into the UK and other countries outside the tropics, usually causing disease in individual persons, but occasionally resulting in clusters of cases of those infections with person-to-person spread. Since there are several different viruses with different geographical distributions, animal vectors and symptoms these details have been collated in Table 38.1 to aid differential diagnosis. Knowledge of the outbreaks occurring in different parts of the world and the recent travel history of returning travellers is very important for initial clinical diagnosis. Malaria should always be considered in the differential diagnosis. If haemorrhagic fever is suspected and malaria is excluded, patients should be initially cared for in the highest-security isolation rooms available and transferred to a specialist haemorrhagic fever facility as soon as possible. No special infection control precautions are required for hantavirus and dengue infections.

Dengue fever virus is the most common of these viruses to be imported into the UK; however, the haemorrhagic form of the disease is relatively rare.

This chapter aims to describe some of the more important haemorrhagic fevers and is not a comprehensive review of all known haemorrhagic fever viruses.

Specimens for Diagnosis

EDTA blood for virus culture or PCR and clotted blood for specific IgM antibody are normally required for laboratory diagnosis. All diagnostic tests should be done in a category 4, high-security facility.

• Lassa Fever

Lassa fever is endemic in many countries in West Africa with seroprevalence rates of 4–55%; incidence is highest in forested areas. Around 100,000–300,000 infections occur per year in West Africa with 5,000 deaths.

There was a major outbreak of Lassa fever in Nigeria in 2017/18 with an estimated case fatality rate of 25%.

Lassa fever virus is an arenavirus. Incubation period is 1–3 weeks. Initial symptoms include fever, retrosternal pain, sore throat, back pain, vomiting, diarrhoea, conjunctivitis, facial swelling, proteinuria and mucosal bleeding. Deafness occurs in up to one-third of patients. Clinical diagnosis is often difficult because symptoms of Lassa fever are so

Table 38.1 Haemorrhagic fever viruses

Disease	Endemic countries	Animal host	Treatment	Person-to-person spread?
Lassa fever	West Africa: Guinea, Liberia, Sierra Leone, Nigeria. The geographic spread may extend to other countries in the region.	The multi-mammate rat, *Mastomys*, which are numerous in the savannas and forests of West, Central and East Africa.	Ribavirin given early in infection. Good supportive care.	YES When a person comes into contact with virus in blood tissue, secretions and excretions from an infected patient. Sexual transmission.
Marburg disease	Marburg disease is indigenous to Africa. The exact geographical spread of infection is unknown. Confirmed cases have been reported from Uganda, Kenya, Zimbabwe, Equatorial Guinea and Republic of Tanzania.	This remains a mystery, but human infection has been acquired after contact with African green monkeys or their tissues.	No antiviral treatment available. Good supportive care.	YES When a person comes into contact with virus in blood, tissue, secretions and excretions from an infected person. Sexual transmission.
Ebola	The disease is maintained in animal host(s) in Africa. Confirmed cases have been reported in the Democratic Republic of the Congo, Gabon, Sudan, the Ivory Coast and Uganda.	The exact geographical spread of the disease in animals is not known, but the first cases in an outbreak become infected through contact with an infected animal.	No antiviral treatment is available. Specific monoclonal antibody treatment and vaccines are available for the Zaire virus. Good supportive care.	YES By contact with blood or secretions of an infected person.
Crimean-Congo haemorrhagic fever	The disease is endemic in many countries in Africa, Europe and Asia.	The virus is transmitted by argasid, hyalomma or ixodid ticks. The virus may infect a wide range of wild and domestic animals and then spread to humans via direct contact with animal tissues and secretions. Ostriches are also susceptible.	No antiviral treatment. Good supportive care.	YES

Table 38.1 (cont.)

Disease	Endemic countries	Animal host	Treatment	Person-to-person spread?
Dengue haemorrhagic fever	Dengue fever and dengue haemorrhagic fever are primarily diseases of tropical and subtropical parts of the world, with a distribution similar to that of malaria.	Dengue is transmitted to humans by *Aedes aegypti* mosquitos, which only bite in the daytime.	No antiviral treatment. Good supportive care.	No
Haemorrhagic fever with renal syndrome and hantavirus pulmonary syndrome	Worldwide in various species of rodents.	Infection occurs through direct contact with faeces, saliva or urine of infected rodents, or by inhalation of aerosolised rodent excretion.	No antiviral treatment. Good supportive care and renal support.	No

varied and non-specific. Eighty per cent of people have mild or asymptomatic infection and 20% have severe multi-system diseases. Fifteen to twenty per cent of hospitalised patients die, but the overall death rate is about 1%. Treatment is supportive but the antiviral drug Ribavirin is suggested for all symptomatic patients with confirmed diagnosis.

There are a number of ways the virus can be transmitted to humans. Virus can be transmitted by direct contact via multi-mammate rat (*Mastomys natalensis*) urine and droppings, especially through contamination of cuts and sores. Contaminated inhaled air in rat-infested households is also another source. Human to human, the virus is transmitted by body fluid and blood contact but is not transmitted through casual contact. Sexual transmission has also been described. Virus is shed in the urine for weeks and can be detected in the semen.

Laboratory diagnosis is normally by demonstration of virus by PCR but also by demonstration of specific IgM/IgG and Lassa antigen in the serum.

• Marburg Disease

Marburg disease virus belongs to the family Filoviridae, genus *Marburgvirus*. Marburg virus was first recognised as causing human disease in Marburg (Germany) when, in 1967, infected non-human primates were inadvertently imported from Uganda into Germany. Since then the virus has caused several outbreaks in sub-Saharan Africa, with an outbreak as recently as in 2023 in Equatorial Guinea and Tanzania.

Marburg virus is often transmitted to humans from bats living in mines and caves. Subsequently, human-to-human transmission is via direct contact with blood and body fluids and with contaminated surfaces and bedding, etc., through broken skin or mucus membrane. Sexual transmission has been described and the virus can persist in the semen for weeks after infection.

Incubation period is 2–21 days. Marburg haemorrhagic fever is a severe disease which affects both humans and non-human primates. Patients present with sudden onset of fever, chills, headache and myalgia. After 5 days, a maculopapular rash appears which is most prominent on the trunk. Nausea, vomiting, chest pain, sore throat, abdominal pain and diarrhoea usually follow. Symptoms become increasingly severe and may include jaundice, severe weight loss, delirium, shock, massive haemorrhage and multi-organ failure. Fatality rate is about 25% but can be as high as 80%. Death occurs most commonly between 8 and 9 days after onset of symptoms.

There is no specific treatment. Research is ongoing for vaccine development.

• Ebola

As with the Marburg virus, the Ebola virus belongs to the family Filoviridae, genus *Ebolavirus*. The genus *Ebolavirus* consists of six species: *Zaire, Sudan, Bundibugyo, Tai forest, Reston* and *Bombali*. The first four of these have been known to cause human disease and all but Reston virus are indigenous to Africa. Until 2014, most outbreaks of Ebolavirus had been small and controlled quickly; however, in 2014 the Zaire virus caused a major epidemic in West Africa with nearly 29,000 cases with a case fatality rate of 40%. Since then there have been several outbreaks in the region of Zaire virus.

Disease is first spread as a zoonosis to humans from bats, porcupines and non-human primates. Human-to-human spread then occurs via direct contact of broken skin and mucous membrane with infected blood, body fluids or via droplet inoculation of virus into the mouth and eyes. Those who provide hands-on medical care and burial are most at risk. In one study it was found that secondary attack rates in those providing nursing care without personal protective equipment (PPE) was 48% as compared to 2% in those household members who had direct contact but did not provide nursing care. Virus can also spread via environmental contamination. The virus has also been detected in semen, and sexual transmission has been described.

Incubation period is 2–21 days. The onset of symptoms is abrupt, characterised by fever, headache, muscle and joint aches and sore throat, followed by diarrhoea and vomiting. A maculopapular rash may develop 5–7 days after onset; internal and external bleeding may also occur. Neurological (occasional meningoencephalitis), ocular (uveitis), cardiac and respiratory involvement can also arise. Infection in pregnancy can lead to premature labour or fetal death. Fatal disease is characterised with more severe early clinical illness with death typically occurring in the second week. The average case fatality rate is 50% and has varied from 25% to 90% in past outbreaks.

Treatment is supportive; specific monoclonal antibody treatment for Zaire virus is available.

As a result of the large Zaire virus epidemic in West Africa, there was accelerated research for effective vaccines and at least two are in use and recommended for those who are at high risk of exposure to Zaire virus.

Diagnosis is by specific PCR or antigen detection in blood samples.

• Crimean-Congo Haemorrhagic Fever

Crimean-Congo haemorrhagic fever (CCHF) virus belongs to the genus *Nairovirus* in the family Bunyaviridae. CCHF was first described in Crimea in 1944. There was then an outbreak in Congo in 1969, hence the name. It is distributed widely and found in Eastern Europe, throughout the Mediterranean, North Western China, Central Asia, the Middle East and the Indian subcontinent. Humans acquire the virus from direct contact with blood or other infected tissue from livestock or an infected person or directly from an infected ixodid tick (which are the vectors of transmission) bite. Domestic animals such as cattle, goats and sheep act as amplifying hosts. The majority of cases have been in agricultural and slaughterhouse workers and vets.

The onset of symptoms is abrupt, characterised by fever, headache, muscle and joint aches and sore throat, followed by diarrhoea, nausea and vomiting. A maculopapular rash, internal and external bleeding, headache, backache, sore eyes and photophobia also occur. A petechial rash may occur with large areas of a purple rash, melena, haematuria, epistaxis and bleeding from gums. Treatment is supportive and case fatality rate in hospitalised patients ranges from 9% to 50%.

• Dengue Haemorrhagic Fever

Dengue haemorrhagic fever (DHF) follows dengue virus infection (see Chapter 2) . Patients with dengue haemorrhagic fever, which is rare, have fever, haemorrhages from gums, bowel and mucosa and thrombocytopaenia. The current four World Health Organization diagnostic criteria for DHF are: fever or history of recent fever for 2–7 days; any haemorrhagic manifestation; thrombocytopenia and evidence of increased vascular permeability. Patients with DHF may go on to develop dengue shock syndrome

(DSS) which is defined by the development of circulatory failure in the patients with DHF. DHF is more likely to occur in persons who have a second infection with a different serotype of virus. DSS has a high mortality. The fatality rates in patients with DSS can be 10% or higher. There is no specific treatment, but fatality rates can be reduced to 1% with good supportive care. Studies from different countries have indicated life-threatening complications from dengue fever in the absence of DHF or DSS. Diagnosis is by detection of viral RNA in the blood by specific PCR or by detection of specific IgM in the serum.

• Haemorrhagic Fever with Renal Syndrome

Haemorrhagic fever with renal syndrome is caused by hantavirus belonging to the family Bunyaviridae including hantaviruses. There are many hantavirus species, at least 10 of which cause human infections. Hantaviruses are divided into two types, the Old World which cause haemorrhagic fever with renal syndrome (HFRS) and New World hantaviruses which cause hantavirus cardiopulmonary/hantavirus pulmonary syndrome (HCPS/HPS). Different rodents transmit the infections to humans in different parts of the world with each pathogenic hantavirus being associated with a wild rodent. The virus is shed in the urine, faeces and saliva of infected rodents and rodent contact is the key to transmission and it is suspected that much of the transmission occurs by the aerosol route.

Old World hantaviruses: Hantaviruses have probably been around for centuries but first came into their own when a large outbreak of infection occurred in the 1950s in United Nations troops posted in Korea during the Korean conflict. The pathogen was later identified as hantavirus. Subsequently, infections and outbreaks have been reported from the Far East, especially China, Korea and Russia. HFRS usually develops 1–2 weeks after exposure. Symptoms start abruptly with fever, headache, back and abdominal pain with nausea and rash. This is followed by low blood pressure, acute shock, vascular leakage and acute kidney failure. The hantavirus species associated with Far Eastern HFRS are *Seoul* and *Hantaan*. A milder form of illness called nephropathica epidemica has been described in Scandinavian and other European countries and is caused by the *Puumala* virus. The case fatality rate varies from 1% to 15% depending on the infecting species and severity of illness.

New World hantaviruses: In May 1993 there was an outbreak of unexplained pulmonary illness with acute respiratory distress syndrome with high fatality rate in the Southwestern United States. Early symptoms were fever, fatigue, muscle aches, headache, chills, nausea, vomiting and diarrhoea. Four to ten days later, coughing and shortness of breath developed. After intensive investigations, the cause was identified as a previously unidentified hantavirus species which was named as the *Sin Nombre* virus. Cases have continued to be reported from the Americas with a reported case fatality rate of 25–50%.

Diagnosis of hantavirus infections is suggested by epidemiology (exposure to rodents). Human to human transmission is rare. Specific diagnosis is by demonstration of virus by PCR or by detection of specific antibodies in the blood.

Treatment for both HFRS and HPS is supportive.

Useful Websites

www.who.int/ith/en

www.cdc.gov/travel

www.traveldoctor.co.uk

www.ukhsa.gov.uk

GOV.UK viral haemorrhagic fevers risk assessment: https://assets.publishing.service
.gov.uk/government/uploads/system/uploads/attachment_data/file/478115/VHF_Algo
.pdf

GOV.UK management of Hazard Group 4 viral haemorrhagic fevers and similar
human infectious diseases of high consequence: https://assets.publishing.service.gov
.uk/government/uploads/system/uploads/attachment_data/file/534002/Management_
of_VHF_A.pdf

39
Infections in Pregnancy and Congenital and Neonatal Infections

Infection in the pregnant woman not only has consequences for the mother but for her unborn child as well. The infection may be transmitted to the fetus in utero (congenital infection), transmitted at or around the time of birth (perinatal infection) or be transmitted sometime after birth in the first few weeks of life (postnatal infection).

Any systemic virus infection in pregnancy may potentially lead to fetal loss, but in this chapter only those infections will be considered which are specifically associated with vertical transmission from the mother to the baby either in utero or in the peri- or postnatal period (see Table 39.1).

Congenital Infection

The following pathogens cause congenital infection of the fetus. Not all are teratogenic (e.g. cause congenital malformation of the fetus).

- Rubella virus
- Cytomegalovirus
- *Toxoplasma gondii*
- Parvovirus B19
- Varicella-zoster virus (chickenpox)
- Zika virus
- *Treponema pallidum* (syphilis)

Perinatal Infection

Most maternal infections are transmitted to the fetus at or around the time of birth as this is the most vulnerable period. Mixing of feto-maternal blood occurs as the placenta ruptures; also, the neonate is exposed to maternal secretions as it comes out of the birth canal. Pathogens which cause perinatal infections are:

- HIV
- Hepatitis B virus
- Hepatitis C virus
- HTLV-1
- Herpes simplex virus
- *Chlamydia trachomatis*
- Varicella-zoster virus (chickenpox)

Table 39.1 Important viral and related congenital infections

Pathogen	Clinical manifestation			Stage of vertical transmission		
	Congenital malformation	Infection without congenital malformation	Chronic infection	In utero	Perinatal	Postnatal
Cytomegalovirus (CMV)	++ (15% babies will have symptoms)	+++	+ (ongoing infection may occur)	++		+++ (breast milk)
Rubella virus	+++ (80% risk of severe malformation if maternal infection in first 6 weeks of gestation)	+ (where maternal infection occurs after first trimester)		+++		
Toxoplasma	++	Where infection occurs in later weeks of pregnancy	Late sequelae as uveitis/ retinitis	++		
Varicella- zoster virus (Chickenpox)	+ (2–3% risk of congenital varicella syndrome after in-utero infection in the first 20 weeks of pregnancy)	+++ (neonatal chickenpox)	Shingles in early childhood	+	+++ (if mother gets chickenpox 7 days before to 7 days after delivery)	
Parvovirus B19		++ (10% risk of fetal loss, hydrops fetalis)		++		
Herpes simplex virus		++ (neonatal herpes simplex infection)		+/-	+++ (80% of all infection acquired at time of birth as a result of primary genital herpes in mother)	++ (20% acquired postnatally from mother or other close relatives via direct contact with infected lesions)

Table 39.1 (cont.)

Pathogen	Clinical manifestation			Stage of vertical transmission		
	Congenital malformation	Infection without congenital malformation	Chronic infection	In utero	Perinatal	Postnatal
Chlamydia trachomatis		+ (ophthalmia neonatorum)			+ (genital chlamydia infection in mother)	
HIV		++	++	+	+++	+++ (breast milk)
Hepatitis B virus		++	+ to +++ Depending on mother's HB e antibody status.	+	+++	
Hepatitis C virus		+	+/-	+/-	+	
HTLV-1		+	++	+	++	+++ (breast milk)

Postnatal Infection

Breast milk is the potential source for transmission to the neonate in the immediate period after birth and breastfeeding is a significant risk factor for vertical transmission of:

- HIV
- HTLV-1
- Cytomegalovirus
- Varicella-zoster virus (chickenpox)

Rubella

Maternal rubella infection in the first trimester invariably leads to transplacental transmission and fetal infection with severe malformation and is an indication for therapeutic termination of pregnancy. The risk of severe fetal malformation is maximum if infection occurs in the first trimester, being about 80% for maternal rubella infection in the first 6–8 weeks of pregnancy. Although fetal infection may occur at any stage of pregnancy it rarely causes severe fetal defects after 17 weeks of gestation.

The classical triad of congenital rubella syndrome (CRS) is congenital bilateral cataract (first associated with congenital rubella infection by an Australian ophthalmologist, Sir Norman Gregg), microcephaly and sensorineural deafness. This is usually accompanied with a purpuric rash (due to thrombocytopenia) and hepatomegaly.

With the introduction of the childhood rubella vaccination programme, rubella and CRS have been virtually eliminated from the UK, USA and other European countries where childhood MMR vaccination programmes are in place. In addition, any pregnant woman found to be susceptible should be offered vaccination in the immediate postpartum period.

Cytomegalovirus

Like rubella, cytomegalovirus (CMV) is a teratogenic virus. Primary CMV infection in pregnancy has an overall 40% risk of transmission to the fetus; however, 85% of these congenitally infected babies will be asymptomatic at birth with only 15% showing congenital stigmata. CMV reactivation in pregnancy has a very low risk of causing congenital infection ($<=1\%$).

Sensorineural deafness is the most common defect. Severe congenital manifestations, such as microcephaly, thrombocytopenic purpuric rash and hepatosplenomegaly, occur but not commonly.

Unlike with rubella, 90% of babies born to mothers who acquire primary CMV infection in pregnancy will not be infected or be asymptomatically infected. Therefore, therapeutic termination is not recommended. Also, CMV infection is asymptomatic in the vast majority of adults, so it is not possible to identify significant contact with a case. Furthermore, there is no effective prophylaxis or vaccination for CMV. For these reasons screening for CMV in pregnancy is not advocated.

Prenatal (fetal) diagnosis by CMV PCR on amniotic fluid (and fetal blood by cordocentesis if indicated) should be offered to patients at high risk of having an affected fetus (primary maternal infection or suggestive findings on ultrasound) and pregnancy should be monitored with serial ultrasound examinations.

Postnatal CMV infection is common with about a third of the babies born to mothers who are positive for CMV antibody acquiring it in the first year of life, mostly via breast milk. It is essential to identify congenitally infected neonates in the first 3 weeks of life as after that, congenital infection cannot be distinguished from postnatally acquired CMV infection.

Recent research suggests some evidence that early treatment with high-dose valaciclovir in the first trimester may reduce the risk of CMV vertical transmission; further research by randomised controlled trials is required.

CMV-specific hyperimmune globulin therapy of pregnant patients with primary CMV infection in early pregnancy to reduce or the risk of symptomatic congenital CMV infection is being investigated; so far, the results are not promising.

Treatment with ganciclovir at birth should be considered for those congenitally infected babies who are symptomatic with end organ disease including central nervous system involvement. Valganciclovir treatment for 6–12 months has been shown to have a beneficial effect, especially on sensorineural deafness. Trials are ongoing for assessment of the efficacy of valganciclovir to treat milder cases of congenital infection, but presently no efficacy data is available. Expert advice should always be sought for management of both mother and baby suspected of having CMV infection.

Varicella-Zoster Virus (Chickenpox)

Fortunately, as the prevalence of varicella-zoster virus (VZV) antibody in the UK is >95% in adults, most women, by the time they get to reproductive age, have evidence of past infection.

Maternal Chickenpox

Chickenpox in pregnancy may be more severe for the mother although there is no clear-cut evidence that pregnant women are at increased risk of complications like primary varicella pneumonia. All pregnant women who have a significant (in the same room for 15 minutes or face-to-face) contact with a case of chickenpox in the infectious period (Chapter 29) should be tested for IgG antibody to VZV and those found to be negative should be given prophylaxis with aciclovir or zoster immunoglobulin (ZIG) preferably within 7 days of contact but not later than 10 days after contact (see latest guidelines). ZIG has a 70% protective efficacy to prevent clinical chickenpox, and in the others, it attenuates clinical disease. There is also some evidence that ZIG may reduce the risk of transmission of infection to the fetus. Aciclovir treatment should be offered to all >= 20 weeks pregnant women who have clinical chickenpox, and treatment should be considered on clinical grounds for those who are <20 weeks' gestation.

Fetal and Neonatal Infection

Infection in the first 20 weeks of gestation has an overall risk of about 2% for fetal malformation as a result of congenital infection. VZV causes infection of the developing neural tube, resulting in rudimentary limbs and scarring.

In addition, if chickenpox develops in the mother in the week before or after delivering, then there is a high risk of the neonate developing chickenpox in the first 10 days of life. This is because the neonate would have been exposed in utero to maternal viraemia in the absence of protective maternal antibodies. Neonatal chickenpox infection has a high mortality rate (approximately 30%). Therefore, all babies born to mothers who develop chickenpox a week before or after birth should be given prophylaxis with ZIG or aciclovir (see latest guidelines).

Live attenuated varicella vaccine is now licensed for use in the UK, and there is a case for identifying chickenpox-susceptible women of reproductive age group and vaccinating them to prevent infection in pregnancy.

Parvovirus B19

There is no evidence that congenital parvovirus B19 infection leads to malformation but infection in the first 20 weeks of pregnancy leads to fetal loss in about 7–10% of infected women. The most serious but fortunately rare complication is hydrops fetalis, which is a result of fetal anaemia due to infection of the fetal red cell precursors. If hydrops is detected and managed in time by in-utero blood transfusion (a sample should be taken at the same time for confirmation of parvovirus B19 infection by PCR), the fetus survives to term with no long-term ill effects. Pregnant women with an acute parvovirus B19 infection should be referred to an obstetrician for follow-up with regular scans.

Toxoplasma

Maternal primary toxoplasma infection can be transmitted to the fetus and often leads to congenital infection and malformation if acquired in the first trimester. Infection can be transmitted throughout pregnancy, but fetal damage occurs much less frequently in the later stages of pregnancy. In the first trimester, transmission of infection occurs in about 25% of cases, most (75%) of which will be severely affected and develop myocarditis, hydrocephalus, mental retardation, retinochoroiditis, etc. Retinochoroiditis may be unilateral and may follow a relapsing course and lead to blindness later in life if untreated.

Pregnant women with acute toxoplasmosis in pregnancy should be treated with the appropriate antibiotic (pyrimethamine + folic acid supplement) to reduce the risk of and to limit fetal damage due to toxoplasmosis. Expert opinion should be sought as pyrimethamine should only be instituted once intrauterine fetal infection is established on the basis of laboratory investigations (Table 39.2). Treatment should also be given to the infected neonate at birth.

Herpes Simplex Virus

There have been rare instances of in-utero herpes simplex virus (HSV) infection as diagnosed by the presence of HSV lesions at birth. A fifth of the cases of neonatal herpes are acquired postnatally by direct contact with maternal skin lesions or from other close relatives and carers. The clinical disease generally tends to be milder in postnatally acquired HSV infection and depends upon the age at infection and whether the neonate has passively transferred maternal antibody for protection.

By far the common route (in 80% of cases) is acquisition of infection at the time of birth from the infected maternal genital lesions. Prolonged rupture of membranes and use of scalp electrodes increase the risk of transmission, so both should be avoided. The risk of transmission to the neonate is greatest (30%) if the mother has genital lesions due to primary infection at the time of delivery; therefore, caesarean section is recommended. HSV reactivation poses a much lower risk (3% or less) as the baby would be protected by passively transferred maternal HSV antibody.

Table 39.2 Diagnosis of congenital infections

Infection	In-utero investigations of fetus			Investigations in the neonate
	Fetal blood obtained by cordocentesis	Amniotic fluid obtained by amniocentesis	Other	
Rubella*	IgM (can get false negative before 24 weeks)	PCR for rubella virus	PCR for rubella on choriovillus biopsy	PCR on urine, throat swab for rubella virus. Rubella IgM tests at birth.
CMV**	CMV PCR and CMV IgM on fetal blood (false negative IgM may occur before 24 weeks)	PCR for CMV	Ultrasound for fetal abnormalities	CMV PCR on urine. CMV PCR on 'Guthrie Blood Spot' which is taken at birth to screen for metabolic disorders.
Parvovirus B19***	Parvovirus B19 IgM and PCR		Ultrasound for monitoring of hydrops fetalis. Parvovirus B19 PCR on fetal tissue in case of miscarriage.	Parvovirus B19 IgM tests
Toxoplasma	Toxoplasma IgM and PCR	Toxoplasma PCR		Toxoplasma IgM and PCR

Notes: * In-utero diagnosis for rubella is rarely indicated as risk to fetus can be assessed on basis of gestational age.
** For a definitive diagnosis of congenital CMV infection, CMV should be demonstrated in a specimen taken by 3 weeks of age as after that, distinction from postnatally acquired CMV cannot be made. In the absence of tests in the first 3 weeks of life 'Guthrie Blood Spot' can be tested retrospectively by CMV PCR. A positive result indicates CMV viraemia at birth and confirms congenital infection but a negative result does not rule it out as not all neonates who are congenitally infected have CMV viraemia at birth.
*** In-utero diagnosis for parvovirus B19 infection is rarely indicated as congenital malformation does not occur.

Very often, it is difficult to distinguish whether the genital herpes lesions, present at the time of labour, are due to primary infection or reactivation (unless previous history of documented genital herpes is present).

Clinical manifestations in the neonate as a result of vertically acquired HSV infection at the time of birth are:

- *Localised skin or eye infection* – usually presents in the second week of life, if not treated then a third of the babies may go on to develop complications.
- *HSV encephalitis* – skin lesions are absent in about 40% of the babies. Presents in second week of life with seizures or other non-specific symptoms. If untreated, this condition has a 50% mortality rate with 70% risk of long-term sequelae in those who survive.
- *Disseminated HSV infection* – presents generally in the first week of life and is the most severe form of neonatal herpes simplex infection. Skin lesions may only be present in 20% of cases so a high clinical index of suspicion is required to diagnose this condition. Infection disseminates to almost all organs with the involvement of the central nervous system (in most cases), liver, kidney, heart, lungs, etc. If untreated it is invariably fatal (80% mortality rate).

Management of Neonatal Herpes Infection

Neonatal herpes simplex infection is a medical emergency and immediate specialist advice should be sought. The neonate should be treated without delay (on clinical suspicion) with high-dose intravenous aciclovir, pending the results of laboratory investigations.

Management of Maternal Genital Herpes Infection

Expert advice should be sought, but here are some general principles that apply:

- Presence of primary genital herpes lesions at the time of delivery is an indication for elective caesarean section.
- Use of fetal scalp electrodes should be avoided if mother has genital lesions or a past history of genital herpes infection.
- Pregnant women who present with primary genital herpes after 34 weeks of gestation should be commenced on aciclovir treatment, which should be continued until term.
- Those presenting before 34 weeks of gestation should be treated with oral aciclovir from 36 weeks onwards (for viral suppression).
- Screening of genital swabs for HSV is not recommended to identify asymptomatic viral shedding.

Although rare, pregnant women can develop fulminant HSV infection, with multi-organ involvement but usually without any skin lesions. Unless treated promptly with high-dose aciclovir this condition is frequently fatal. Women often present with abdominal tenderness and raised liver enzymes.

Chlamydia trachomatis

Maternal genital chlamydia infection at the time of birth classically presents as ophthalmia neonatorium. Infection should be treated with systemic antibiotics as a third of

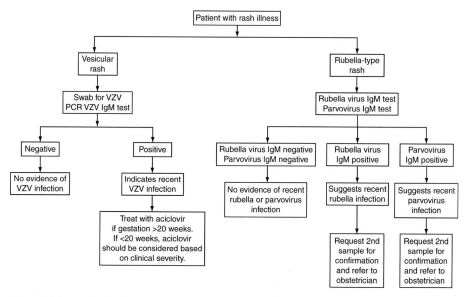

Figure 39.1 Investigations in a pregnant woman suspected of having a viral rash

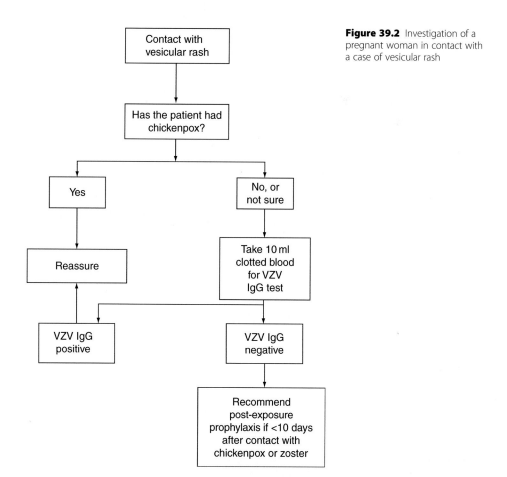

Figure 39.2 Investigation of a pregnant woman in contact with a case of vesicular rash

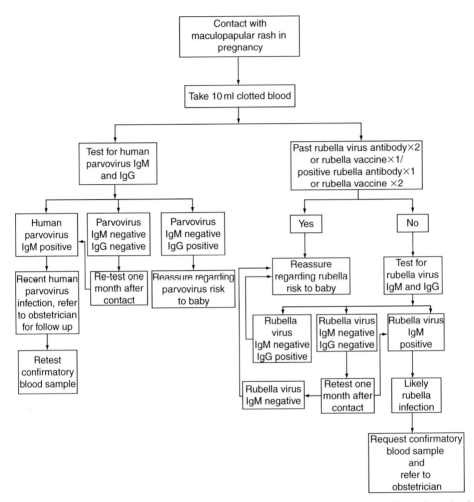

Figure 39.3 Investigation of a pregnant woman in contact with a case of suspected maculopapular viral rash

babies will also have nasopharyngeal infection which if untreated may lead to pneumonitis (see Chapter 30).

Maternal and neonatal infection with HIV, hepatitis B, hepatitis C and HTLV-1 are discussed in detail under the individual chapter headings and the reader is referred to these chapters.

Follow-up of Babies Suspected of Vertically Acquired Infection

Many congenital infections are not clinically apparent at birth and others manifest late as they are acquired at the time of birth. It is therefore important to follow the newborn clinically and by laboratory investigations to ensure that infection has not occurred, if the mother has had a proven or suspected infection during pregnancy. For blood-borne viruses like HIV, long-term follow-up for a year or 18 months may be required. For others like CMV and toxoplasmosis some of the long-term sequelae may appear only in the teenage years.

Laboratory Diagnosis and Management
Refer to Table 39.2 and Figures 39.1–39.3.

Always refer to the latest local and national guidelines for diagnosis and management of infections in pregnancy.

Useful Website
Royal College of Obstetricians and Gynaecologists, Chickenpox in Pregnancy (Green-top Guideline No. 13): https://www.rcog.org.uk/guidance/browse-all-guidance/green-top-guidelines/chickenpox-in-pregnancy-green-top-guideline-no-13/

Respiratory Virus Infections

Individual respiratory virus infections are difficult to diagnose clinically because they all cause similar symptoms. They often occur in outbreaks, at certain times of the year and in certain age groups, which increases the accuracy of clinical diagnosis. For example, respiratory syncytial virus (RSV) infection most frequently occurs in children under the age of 18 months from November to February each year and is associated with bronchiolitis, sometimes requiring hospital admission.

Several viruses, such as rhinoviruses, coronaviruses, enteroviruses, respiratory adenoviruses and parainfluenza viruses, are causes of the 'common cold'. It is interesting that parainfluenza virus types 1 and 2 cause outbreaks in the winter months while parainfluenza virus type 3 causes 'summer colds'.

Several of these viruses (especially parainfluenza viruses, RSV and Covid-19) can cause pneumonia. See Table 40.1 for clinical presentation of respiratory virus infections in different groups of patients.

Influenza

Influenza viruses are the most significant respiratory virus infection (currently alongside SARS-CoV-2). As a result of the profound malaise and myalgia associated with influenza, clinical diagnosis is more accurate than with other respiratory virus infections. Seasonal influenza occurs each year in the UK from October to April. Nobody can predict exactly when an outbreak of influenza will occur each year, which influenza virus will be involved, how severe the symptoms will be and which age group will be worst affected. If persons acquire a bacterial lung infection on top of influenza, this can result in severe or fatal infection. There is an extensive surveillance programme in the UK for influenza, which involves general practitioners, the UK Health Security Agency and the Department of Health. This gives impending warning of the first influenza cases of the season and monitors each evolving national outbreak. There are two influenza viruses (influenza A virus and influenza B virus) that cause influenza outbreaks. Influenza B virus is genetically fairly stable and does not change antigenically significantly from year to year. By contrast, influenza A virus is constantly mutating and the virus strain(s) causing infections one year are unlikely to be the ones causing influenza A outbreaks the following year. There are currently two types of influenza A viruses circulating in the world – H3N2 (haemagglutinin type 3 and neuraminidase type 2) and H1N1 (haemagglutinin type 1 and neuraminidase type 1) viruses. The haemagglutinin and neuraminidase are antigens on the virus surface against which neutralising protective antibodies are made. These are the vital constituents of influenza vaccines (which

Table 40.1 Respiratory virus symptoms in different groups of patients

Virus	Children	Adults	Elderly	At-risk groups
Adenoviruses	Cough, sore throat, pharyngitis (hepatitis)	Cough, sore throat, pharyngitis	Cough, sore throat, pharyngitis	Organ transplant recipients can have measles-like symptoms. Haematopoeitic stem cell transplant recipients have a higher risk of severe/fatal pneumonia.
Coronaviruses (common cold)	Upper respiratory tract 'cold' symptoms, bronchiolitis, pneumonia	Upper respiratory tract 'cold' symptoms, pneumonia	Upper respiratory tract 'cold' symptoms, bronchiolitis, pneumonia	
SARS-CoV-2	Less severe respiratory symptoms	Cough, fever, sore throat, pneumonia. More severe with increasing age.	Cough, fever, sore throat, pneumonia. More severe with increasing age. More likely to have severe/fatal infection.	Immunosuppressed persons, pregnant women, elderly, ethnic minorities, high BMI at greater risk of severe/fatal infection.
Enteroviruses	Upper respiratory tract symptoms (often with a maculopapular rash), pharyngitis, bronchiolitis, pneumonitis.	Upper respiratory tract symptoms (often with a maculopapular rash), pharyngitis, bronchiolitis, pneumonitis.	Upper respiratory tract symptoms (often with a maculopapular rash), pharyngitis, bronchiolitis, pneumonitis.	Low birthweight and premature babies at greater risk of severe/fatal infection.
Human metapneumoviruses	Usually, mild self-limiting upper respiratory tract symptoms – cough, fever, rhinitis. Some can develop pneumonia.	Usually, mild self-limiting upper respiratory tract symptoms – cough, fever, rhinitis. Some can develop pneumonia.	Usually, mild self-limiting upper respiratory tract symptoms – cough, fever, rhinitis. Some can develop pneumonia.	In immunocompromised persons, pneumonia is more likely, especially lung transplant recipients (chronic lung allograft dysfunction).
Influenza	Fever, headache, influenza-like symptoms. Less likely to have severe symptoms.	Fever, headache, influenza-like symptoms	Fever, headache, influenza-like symptoms. Greater risk of pneumonia and severe/fatal symptoms.	Immunocompromised persons, pregnant women, elderly persons, those with high BMI, and those with chronic renal, respiratory, heart, liver and kidney disease.

Table 40.1 (*cont.*)

Virus	Children	Adults	Elderly	At-risk groups
Parainfluenza viruses	Mostly upper respiratory tract symptoms, croup (PIV-1&2), bronchiolitis, lower respiratory tract symptoms (PIV-3).	Fever, cough, sore throat, runny nose, bronchitis, pneumonia	Fever, cough, sore throat, runny nose, bronchitis, pneumonia	Immunocompromised persons are at greater risk of pneumonia. Transplant recipients are at a greater risk of organ rejection and allograft dysfunction.
Rhinoviruses	Usually 'common cold' symptoms – sneezing, nasal discharge and cough.	Usually 'common cold' symptoms – sneezing, nasal discharge and cough.	Usually 'common cold' symptoms – sneezing, nasal discharge and cough.	Immunocompromised persons at greatly increased risk of pneumonia and fatal infection.
RSV	Bronchiolitis, pneumonia, croup	Most have 'cold'-type symptoms but 25% have lower respiratory tract symptoms.	Similar symptoms to younger adults. Increased risk of lower respiratory tract symptoms and death.	Children <24 months old with severe combined immunodeficiency syndrome, bronchopulmonary dysplasia or congenital heart disease at higher risk of severe/fatal infection. Immunocompromised persons at significantly greater risk of lower respiratory tract symptoms. Patients with haematopoietic stem cell transplant, intensive chemotherapy or lung transplant at greater risk of severe/fatal disease.

currently contain influenza A H1N1 and H3N2 and influenza B components). The influenza viruses circulating in the southern hemisphere in our summer determine the influenza virus strains in our UK vaccine for the next winter.

Influenza can be treated with antivirals such as oseltamivir and zanamivir, but to be most effective, treatment should be started less than 48 hours after the onset of symptoms. Influenza vaccine is available each year and is offered to those members of the community most susceptible to severe infection (the elderly, immunosuppressed persons, pregnant women and those with chronic conditions such as renal and heart disease and diabetes). Healthcare workers in patient contact should be offered annual influenza vaccination, in order to minimise the risk of infecting vulnerable patients.

Parainfluenza Viruses

Most people experience several parainfluenza virus illnesses during their lifetime. There are no particular distinguishing features to enable accurate clinical diagnosis. Infection can be severe or fatal in immunocompromised persons, especially in those having received a haematopoietic stem cell transplant. Parainfluenza virus types 1 and 2 cause infections in the colder months of the year and are associated with croup, while parainfluenza type 3 infections are normally more common in the summer and cause bronchiolitis, bronchitis and pneumonia. There is no specific antiviral treatment, except in immunocompromised children, who can be treated with ribavirin.

Respiratory Syncytial Virus

Respiratory syncytial virus (RSV) causes respiratory symptoms in people of all ages, usually between November and February, but most characteristically, it causes bronchiolitis in young children less than 2 years old. Infection can be more severe and fatal in immunocompromised persons, especially in those having received a haematopoietic stem cell transplant. Ribavirin is available for treatment in children and immunocompromised patients and palivizumab can be used for prophylaxis for the prevention of serious lower respiratory tract disease caused by RSV in children (1–23 months of age) at high risk of disease (e.g. premature babies born at <35 weeks' gestation with bronchopulmonary dysplasia).

SARS-CoV-2

SARS-CoV-2 is the etiological agent for Covid-19 and a novel coronavirus which was first identified in Wuhan, China in 2019 and quickly spread around the world, causing a major pandemic and killing millions of people. It is a member of the coronavirus family – most of which cause 'common colds'. As SARS-CoV-2 has evolved and the population has gained some immunity via natural infection or vaccination, the severity of disease and presenting symptoms have changed, but common symptoms include sore throat, fever, cough, shortness of breath, loss of taste and smell, and fatigue. Some people continue to experience a range of effects (long Covid) for many months. Mortality rates are higher in the elderly. Several vaccines are in widespread use. Antiviral drugs (e.g. nirmatrelvir/ritonavir) as well as antibody preparations are available for treatment, but supportive care (including oxygen support and dexamethasone) and intensive care (including ventilation and extracorporeal membrane oxygenation) are the main forms of treatment.

Other Respiratory Viruses

Rhinoviruses, enteroviruses and adenoviruses can also cause respiratory symptoms. It is difficult to clinically diagnose infection with these viruses specifically, unless there are other symptoms present.

Adenoviruses can cause respiratory symptoms as well as other symptoms (e.g. conjunctivitis, maculopapular rash or lymphadenopathy). Infections can be severe and may be fatal in immunocompromised persons, especially in children and in haematopoietic stem cell transplant recipients. Immunosuppressed patients with life-threatening illness have been treated off-licence with cidofovir.

Enteroviruses can also cause respiratory symptoms as well as maculopapular rashes, meningitis and conjunctivitis.

There are no licensed antivirals for treatment of these viruses.

Laboratory Diagnosis

In hospitalised young children under 2 years of age, the best sample to take is a nasopharyngeal aspirate. Respiratory viruses are most commonly diagnosed by testing a viral nose and throat swab, but in some patients (notably those with lower respiratory tract symptoms in ICU) bronchoalveolar lavage is a superior specimen. In bygone days, immunofluorescence and virus culture was used for diagnosing respiratory viruses, but these days, molecular tests such as PCR are almost universally employed alongside rapid test kits (which are very helpfully employed in many accident and emergency departments during the winter months).

Infection Control

Persons with respiratory symptoms in hospitals and nursing homes should be isolated, if possible, to prevent infection in others. Special care should be taken in immunocompromised (e.g. haematopoietic stem cell transplant recipients) and elderly persons, in whom these infections can be fatal. Prophylactic antiviral agents are available to protect against influenza virus and RSV infections in persons at high risk of severe disease, and influenza and Covid-19 vaccines are available for staff and higher-risk persons.

Travel-Related Infections

There has been a rapid increase in international travel in the last 40 years (until the Covid-19 pandemic decimated the industry for a while). Travel, in the past, was the domain of the rich, but due to the availability of cheaper air travel and 'package' holidays, it has come within the grasp of most people in the developed world. People are travelling far, and to parts of the world that were previously inaccessible to them. The desire to visit far-flung 'exotic' locations is insatiable. With this exotic travel comes the danger of being exposed to infections outside one's routine experience. There is also a tendency to throw caution to the wind, not to take the usual precautions and to expose oneself to risks. One of the aims of a holiday, after all, is to relax and try new experiences; it is not surprising therefore that many travellers become ill on holiday or soon after they return home. In this chapter we list some common (and not so common) clinical illnesses due to infections that are seen in returning travellers in the UK (see Table 41.1). The reader should consult the individual virus chapters for details of individual infections.

Gastroenteritis

Diarrhoea is by far the most common complaint in travellers. Most of the infections are caused by bacteria. However, noroviruses are important viral pathogens, especially in those who indulge in eating raw shellfish such as oysters. Impressive outbreaks of norovirus gastroenteritis have occurred in hotels and cruise ships, where a large number of people are confined in an enclosed space; there are many horror stories of holidays being ruined because of this.

Pyrexia of Unknown Origin (PUO)

In travellers who return to the UK with a febrile illness, there is a need for them to reveal an accurate travel history and activities undertaken while on holiday, as often these are valuable clues which aid clinical diagnosis. Malaria and typhoid should be considered first and need to be ruled out. Dengue virus infection may present as a non-specific febrile illness. The most dangerous infections in persons returning to the UK with PUO are the haemorrhagic fevers (see Chapters 2 and 38). The Advisory Committee on Dangerous Pathogens has produced guidelines for risk assessment (see website link at the end of this chapter). Prompt specialist advice from an infectious diseases physician should always be sought in cases of suspected haemorrhagic fever.

Respiratory Infections

The most likely cause of these will be the common respiratory viruses prevalent at the time of travel. However, persons returning from certain travel locations (e.g. Saudi

Table 41.1 Viral infections associated with travel outside the UK

	Virus	Clinical presentation	Transmission routes
Viruses occurring in the UK and also imported by returning travellers from endemic countries	Hepatitis A	Hepatitis	Consumption of contaminated food or water
	Hepatitis B	Hepatitis	Unprotected sexual intercourse, medical intervention, blood contact
	HIV	HIV seroconversion illness	Unprotected sexual intercourse, medical intervention, blood contact
	Norovirus	Diarrhoea and vomiting	Consumption of contaminated food or contact with a case
	Hepatitis E	Hepatitis	Consumption of contaminated food or water
Viruses not endemic in the UK and imported by returning travellers	Dengue and other arboviruses	See Chapters 2 & 38	See Chapters 2 & 38
	Viral haemorrhagic fevers	See Chapter 38	See Chapter 38
	Rabies	History of dog or animal bite. See Chapter 24	A dog or animal bite

Arabia), especially if they are immunocompromised, need special consideration and advice (e.g. to discuss the likelihood of them having acquired the potentially fatal Middle East respiratory syndrome virus, or MERS). See Chapter 12.

Hepatitis

Hepatitis A and E are the most common causes of hepatitis in returning travellers from countries where these infections are endemic. The infections are spread by the faecal-oral route by consuming contaminated food or water. While in endemic countries, it is therefore advisable to avoid eating salads and other uncooked food and to drink only bottled water. There is effective vaccination for hepatitis A and all travellers to endemic countries should be immunised prior to travel.

Hepatitis B infection abroad should be considered in the differential diagnosis in persons presenting with hepatitis after returning from abroad up to 6 months previously, especially if they have engaged in sexual intercourse while abroad. There is also effective vaccination for hepatitis B and travellers to endemic countries should consider being immunised prior to travel, especially if travelling as a 'medical tourist' or likely to be in blood contact or engage in sexual intercourse while abroad.

Rabies

A dog bite or animal bite or lick on an open wound in countries where rabies is still endemic is a medical emergency and post-exposure vaccine (and sometimes rabies immunoglobulin) prophylaxis should be given as soon as possible, since rabies in humans is invariably fatal. In order to ascertain if the country visited is rabies-free, low risk or high risk and to obtain advice about appropriate management in the UK, consult the rabies GOV.UK website listed at the end of this chapter.

Infections Associated with Medical Tourism

The term 'medical tourism' is used for people who travel abroad with the express purpose of receiving medical treatment (e.g. dental procedures or plastic surgery). Most of these infections are caused by blood-borne viruses. Patients with chronic renal failure usually receive their regular haemodialysis treatment from a local unit. If they travel and require haemodialysis treatment while abroad, there is often an increased risk of them acquiring hepatitis B or C infection and transmitting infection to other patients in their local unit. Some overseas dialysis units are well run and offer minimal risk of infection, but many are not. There is an agreed protocol for testing returning travellers who have recently been dialysed while abroad (Good Practice Guidelines for dialysis away from base – see the website address at the end of this chapter). Transfusion of blood or blood products while abroad may, in some countries, be associated with an increased risk of acquiring HIV, HBV or HCV infection.

Miscellaneous Infections

Infections in the returning traveller are not limited to those mentioned and the differential diagnosis will depend on the presenting clinical features and epidemiological history. The clinician must not be misled by the history of travel and forget to think of common infections such as Epstein–Barr virus and cytomegalovirus, which could also have been acquired in the UK. Sexual history, if relevant, should be sought to rule out any sexually transmitted infections.

Useful Websites

GOV.UK: Viral haemorrhagic fevers risk assessment: https://assets.publishing.service .gov.uk/government/uploads/system/uploads/attachment_data/file/478115/VHF_Algo .pdf

GOV.UK: Management of hazard group 4 viral haemorrhagic fevers and similar human infectious diseases of high consequence: https://assets.publishing.service.gov .uk/government/uploads/system/uploads/attachment_data/file/534002/Management_ of_VHF_A.pdf

GOV.UK: Rabies: risk assessment, post-exposure treatment, management: www.gov .uk/government/collections/rabies-risk-assessment-post-exposure-treatment- management

UK Department of Health Good Practice Guidelines for renal dialysis/translation units: https://assets.publishing.service.gov.uk/government/uploads/system/uploads/ attachment_data/file/382208/guidelines_dialysis_away_from_base.pdf

Chapter

42

Viral Eye Infections

There are several viruses which can cause infections in or around the eye. These are best considered according to what symptoms they cause. For chlamydial eye infections, see Chapter 30.

Conjunctivitis

Conjunctivitis is inflammation of the conjunctiva and is sometimes called 'red eye'. Virus infections can cause these symptoms, but it can also be caused by other conditions, such as allergies like hay fever. Viral conjunctivitis is very infectious and can cause sizeable outbreaks. Although several viruses can cause these symptoms, adenoviruses and entero-viruses are the most likely causes.

Adenovirus conjunctivitis used to be called 'shipyard eye' because one of the earliest outbreaks of this condition occurred in a shipyard in the north of England. Occupational health staff inadvertently spread the infection between metal workers, who were attending to have pieces of metal removed from their eyes. The forceps used for this purpose were inadequately sterilised between patients, thus causing an outbreak.

Several enteroviruses (especially enterovirus 70 and coxsackie virus A24) can cause conjunctivitis. These viruses can cause extensive outbreaks and are very infectious. Enterovirus 70 used to be called 'Apollo eye' after a large outbreak in Africa which it was alleged was a result of people staring at the sky to look at the Apollo spacecraft.

Keratitis

Keratitis is corneal inflammation and ulceration, which can lead to blindness. Herpes simplex virus (HSV) is the most significant virus associated with keratitis. Primary infection can produce ulcers on the cornea, which should be treated with aciclovir. When the primary infection subsides, the virus becomes latent. The virus can reactivate, producing another episode of corneal ulceration. Successive episodes of corneal ulcer-ation can produce extensive corneal scarring and even blindness. Prompt diagnosis and treatment is essential.

Herpes Zoster Ophthalmicus

This is defined as herpes zoster involvement of the ophthalmic division of the fifth cranial nerve. About 50% of patients will have ocular involvement if antiviral therapy is not used. With the onset of the rash, conjunctivitis, uveitis and keratitis may occur with acute retinal necrosis. Vesicular lesions on the side or tip of the nose correlate highly with eye involvement.

Table 42.1 Diagnosis and treatment of viral eye infections

Symptoms	Virus	Special clinical features	Diagnosis	Treatment
Conjunctivitis	Adenovirus	Follicular and pseudomembranous conjunctivitis	Conjunctival swab for PCR	None
	Enteroviruses Enterovirus 70 and Coxsackie A24	Acute haemorrhagic conjunctivitis (very infectious)	Conjunctival swab for PCR	None
	HSV	Follicular conjunctivitis	Conjunctival swab for PCR	Aciclovir ointment and oral aciclovir if severe infection
	Measles virus	Mucopurulent keratoconjunctivitis	Conjunctival swab for PCR	None
	Influenza A	Follicular conjunctivitis (especially Avian influenza)	Conjunctival swab for PCR	Oseltamivir
Corneal inflammation and keratitis	HSV	Dendritic and geographic corneal ulcers and disciform keratitis	Conjunctival swab for PCR	Aciclovir ointment and oral aciclovir if severe infection
	VZV	Epithelial disease and disciform keratitis	Conjunctival swab for PCR	Aciclovir ointment and oral aciclovir if severe infection
	Adenoviruses	Keratitis	Conjunctival swab for PCR	None
	Measles virus	Epithelial keratitis	Conjunctival swab for PCR	None
Scleritis	HSV	Scleritis	Conjunctival swab for PCR	Aciclovir ointment and oral aciclovir if severe infection
	VZV	Scleritis	Conjunctival swab for PCR	Aciclovir ointment and oral aciclovir if severe infection
Retinitis and neuritis	CMV	Nectrotising retinitis and optic neuritis especially in HIV infection (AIDS)	Clotted blood for CMV IgM and IgG or retinal biopsy for CMV PCR	Iv or intra-ocular ganciclovir (foscarnet, cidofivir if ganciclovir is not indicated)
	VZV	Retinitis	Clotted blood for VZV IgM and IgG or retinal biopsy for VZV PCR	Iv aciclovir

Table 42.1 (cont.)

Symptoms	Virus	Special clinical features	Diagnosis	Treatment
	Toxoplasma gondii	Retinitis, choroiditis and uveitis	Retinal biopsy for *Toxoplasma gondii* PCR	Pyrimetahmine + Sulphadiazine
Eyelid and periocular skin infection	Molluscum contagiosum	Molluscum nodules	Histology or PCR	
	VZV	Ophthalmic zoster	Vesicle fluid or swab for VZV PCR	Aciclovir, famciclovir or valaciclovir
	HSV	Vesicular blepharo-conjunctivitis	Vesicle fluid or swab for HSV PCR	Aciclovir, famciclovir or valaciclovir
	Papillomaviruses	Papillomata on lid and conjunctiva	Clinical but if unsure biopsy for papilloma virus PCR	
	Human herpes virus 8 (HHV-8)	Kaposi's sarcoma in HIV-positive patients	Clinical but if unsure biopsy for HHV-8 PCR	

Retinitis: Varicella-zoster virus (VZV) retinitis can occur in both immunocompetent and immunocompromised patients. In the immunocompromised (especially AIDS patients) cytomegalovirus (CMV) retinitis and *Toxoplasma gondii* uveitis and retinitis also occur.

These and other eye conditions associated with virus infection are shown in Table 42.1. In addition, *Chlamydia trachomatis* causes both conjunctivitis and keratitis (in trachoma). These are discussed in Chapter 30.

Chapter

43

Viral Gastroenteritis

Clinical

Gastroenteritis can be caused by bacteria or viruses. Many different viruses can cause viral gastroenteritis. Viral infection can be associated with either diarrhoea or vomiting, or both. Bacterial infections often have a longer incubation period unless illness is caused by bacterial toxins, when the onset is shorter (e.g. 12 hours). Within hospitals, outbreaks involving diarrhoea and vomiting, especially if staff are symptomatic, should be regarded as norovirus outbreaks until proved otherwise. In food-borne infections (e.g. norovirus) symptoms occur 12–48 hours after eating contaminated food.

Epidemiology

Rotaviruses (see Chapter 27)

In young children under the age of 18 months, rotavirus infection is the most common cause of diarrhoea and vomiting. Infection in very young children occurs every winter from December to March. Mild infection occurs in adults, but is more severe in the elderly. Rotavirus symptoms usually begin about 2 days after infection with the virus and last for 3–8 days, but may last longer. Rotaviruses are infrequently associated with outbreaks, but outbreaks can occur in hospitals and nursing homes in the elderly or in very young persons (e.g. in nurseries and playgroups).

Noroviruses (see Chapter 19)

Noroviruses are the most common causes of diarrhoea and vomiting outbreaks in all ages. Symptoms usually begin 12–48 hours after infection with the virus and last 1–3 days. Hospitals, care homes, holiday camps and cruise ships are frequent outbreak locations. Outbreaks should be managed with strict infection control procedures such as patient isolation or cohorting, symptomatic staff exclusion and thorough cleaning when the outbreak is over (see local guidelines). Noroviruses mutate frequently, which results in the emergence of new epidemic strains and more extensive outbreaks of diarrhoea and vomiting, every few years.

Other Enteric Viruses

Adenoviruses, astroviruses, sapoviruses and caliciviruses can cause diarrhoea and vomiting in all age groups. They tend to be associated with sporadic cases, but rare outbreaks do occur.

- Adenovirus symptoms usually begin 3–10 days after infection with the virus and last 1–2 weeks.
- Astroviruses cause gastroenteritis in all ages, but children, the elderly and immunocompromised persons are most susceptible. Symptoms begin 4–5 days after infection and last for 1–4 days.
- Sapovirus infections usually occur in children and infants and are associated with outbreaks in nurseries and care centres. There is an incubation period of 1–4 days. Symptoms are similar to those of noroviruses.
- Caliciviruses cause symptoms similar to noroviruses and have an incubation period of 2 days and the symptoms usually last for 3–4 days.

Food-Borne Infection

Viral food-borne infection is usually caused by noroviruses. Contaminated shellfish (e.g. cockles, oysters and mussels) and vegetables eaten uncooked and grown on land fertilised with human faecal waste are frequently the cause, but infection can be transmitted via food when infected symptomatic food handlers do not wash their hands properly before handling food. Hepatitis A and hepatitis E viruses can also be spread via contaminated food, but they principally cause jaundice and are not usually associated with gastroenteritis.

Laboratory Diagnosis

Laboratory diagnosis is performed on faeces samples, preferably taken in the first 3 days after the onset of symptoms. See the website (in the Useful Website section) for details of how to diagnose gastroenteritis outbreaks. Laboratory diagnostic techniques include RT-PCR, enzyme immunoassay, agglutination and electron microscopy. Figure 43.1 shows electron microscope pictures of noroviruses, rotaviruses and adenoviruses.

Current UK advice is to consider testing for viruses in certain circumstances following discussion with the local laboratory. Norovirus testing is not recommended as frontline testing in sporadic cases except in patients who are immunocompromised. Testing is dependent on local laboratory policies. However, if a norovirus outbreak is suspected, consider submitting stool samples as early as possible during the acute phase of the illness.

Treatment

There is no antiviral treatment for viral gastroenteritis; replacement of fluids in severe cases is important.

Prophylaxis

There is a vaccine for rotavirus infection, offered as part of the UK national childhood immunisation programme. It is a live attenuated vaccine administered orally and is over 85% effective in protecting against severe rotavirus gastroenteritis in the first 2 years of life.

Infection Control

Gastroenteritis viruses (especially noroviruses) are very infectious, especially when the environment is contaminated with vomit and faeces. Symptomatic persons should be

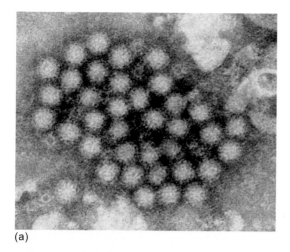

(a)

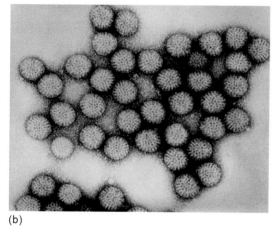

(b)

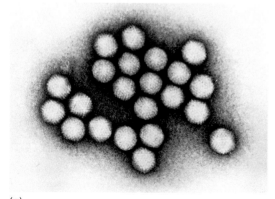

(c)

Figure 43.1 Electron micrograph photographs of some viruses causing gastroenteritis (courtesy of CDC)
a Norovirus.
b rotavirus.
c adenovirus.

isolated as much as possible and in cases of norovirus infection, persons should not mix socially or for work until 48 hours after the symptoms stop. Contaminated environments should be cleaned thoroughly with chlorine-based disinfectants (especially in hospitals, where terminal deep cleans should be done at the end of an outbreak).

Useful Website

National Health Service UK standards for microbiology investigations – gastroenteritis: https://assets.publishing.service.gov.uk/government/uploads/system/uploads/attachment_data/file/930517/S_7i2_FINAL-UKSMI.pdf

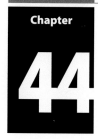

Chapter

Viral Hepatitis

44

Viral hepatitis is a clinical diagnosis and presents as a systemic infection primarily affecting the liver. Hepatitis A, B, C, D and E viruses are all hepatotropic viruses and primarily cause hepatic infection, whereas Epstein–Barr virus (EBV), cytomegalovirus (CMV) and other viruses may cause hepatitis as part of a more generalised systemic infection. The differential diagnosis, in persons presenting with hepatitis, should also include non-viral causes, such as leptospirosis.

Clinical

The clinical features of hepatitis include nausea, vomiting, lack of appetite, dark urine, pale stools and pain in the right upper quadrant of the abdomen. This is normally preceded by prodromal symptoms, which may include fever, arthralgia, myalgia, headache and rash. Clinically, it is not possible to determine the etiological agent, although there may be clues in the epidemiology (Table 44.1). Many cases of acute viral hepatitis, especially in children, may be asymptomatic (e.g. not accompanied by jaundice). About 70% of persons with acute hepatitis C virus (HCV) infection develop an asymptomatic infection initially, but some will develop severe symptomatic liver disease in later life. Diagnosis is only made by chance or due to investigations of non-specific symptoms or during follow-up after known exposure. The main abnormal laboratory blood test results are elevated liver function test values, with peak alanine aminotransferase (ALT) levels of >1000 U/L, especially in hepatitis A and B virus infections. Peak ALT levels tend to be lower in acute HCV infections.

Both hepatitis B virus (HBV) and HCV may fail to clear after acute infection, leading to persistent/chronic hepatitis, cirrhosis and, in some cases, hepatocellular carcinoma. Chronic infection with hepatitis A virus (HAV) or hepatitis E virus (HEV) does not occur in immunocompetent persons, although HEV can be associated with chronic infection in immunocompromised patients. Hepatitis D or Delta virus (HDV) causes both acute and chronic infections, but only in conjunction with HBV co-infection as it requires HBV to infect humans.

Differential Diagnosis

Other non-viral organisms can cause hepatitis in humans (e.g. leptospira, rickettsia, *Coxiella burnetii* and bacteria). Other non-infective causes of hepatitis should be considered, including drugs, alcohol, metabolic liver disease, autoimmune liver disease, cryptogenic hepatitis and obstructive hepatitis.

Table 44.1 Clinical and epidemiological features of viral causes of hepatitis

Virus	Clinical	Route of transmission	Risk groups
Hepatitis A virus	Incubation period 2–6 weeks, acute onset, no chronic infection	Food- and water-borne, faecal-oral	Travellers to endemic countries, sewage workers, poor hygiene standards
Hepatitis B virus	Incubation period 2–6 months, acute or insidious onset, can become chronic infection	Sexual, blood, IV drug use, mother to baby	IV drug users, healthcare workers, sex workers, men who have sex with men, piercing/tattoo
Hepatitis C virus	Incubation period 2–12 weeks, insidious onset, 80% develop chronic infection	Sexual, blood, IV drug use, mother to baby	IV drug use, healthcare workers, piercing/tattoos
Hepatitis D virus	Incubation period 1–6 months, acute or insidious onset, can be chronic infection	Sexual, blood, IV drug use, mother to baby	IV drug use, healthcare workers, piercing/tattoos
Hepatitis E virus	Incubation period 2–8 weeks, acute onset, no chronic infection	Food- and water-borne, faecal-oral	Travellers, eating undercooked infected meat. Pregnant women and their unborn children. Immunocompromised persons.
Cytomegalovirus	Incubation period 3–6 weeks, usually asymptomatic, can be severe, chronic infection in the immunocompromised, who can experience reactivated infection	Sex, saliva, mother to baby, via blood and donated organs in transplant recipients	Unborn babies of infected mothers in utero, transplant recipients, HIV-positive persons
Epstein–Barr virus	Incubation period 2–3 weeks, typically causes glandular fever	Saliva and sexual contact, 'kissing disease'	Immunocompromised persons
Exotic viruses: Yellow fever virus, hantavirus, Lassa fever virus, Marburg/Ebola viruses, Junin and Machupo viruses, Kyasanur Forest virus	Various symptoms including haemorrhagic fever	Different routes involving mosquitos, monkeys, small mammals, ticks	Travellers to different endemic countries. Since these viruses have distinct geographical areas of endemicity, knowing which countries have recently been visited narrows down the likely viral cause.

Table 44.2 Laboratory markers of hepatitis viruses A–E and clinical interpretation

Virus	Acute infection	Chronic infection	Resolved infection
Hepatitis A	HAV IgM +ve HAV IgG +ve or −ve	Not applicable	HAV IgM −ve HAV IgG +ve
Hepatitis B	HBsAg +ve Anti-HBc IgM +ve*	HBsAg +ve Anti-HBc IgM −ve* Anti-HBc +ve	HBsAg −ve Anti-HBc +ve Anti-HBs +ve
Hepatitis C	Anti-HCV +ve HCV RNA +ve	HCV RNA +ve	Anti-HCV +ve or −ve HCV RNA −ve
Hepatitis D	HDV antigen +ve Anti-HDV +ve	HDV antigen +ve Anti-HDV +ve	HDV antigen −ve Anti-HDV +ve or −ve
Hepatitis E	HEV IgM +ve HEV IgG +ve or −ve	Not applicable in immunocompetent	HEV IgM −ve HEV IgG +ve

Note: * Anti-HBc IgM results can be difficult to interpret. Only reliable high anti-HBc IgM values are suggestive of recent primary HBV infection. Low anti-HBc IgM values can be found in persons with chronic HBV infection, especially after a disease 'flare'.

Epidemiology

Hepatitis B and C infections occur worldwide, with the main route of spread being via exposure to infected blood and blood-contaminated secretions, sexual and vertical (mother to baby). Hepatitis C is much less efficiently transmitted by sexual or vertical routes (<5%) as compared to hepatitis B.

Hepatitis A and E viruses are transmitted by the faecal-oral route, which may be person-to-person (less likely with HEV) or via contaminated food or water. Both of these infections are more prevalent in developing countries with poor enteric hygiene (e.g. the Indian subcontinent, Southeast Asia, Africa and some parts of eastern Europe). Food- and water-borne outbreaks, especially of HEV, are not uncommon in these countries. Travellers to endemic countries from low-risk countries (e.g. UK, USA, Australasia) are at particular risk of infection due to lack of immunity.

Laboratory Investigations

Diagnosis is by serology; a 5–10 ml clotted blood sample should be submitted to the laboratory with clinical details, a date of onset of symptoms and appropriate epidemiological information, including history of foreign travel and at-risk exposure, if any. The serological screening tests are usually based on enzyme-linked immunosorbent assays. In addition, molecular nucleic acid amplification test diagnostic tests, such as the PCR test are used to detect viral RNA (HAV, HCV, HEV) or DNA (HBV). Quantitative PCR assays are used to determine infectivity and monitor treatment progress. A negative PCR result is indicative of viral clearance. Table 44.2 shows the interpretation of laboratory results for hepatitis viruses A–E.

For details of which virology laboratory tests to request in patients presenting with acute or chronic hepatitis, see Table 44.3.

Table 44.3 Tests to request in patients presenting with acute or chronic hepatitis

	Acute hepatitis	Chronic hepatitis
First-line tests	HAV IgM HBsAg Anti-HBc IgM Anti-HCV HEV IgM CMV IgM EBV VCA IgM EBNA antibody	HBsAg Anti-HBc HBeAg Anti-HBe Anti-HCV HCV RNA
In immunocompromised persons	HCV RNA	
If drug user	Anti-HDV	Anti-HDV
Other tests to consider if first-line tests are negative	Leptospira antibody *Coxiella* *burnetii* antibody	

Table 44.4 Management of viral hepatitis

Virus	Available antiviral treatment*	Pre-exposure prophylaxis	Post-exposure prophylaxis	Control of infection
Hepatitis A	No treatment	HAV vaccine	HAV vaccine Human normal immunoglobulin	Enteric precautions, avoid contaminated food and water, handwashing
Hepatitis B	Entecavir, peginterferon alfa, tenofovir alafenamide tenofovir disoproxil	HBV vaccine	HBV vaccine Hepatitis B immunoglobulin	Avoid sexual percutaneous or mucous membrane exposure to blood or blood-stained secretions
Hepatitis C	Sofosbuvir, ribavirin, peginterferon alfa, velpatasvir, voxilaprevir, glecaprevir, pibrentasvir	None	Antiviral treatment is recommended for those persons who acquire HCV infection	As for HBV
Hepatitis D	As for HBV	As for HBV	As for HBV	As for HBV
Hepatitis E	Ribavirin for chronic infection in the immunocompromised	None	None	Enteric precautions, avoid contaminated. food and water, handwashing

Note: * There are many antiviral drugs and antiviral drug combination treatments for treating chronic HBV, HCV and HDV infection – always seek expert medical advice before administering treatment, which may need to last for 6 months or more.

Management

Treatment for chronic hepatitis B and C infections has improved in recent years, with the availability of more effective antiviral drugs and drug combination regimes, with most patients clearing the viruses or achieving a sustained viral response. There is no treatment for acute HAV or HEV infection. Since acute symptomatic HBV infection is almost always self-limiting in immunocompetent persons, treatment of acute infection is not warranted.

The mainstay of management of viral hepatitis remains the prevention of transmission by control of infection measures and by encouraging those persons at increased risk of infection to have pre-exposure vaccination or by giving prompt post-exposure prophylaxis (see Table 44.4).

Chapter 45

Virus Infections in Immunocompromised Patients

There are several categories of immunocompromised patients, such as:

- those with cellular immune deficiencies like severe combined immunodeficiency;
- those with immunosuppression due to acute and chronic leukaemia and lymphomas;
- solid organ transplant recipients on immunosuppressant drugs;
- bone marrow transplant recipients;
- patients with HIV/AIDS;
- patients on immunosuppressive drugs, especially biological therapies (such as B-cell, interleukin and tumour necrosis factor -alpha (TNF) inhibitors for management of their illness).

Individual risk of infection depends on patients' risk of exposure to infections in the past and in future and their reason for and level of immunosuppression. All immunosuppressed patients are vulnerable to community-acquired virus infections; however, these infections are generally more severe with associated complications and mortality, persist for longer and may be intractable to treat. Reactivation of infection (especially of viruses belonging to the herpes virus group) is a particular issue in immunosuppressed patients.

Different viruses cause different clinical symptoms in these patients. HIV-positive/ AIDS patients often have different symptoms to transplant recipients and need different treatment and prophylactic strategies.

This chapter brings together some of the viral infections that are especially problematic in immunosuppressed patients and may need a different approach to management as compared to immunocompetent individuals. Readers should also refer to chapters in the book on individual viruses. Tables 45.1 and 45.2 give details of virus infections in transplant recipients and in HIV-antibody positive/AIDS patients respectively.

Cytomegalovirus

Cytomegalovirus (CMV) is the most important virus infection in transplant recipients. In solid organ transplants infection acquired from the donor organ is usually most severe and can be fatal. Eighty per cent of CMV antibody–negative patients who receive an organ from a CMV antibody–positive donor will acquire primary CMV infection. Between 30% and 60% of CMV antibody–positive organ recipients will experience CMV reactivation from 1 to 3 months after transplantation. The severity of the symptoms will depend on the amount and type of immunosuppressive treatment they are receiving. Lung transplant recipients usually have more severe CMV disease than heart, liver or kidney transplant recipients. In bone marrow transplants (BMT) the risk is related to the recipients' CMV status, being highest in CMV-positive recipients who

Table 45.1 Virus infections in transplant recipients

Viruses	Symptoms and signs	Diagnosis and samples	Strategies to reduce risk of severe symptoms
CMV	• Pneumonitis • Fever • Malaise • ↑ LFTs • ↓ WBC • GI tract lesion • Retinitis	• EDTA blood for CMV PCR and quantitative CMV PCR • Clotted blood for CMV IgM in organ recipients (CMV PCR is preferred in other groups as serology is not reliable due to poor immune response).	• Identify CMV antibody–negative organ recipients who have received organ(s) from a CMV antibody–positive donor and bone marrow transplant recipients at high risk of reactivation and give oral valganciclovir prophylaxis. • Monitor transplant recipients for CMV infection and treat infected patients with ganciclovir.
HSV	• Skin lesions • Pneumonitis (especially in lung and heart and lung recipients) • Encephalitis	• Vesicle fluid or skin lesion swab for PCR • CSF (if encephalitis) • Bronchioalveolar lavage (BAL) or lung biopsy (if pneumonitis)	• Identify HSV antibody–positive organ and bone marrow transplant recipients at high risk of potentially fatal HSV pneumonitis (e.g. lung and heart and lung recipients) and give oral aciclovir prophylaxis.
VZV	• Chickenpox • Shingles • CNS symptoms in the absence of skin lesions	• Vesicle fluid or skin lesion swabs for PCR • CSF if encephalitis or meningitis	• Identify VZV antibody–negative patients and warn them to avoid contact with persons with chickenpox or shingles. If they do come in contact, give zoster immunoglobulin (ZIG) or oral aciclovir prophylaxis promptly. • Good infection control to prevent infection in other VZV antibody–negative patients.
EBV	• Vague symptoms such as fever, malaise, respiratory • Lympho-proliferative syndrome/ lymphoma	• EDTA blood for EBV PCR or quantitative EBV PCR • Clotted blood (paired samples) for EBV IgM and VCA antibody tests	• If severe EBV infection (especially lymphoproliferative syndrome (PTLD) or lymphoma reduce immunosuppression as much as possible and consider treatment with rituximab.

Table 45.1 (cont.)

Viruses	Symptoms and signs	Diagnosis and samples	Strategies to reduce risk of severe symptoms
HHV-6, -7 and -8	HHV-6 encephalitis. Kaposi sarcoma associated with HHV-8.	• PCR on EDTA blood for HHV-6. Histology and PCR on biopsy for HHV-8.	• No specific antiviral treatment. Chemotherapy for Kaposi sarcoma.
Adenoviruses	• Pneumonia • Diarrhoea and vomiting • Measles-like rash in children	• Nose and throat swabs for PCR • Nasopharyngeal aspirate (NPA) for PCR • EDTA blood for PCR • Stools for PCR	• Good infection control to prevent infection in other patients. • Treat with cidofovir (or brincidofovir) if clinically indicated.
Respiratory viruses	• Pneumonia	• Nose and throat swabs for NAAT*/PCR • NPA for NAAT/PCR or for point of care testing	• Good infection control to prevent infection in other patients. • Consider reducing immunosuppression if possible.
Hepatitis B	• Fulminant and chronic hepatitis	• HBV viral load and hepatitis B serology	• Monitoring for HBV DNA levels and prophylaxis/treatment with specific antiviral drugs.
Hepatitis E	• Fulminant and chronic hepatitis	• HEV PCR in stool and blood	• Reduce immunosuppression, treat with ribavirin.
Polyomaviruses	• CNS symptoms (PML) with JC virus • Nephropathy and haemorrhagic cystitis with BK virus	• CSF for JC virus PCR • Urine and blood for BK virus PCR	• Reduce immunosuppression if possible.
Papillomaviruses	• Skin warts • Genital warts	• Clinical diagnosis but lesion biopsy for PCR may be done if unsure of diagnosis.	• None
Parvovirus B19	• Intractable aplastic anaemia	• Parvovirus B19 IgM (may be false negative) • Parvovirus B19 PCR on blood	• No specific treatment. • Try to reduce immunosuppression.

Table 45.1 (cont.)

Viruses	Symptoms and signs	Diagnosis and samples	Strategies to reduce risk of severe symptoms
Toxoplasma gondii	• Fever • Pneumonia • Encephalitis • Myocarditis	• Clotted blood for *T. gondii* IgM in organ recipients • EDTA blood or CSF for *T. gondii* PCR	• Identify *T. gondii* antibody–negative liver, heart and heart–lung organ recipients who receive organs from *T. gondii* antibody–positive donor and give 6 weeks' co-trimoxazole or pyrimethamine after transplantation.

Note: * NAAT – nucleic acid amplification test; of which PCR is most commonly used.

Table 45.2 Virus infections in HIV antibody–positive/AIDS patients

Viruses	Symptoms and signs	Diagnosis and samples	Strategies to reduce risk of severe symptoms
CMV	• Fever • Malaise • GI tract lesion • Retinitis • Encephalitis	• EDTA blood for CMV PCR and quantitative CMV PCR	• Oral valganciclovir prophylaxis to prevent CMV retinitis for those with advanced HIV infection and low white cell blood counts.
HSV	• Skin lesions • Genital herpes • Pneumonitis • Encephalitis	• Vesicle fluid or skin lesion swab for PCR • CSF (if encephalitis) • Bronchioalveolar lavage (BAL) or lung biopsy (if pneumonitis)	• Some severely immunocompromised patients with frequent recurrent HSV infections require continuous oral aciclovir prophylaxis.
VZV	• Chickenpox • Shingles • CNS symptoms in the absence of skin lesions	• Vesicle fluid or skin lesion swabs for PCR • CSF if encephalitis or meningitis	• Identify VZV antibody–negative patients and warn them to avoid contact with persons with chickenpox or shingles. If they do come in contact, give zoster immunoglobulin (ZIG) or oral aciclovir prophylaxis promptly. • Good infection control to prevent infection in other VZV antibody–negative patients.

Table 45.2 (cont.)

Viruses	Symptoms and signs	Diagnosis and samples	Strategies to reduce risk of severe symptoms
EBV	• Vague symptoms such as fever, malaise, respiratory • Hairy leukoplakia on the tongue	• EDTA blood for EBV PCR or quantitative EBV PCR	• None
HHV-8	• Kaposi's sarcoma	• Biopsy for histology and HHV-8 PCR	• Effective antiretroviral therapy to control HIV replication; chemotherapy for Kaposi's sarcoma
JC polyomavirus	• CNS symptoms as PML	• CSF for PCR	• None
Papillomaviruses	• Genital warts • Skin warts	• Clinical diagnosis, lesion biopsy for PCR if unsure	• Symptomatic treatment
Toxoplasma gondii	• Encephalitis • Fever • Retinitis • Myocarditis	• CSF and EDTA blood for *T. gondii* PCR	• Co-trimoxazole or pyrimethamine prophylaxis for very immunosuppressed patients

receive bone marrow from a CMV-negative donor; this is due to the infection of engrafted bone marrow with the recipients' virus.

Symptoms in HIV antibody–positive patients are different to those in transplant recipients due to the different nature of the immunosuppression in these patients. Transplant patients are given immunosuppressive drugs to eliminate the T-cell response related to organ rejection. HIV antibody–positive/AIDS patients have a far more extensive T-cell immunosuppression. Most infections result from reactivation of latent infection. CMV retinitis is the most common complication and may lead to blindness if untreated.

Management of CMV infection involves establishment of CMV serostatus, prophylaxis and treatment.

Pre-transplant CMV antibody screening to establish the donor and recipient serostatus allows assessment of the risk of post-transplant infection. The risk of severe CMV disease is highest in donor-positive, recipient-negative solid organ transplant recipients and donor-negative, recipient-positive bone marrow transplant recipients. In HIV/AIDS and other immunosuppressed patients CMV serostatus helps to predict the risk of reactivation as severity of immunosuppression increases either due to their underlying illness or due to immunosuppressive treatments.

CMV prophylaxis with oral valganciclovir is now the mainstay of prophylaxis in transplant recipients. The duration of antiviral prophylaxis depends upon the organ transplanted, the specific risk status of the patient and local/national recommendations. This approach has resulted in a major reduction of morbidity and mortality of transplant-related CMV disease in those at risk of donor-acquired primary CMV infection or at risk of reactivation of their latent infection. All patients should be regularly monitored either weekly or fortnightly for CMV viraemia so early treatment with either oral valganciclovir or I/V ganciclovir can be started. A hybrid approach of regular monitoring for CMV infection with pre-emptive treatment with oral valganciclovir or I/V ganciclovir has been shown to be as effective as universal antiviral prophylaxis.

Antiviral treatment for CMV disease is oral valganciclovir or I/V ganciclovir (foscarnet or cidofivir for resistant virus or if ganciclovir is contraindicated). The aim of treatment should be to clear the infection as shown by clearance of CMV viraemia, that is, a negative CMV PCR result on blood. The minimum duration of treatment is usually 2–3 weeks but may be longer depending upon virus clearance and may also require the reduction of immunosuppression if clinically possible.

Intra-ocular ganciclovir is used to treat CMV retinitis.

Epstein–Barr Virus

Primary Epstein–Barr virus (EBV) infection is rare in adult transplant recipients. It is more common in children and is usually acquired with the donor organ.

EBV causes glandular fever in immunocompetent persons but not in transplant recipients, who usually have vague symptoms (fever, headache). About 60% of organ transplant recipients who have experienced EBV infection in the past will have reactivation of EBV latent infection in the first few years after transplantation (most in the first year). The most important symptoms associated with EBV infection are post-transplant lymphoproliferative syndrome (PTLD) or lymphoma, which occur in 2–5% of UK organ recipients (with a higher percentage in the USA because higher levels of immunosuppression are given there). It is recommended that pre-transplant EBV serostatus of both donor and recipient should be established.

Since the development of PTLD is associated with the degree of immunosuppression, management largely relies on, where possible, tapering or withdrawing immunosuppressive drugs. In addition, EBV monitoring by PCR on blood for routine evaluation of patients at high risk of PTLD with pre-emptive treatment with rituximab is another approach.

There is no specific antiviral drug recommended for treating EBV, but the use of humanised monoclonal antibody (rituximab) directed against the CD20 epitope of infected B-cells has some success in treating PTLD. Recent advances in adoptive immunotherapy with EBV-specific cytotoxic T-cells also show promise. Lowering the doses of immunosuppressive drugs should always be attempted in patients with PTLD or lymphoma.

In HIV antibody–positive/AIDS patients EBV infection is also associated with hairy leukoplakia, which presents with lesions on the tongue. Primary EBV infection is rare because 95% of persons have had EBV infection by their late teenage years.

Herpes Simplex Virus

Herpes simplex virus (HSV) infection in transplant recipients is almost always a reactivation of latent infection, which occurs from a few weeks to a few months after transplantation. Symptoms can vary from a small cold sore, genital or skin lesion to extensive skin eruptions and, rarely, encephalitis.

Since patients are often very immunosuppressed, especially in the first few months after transplantation, lesions can be extensive.

HSV infection in HIV-positive patients is almost always a reactivation of latent infection, which occurs when white blood cell levels fall and can be one of the earliest signs that a patient is developing AIDS.

Antiviral prophylaxis with aciclovir or valaciclovir in the first few months after transplant is recommended in those at risk of HSV reactivation.

Active infection should be treated with oral or I/V aciclovir or oral valaciclovir (depending on the severity of the symptoms). Foscarnet or cidofovir can be used in case of infection with resistant HSV.

Varicella-Zoster Virus

Primary varicella-zoster virus (VZV) infection causes chickenpox; reactivation of latent VZV infection gives rise to zoster (shingles), usually presenting in one dermatome served by a sensory nerve on one side of the body, but widespread vesicular lesions do occur in immunocompromised patients due to more severe infections.

Primary VZV infection (chickenpox) is rare in adults, but, if it occurs, it can lead to widespread lesions and multisystem involvement in both children and adults (haemorrhagic chickenpox) and has a high mortality. Reactivation of latent VZV infection (zoster or shingles), usually presenting in one dermatome served by a sensory nerve on one side of the body, is more common. Widespread vesicular lesions in more than one dermatome occur in the most severe infections. Zoster is most common from 1 to 4 months after transplantation.

Zoster is the most frequent VZV infection in HIV antibody–positive/AIDS patients. It usually presents when white cells fall and before patients develop AIDS. Patients can have several episodes of zoster.

Antiviral prophylaxis with valaciclovir or aciclovir in the first few months after transplant in those who are VZV-antibody positive is recommended in transplant setting.

Severe VZV infections are treated with I/V aciclovir, but less severe infections can be treated with oral valaciclovir or famciclovir.

Human Herpesviruses Types 6, 7 and 8 (HHV-6, -7 and -8)

In immunosuppressed individuals there can be serious complications from HHV-6B reactivation resulting in severe disease in transplant recipients with clinical manifestations, such as encephalitis, bone marrow suppression and pneumonitis, as well as graft rejection, often in association with other beta-herpesviruses. In people with HIV/AIDS, HHV-6 reactivations cause disseminated infections leading to end organ disease and death.

HHV-8 causes Kaposi's sarcoma, a cancer more commonly occurring in AIDS patients, as well as primary effusion lymphoma, which is a large B-cell lymphoma, and HHV-8-associated multicentric Castleman's disease.

Adenoviruses

Organ transplant recipients, especially children, infected with respiratory adenoviruses can have measles-like rash and conjunctivitis but no Koplik's spots. Bone marrow transplant recipients can experience severe or fatal infection. Enteric adenoviruses can cause prolonged symptoms and viral excretion in transplant recipients, especially children. Many paediatric centres therefore follow their high-risk bone marrow transplant recipients with regular laboratory screens for adenovirus infection. Adenoviruses may cause myocarditis, meningoencephalitis or hepatitis in immunocompromised people.

Excretion of the virus in stool and respiratory secretions can be prolonged and patients may need regular monitoring after infection to check their infectivity and prevent spread to other vulnerable patients. Risk factors for adenovirus disease are T-cell depletion, unrelated and cord blood hematopoietic stem cell transplantation, and severe graft-versus-host. High-risk patients should be monitored by testing of stool and blood by virus-specific PCR. Although no controlled trials have been performed cidofovir is the drug of choice for treating systemic adenovirus infection in immunocompromised patients. If cidofovir is contraindicated because of renal insufficiency, brincidofovir should be considered because it is less renal toxic.

Respiratory Viruses: Influenza, Parainfluenza, Respiratory Syncytial (RSV) Viruses and SARS-CoV-2

All of these respiratory viruses can cause severe infection in the transplant setting (especially in bone marrow transplant recipients). Viral pneumonitis is the most serious complication and has high morbidity and may have a fatal outcome as patients are not able to clear the virus. These viruses can spread easily in bone marrow transplant units and careful infection control precautions are necessary in order to limit their transmission to other vulnerable patients. Bone marrow transplant patients appear to be at highest risk, especially prior to marrow engraftment, when RSV infection carries an 80% risk of pneumonia and death. Treatment is supportive with reduction in immunosuppression where clinically possible. Antiviral treatment is dependent on the infecting virus (see individual virus chapters).

Hepatitis B Virus

Hepatitis B vaccine is recommended for all those who are susceptible, especially pre-transplantation in those who are being considered for solid organ transplants.

All patients who are positive for HBsAg should be on treatment or started on treatment with a specific nucleoside analogue (NA) like entecavir or one of the tenofovir compounds to control viral replication and their viral load should be monitored regularly. HBsAg negative but HBcore antibody–only positive patients should be regularly monitored as these patients have a high risk of HBV reactivation. Prophylactic treatment with an NA should be considered along with monitoring in those who are being aggressively immunosuppressed.

Hepatitis E Virus

Chronic hepatitis E virus (HEV; defined as persistence of HEV in blood or stool for more than 3 months) occurs in immunocompromised persons, especially organ transplant recipients. Chronic infection may result in a life-threatening illness such as fulminant liver failure or liver cirrhosis. Reduction in immunosuppression will generally help clear the virus, but ribavirin treatment in those with persistent viraemia should be considered with the aim of achieving sustained virological response. Patients on treatment should be regularly monitored for the virus in blood and stool and treatment should continue until negative PCR results are obtained.

Polyomaviruses

Human polyomavirus 1(BK virus) causes nephropathy in renal transplant recipients and haemorrhagic cystitis and central nervous system symptoms in organ transplant recipients (especially in bone marrow transplant recipients). Polyomavirus 2 (JC virus) causes lesions in the brain (progressive multifocal leukoencephalopathy, or PML). See also Chapter 20.

Papillomaviruses

Papillomaviruses cause wart lesions in transplant recipients. Transplant patients can have extensive lesions. Patients with AIDS develop difficult-to-treat and extensive wart lesions as a result of infection with papillomaviruses. They are also more prone to develop malignancies related with the oncogenic papillomaviruses (genotype 16, 18).

Parvovirus B19

Infection in the immunocompromised may result in chronic parvovirus infection due to the failure of the immune system to clear the virus. This can lead to hypoplasia or aplasia of erythroid cells and precursors leading to the patient developing chronic intractable aplastic anaemia. The blood picture shows significant reduction of reticulocytes. Besides anaemia, leukopenia and thrombocytopenia has also been reported. Other complications, such as hepatitis, myocarditis, encephalitis and pneumonitis associated with parvovirus B19 infection have also been reported in the immunocompromised.

Toxoplasma gondii

Toxoplasma gondii infection can be acquired from organ donors. Sixty per cent of heart, 20% of liver and <1% of kidney *Toxoplasma gondii* antibody–negative transplants acquire primary infection from antibody-positive organ donors. Infection can be life-threatening, but sulphadiazine and pyrimethamine treatment is available. For those at risk of donor-acquired infection, cotrimoxazole or pyrimethamine prophylactic treatment can prevent symptomatic infection. Between 1% and 2% of patients experience symptomatic *Toxoplasma gondii* reactivation after transplantation.

Toxoplasma gondii infection in HIV antibody–positive/AIDS patients is usually reactivation of latent infection. The most likely symptoms are fever, malaise, retinitis and space-occupying lesions in the brain, which need to be differentiated from lymphoma. Infection can be life-threatening, but sulphadiazine and pyrimethamine are available for treatment and continuous prophylaxis in those severely immunosuppressed patients at risk of reactivation.

Management

Depends on prophylaxis, monitoring and treatment of various infections.

A thorough epidemiological assessment of the patients will provide clues to the infections that have occurred in the past and which might potentially reactivate with immunosuppression and for which the patient may require prophylaxis and monitoring or both.

For transplantation a major consideration is donor-acquired infections.

Before transplantation a thorough assessment is required which should include, at minimum, baseline testing for HIV, hepatitis B and C viruses, and antibody testing to establish serostatus for CMV, EBV, *Toxoplasma gondii*, HSV and VZV. Screening for other viruses may be indicated depending on the epidemiological and clinical context.

Prophylaxis

Ensure that all immunocompromised patients or those being considered for immuno-suppressive therapy, for example potential transplant recipients, are immunised for all preventable viral infections for which effective vaccines are available. As live vaccines are contraindicated in immunosuppressed patients these should be avoided.

In addition, chemoprophylaxis with specific antiviral agents for CMV, VZV, HSV and hepatitis B helps to reduce the risk of serious disease in transplant recipients and other severely immunocompromised patients.

Monitoring and Treatment

As infections are more difficult to treat when patients are immunosuppressed, any active infection identified pre-transplantation or prior to start of immunosuppressive therapy should be treated first. Clinical judgement to go ahead irrespective is required for life-saving transplants and immunosuppressive treatments.

Management of some viral infections, for example CMV, EBV and hepatitis B, requires regular viral monitoring to identify those at maximum risk of serious disease so early treatment can be instituted.

Useful Websites

British Transplantation Society: www.bts.org.uk

British Society of Blood and Marrow Transplantation and Cellular Therapy: www.bsbmtct.org

GOV.UK: Guidance on SaBTO microbiological safety guidelines: www.gov.uk/government/publications/guidance-on-the-microbiological-safety-of-human-organs-tissues-and-cells-used-in-transplantation

Viral Malignancies

46

Cell growth, differentiation and death are controlled by genes. Mechanisms are needed for both stimulating and suppressing growth. Breakdown in the mechanism for control of cell growth leads to uncontrolled growth and malignancy. There are many ways in which cells may lose this intrinsic control – viral infections being one of them. Not all viruses are oncogenic (i.e. able to induce cancer in humans). It is mainly, although not exclusively, DNA viruses that have this potential. Human T-cell lymphotropic virus types 1 and 2 and hepatitis C virus are examples of RNA viruses that are able to induce malignancy. Oncogenic viruses cause 20% of all human cancers.

How Do Viruses Cause Cancer?

Infection with certain types of viruses can increase the risk of a person acquiring cancer, although not everyone who is infected with the virus will develop cancer. These viruses can either insert additional viral oncogenic genes into the host cell or enhance already existing oncogenic genes (proto-oncogenes) in the genome. These viruses must have at least one virus copy in every tumour cell expressing at least one protein or RNA that is causing the cell to become cancerous. DNA oncoviruses transform infected cells by integrating their DNA into the host cell's genome.

An oncogene is a mutated gene that has the potential to cause cancer. Before an oncogene becomes mutated, it is called a proto-oncogene, and it plays a role in regulating normal cell division. Cancer can arise when a proto-oncogene is mutated, changing it into an oncogene and causing the cell to divide and multiply uncontrollably. Initially, oncogenes were identified in viruses, which could cause cancers in animals. Later, it was found that oncogenes can be mutated copies of certain normal cellular genes. Intact proto-oncogenes play important functions, regulating normal cellular growth, division and apoptosis (programmed or controlled cell death). Oncogenes or mutated copies of the proto-oncogenes may lead to uncontrolled cell growth and the escape from cell death, which may result in cancer development.

Viral oncogenicity can also involve chronic non-specific inflammation occurring over decades of infection (e.g. as in hepatitis C–induced liver cancer). Some viruses initiate persistent infections and manipulate host cellular signalling and DNA damage responses, which promotes the initiation of and development of cancer. They may also disrupt the person's immune system, thus increasing the risk of cancer developing.

Human Malignancies Caused by Viruses

Often, it is difficult to associate directly a viral aetiology with a human malignancy, because of the long latent period between infection and the development of cancer.

Table 46.1 Human oncogenic viruses and the cancers they cause

Virus	Associated malignancy	Higher prevalence
Epstein–Barr virus (EBV)	Burkitt's lymphoma, Hodgkin's lymphoma, gastric carcinoma, nasopharyngeal carcinoma	
Hepatitis B virus (HBV)	Hepatocellular carcinoma	Persons with chronic HBV infection
Human T-cell lymphotropic virus 1 (HTLV-1)	Adult T-cell leukaemia	
Human papillomaviruses (HPVs)	Cervical carcinoma, oropharyngeal carcinoma, other anogenital carcinomas	
Hepatitis C virus (HCV)	Hepatocellular carcinoma	Persons with chronic HCV infection
Human herpesvirus 8 (HHV-8)	Kaposi's sarcoma	HIV-infected persons, immunosuppressed persons, persons indigenous to the Mediterranean, Middle East and sub-Saharan Africa
Merkel cell polyomavirus	Merkel cell carcinoma (skin cancer)	Immunosuppressed and elderly persons

Table 46.1 provides details of human oncogenic viruses which have been proven to cause the cancers we list next.

Adult T-Cell Leukaemia/Lymphoma

Adult T-cell leukaemia/lymphoma (ATL) is an aggressive form of adult leukaemia/ lymphoma associated with the human T-cell lymphotropic virus HTLV-1 (see Chapter 15). HTLV-1 possesses a reverse transcriptase enzyme which converts the viral RNA into DNA in the first step of replication cycle. This pro-viral DNA is capable of integrating in the cellular DNA, and the virus's oncogenicity is mediated through interaction between viral and host proteins, leading to T-cell proliferation and trans-formation. HTLV-1 can be transmitted sexually, by blood-to-blood contact (e.g. by blood transfusion or sharing needles) and via breastfeeding. An estimated 5–10 million people globally are infected with HTLV-1; most infections are asymptomatic. The vast burden of infection is in Japan, the Caribbean, Central and South America and Africa. The prevalence of antibody in Japanese blood donors is about 1% but is higher in southern Japan and in older age groups. The lifetime risk of developing ATL in people with proven HTLV-1 infection is estimated to be about 5%. ATL has a much higher prevalence in Japan or people of Japanese descent. ATL presents as four clinical subtypes: acute, lymphomatous, chronic and smouldering, with the more aggressive subtypes (acute and lymphomatous) representing the majority of cases. Clinical presentation depends on the subtype. People may present with lymphadenopathy, hepatosplenomegaly and hypercalcaemia through involvement of the skin, lung, bones and other organs.

Treatment is not indicated for asymptomatic people living with HTLV-1. Although anti-HIV drugs, which have activity against the HTLV-1 reverse transcriptase and integrase enzymes, have been tested in limited clinical trials, HTLV-1 proviral DNA levels were not reduced. Anti-HIV protease inhibitors and non-nucleoside reverse transcriptase inhibitors have no anti- HTLV activity. Reverse transcriptase and integrase inhibitors may have a role in prevention of HTLV infection, but further studies are required to confirm this. ATL can be treated with chemotherapy, monoclonal antibodies or bone marrow transplant, but treatment outcomes are often poor. Zidovudine and interferon-alpha is the recommended first-line treatment for leukaemic forms of ATL. Prophylaxis against opportunistic infections is important. In 2021, mogamulizumab was approved for relapsed/refractory treatment of ATL in Japan.

Burkitt's Lymphoma

Burkitt's lymphoma is a cancer of the lymphatic system, particularly B lymphocytes. It is named after Denis Burkitt, the Irish surgeon who first described the disease in 1958 while working in equatorial Africa. Burkitt's lymphoma is usually a disease seen in childhood and is uncommon in adults, in whom it has a worse prognosis. The overall cure rate for Burkitt's lymphoma in developed countries is about 90%, but it is worse in low-income countries.

The endemic (African) variant is mainly seen in children living in malaria-endemic regions of the world (e.g. equatorial Africa, Brazil and Papua New Guinea) and EBV infection is found in nearly all patients. Chronic malaria is believed to reduce resistance to EBV, allowing it to proliferate. The disease often involves the jaw or other facial bones, distal ileum, caecum, ovaries or kidneys. EBV promotes the development of malignant B-cells via proteins that limit apoptosis in cells that have the c-myc translocation. Apoptosis is limited by EBV through various means such as the EBNA-1 protein. Malaria has been found to cause genomic instability in endemic Burkitt's lymphoma. Malaria can lead to the reactivation of latent EBV and also myc translocations via activation of the toll-like receptor 9. Malaria also promotes B-cell proliferation by altering the regular immune response.

The sporadic (non-African) type of Burkitt's lymphoma is the most common variant found in places where malaria is not prevalent (e.g. North America and parts of Europe). The tumour cells have a similar appearance to the cancer cells of the endemic (African) Burkitt's lymphoma, but cases are rarely associated with the EBV infection.

Immunodeficiency-associated Burkitt's lymphoma is usually associated with HIV infection or in patients who have received a transplant. EBV has not been shown to have a causal link in this form of Burkitt's lymphoma.

Cervical Cancer

Cervical cancer is caused by the abnormal growth of cells that have the ability to invade or spread to other parts of the body. Usually, no symptoms are seen in the early stage of the disease; later symptoms can include abnormal vaginal bleeding, pelvic pain or pain during sexual intercourse.

Human papillomavirus (HPV) infection causes more than 90% of cases. However, most women who have had HPV infections do not develop cervical cancer. HPV types 16 and 18 strains are responsible for nearly 50% of high-grade cervical pre-cancers.

HPV types 16 and 18 are the cause of 75% of cervical cancer cases, with types 31 and 45 causing 10%. The HPV types most associated with a high risk for the development of cervical cancer are types 16, 18, 31, 33, 35, 39, 45, 51, 52, 56, 58, 59, 68, 73, and 82.

Other risk factors include smoking, a weak immune system, birth control pills, starting sex at a young age and having many sexual partners, but these are less important. Genetic factors also contribute to cervical cancer risk.

Genital warts are caused by various types of HPV, but these are usually not linked with cervical cancer.

There are several HPV vaccines that can protect against HPV-induced cervical cancer. Girls and boys aged 12–13 years in the UK are offered the HPV vaccine as part of the National Health Service vaccination programme. The bivalent vaccine Cervarix® was the HPV vaccine offered initially in 2008 but subsequently from 2012 the quadrivalent vaccine Gardasil® has been offered. In February 2014, the UK Joint Committee on Vaccination and Immunisation concluded that a two-dose schedule in adolescents could be recommended up to (and including) 14 years of age for both Cervarix® and Gardasil®. Since 2023, the UK recommendation is for a one-dose Gardasil®9 regime for the vaccination of adolescents. Since different countries may have varying vaccination schedules, which may change over time, it is important to check the latest national and local guidelines.

More than a decade after the introduction of the national HPV immunisation programme, evidence of the impact of vaccination has shown reductions in HPV type 16/18 infection, genital warts, precancerous lesions and cervical cancer among vaccinated cohorts.

Hepatocellular Carcinoma

Hepatocellular carcinoma is the most common type of primary liver cancer in adults and is currently the most common cause of death in people with cirrhosis. It can result from chronic liver inflammation (cirrhosis) and is often caused by chronic HBV or HCV infection or following exposure to toxins such as alcohol, aflatoxin or pyrrolizidine alkaloids. The impact of these risk factors varies in different regions of the world. In regions where hepatitis B infection is endemic (e.g. south-east China), hepatitis B is the predominant cause of hepatocellular carcinoma, whereas in countries where the population is protected by routine hepatitis B vaccination (e.g. UK, USA) cases are more likely to be caused by cirrhosis, linked with chronic hepatitis C disease, obesity and excessive alcohol consumption.

Chronic HBV and HCV infections can stimulate the development of hepatocellular carcinoma by repeatedly causing the body's immune system to attack the hepatocytes. Activated immune-system inflammatory cells release free radicals, such as reactive oxygen species and nitric oxide reactive species, which can cause DNA damage and lead to carcinogenic gene mutations. This constant cycle of damage followed by repair can lead to replication errors, which in turn lead to carcinogenesis (e.g. in chronic HCV infection causing cirrhosis), whereas in chronic hepatitis B, the integration of the viral genome into infected cells can directly induce a non-cirrhotic liver to develop hepatocellular carcinoma.

Hodgkin's Lymphoma

Hodgkin's lymphoma is named after the English physician Thomas Hodgkin, who first described it in 1832. It is a lymphoma which develops from mutated lymphocytes. There are two types of Hodgkin's lymphoma (classic and nodular). Approximately 50% of cases of classic Hodgkin's lymphoma are caused by EBV infection. Symptoms may include fever, night sweats and weight loss, often with non-painful enlarged lymph nodes in the neck, in the groin or under the arm.

Kaposi's Sarcoma

Kaposi's sarcoma is an endothelial cell carcinoma which causes lesions in the skin, in lymph nodes, in the mouth or in other organs. The skin lesions are usually painless, purple and may be flat or raised. Lesions can occur singly, in clusters or may be widespread. It is not a true sarcoma. It is a cancer of lymphatic endothelium and forms vascular channels that fill with blood cells, giving the tumour its characteristic purple bruise-like appearance. HHV-8 can be found in almost 100% of Kaposi's sarcoma lesions.

There are four types of Kaposi's sarcoma:

- *Classic* – usually affects older men in regions where HHV-8 is highly prevalent (Mediterranean, Eastern Europe, Middle East), is usually slow-growing and usually only affects legs.
- *Endemic* – most common in sub-Saharan Africa and is more aggressive in children, while older adults present similarly to the classic form.
- *Immunosuppression related* – occurs in people following organ transplantation and usually affects the skin.
- *Epidemic (also referred to as AIDS-related)* – occurs in people with AIDS and lesions, often extensive, and can be seen on many parts of the body.

Merkel Cell Carcinoma

Merkel cell carcinoma is a rare, aggressive skin cancer which usually presents as a single, painless, skin-coloured or red-coloured lump on sun-exposed skin, which may grow rapidly over several weeks and may spread quickly to surrounding tissues or to other parts of the body. Factors associated with developing Merkel cell carcinoma include having fair skin colour, older age, a history of excess sun exposure, chronic immunosuppression and being infected with the Merkel cell polyomavirus. The Merkel cell polyomavirus has been detected in most people who have Merkel cell carcinoma.

Nasopharyngeal Carcinoma

This is another EBV-related cancer. It occurs in children and adults and is more common in certain regions of East Asia and Africa than elsewhere, with viral (EBV), dietary (e.g. nitrosamines in salted fish) and genetic (e.g. having Chinese ancestry) factors implicated as causes. EBV is associated with types 2 and 3 nasopharyngeal carcinomas. EBV can infect epithelial cells and is associated with their transformation.

Post-transplant Lymphoproliferative Disease

Post-transplant lymphoproliferative disease (PTLD) is an aggressive form of lymphoma caused by uncontrolled B-cell proliferation due to immunosuppressive treatment after organ or hematopoietic stem cell transplantation. The incidence of PTLD depends on the type of transplant received and the immunosuppressive treatment that patients are given (both type of drugs and amount). There is a wide variation in incidence from 1% to 10%. The main risk factors for PTLD are the extent of immunosuppression and EBV infection (although EBV infection is not linked to all cases). These patients may develop polyclonal polymorphic B-cell hyperplasia. EBV infection in immunosuppressed patients leads to uncontrolled proliferation of the infected B-cells and subsequently to lymphoma. The initial B-cell proliferation is polyclonal; transformation of one or more B-cell clones leads to the development of lymphoma. In the initial stages of PTLD, proliferation is polyclonal. With mutation and selective growth the lesion becomes oligoclonal and, later, monoclonal. EBV-naïve patients who receive a donation from an EBV-positive donor are at the highest risk of developing a lymphoma and the risk of developing PTLD is highest in the first transplant year, when immunosuppression is at its most intense. Symptoms of PTLD are non-specific and highly variable and may include night sweats, malaise, fever and weight loss. The digestive tract, central nervous system or transplanted organ are often involved. This syndrome first came to light in the transplant community with the first use, by Sir Roy Calne, of ciclosporin, a calcineurin inhibitor used as immunosuppressant in organ transplantation to inhibit T-cell function. The continued use of other calcineurin inhibitors besides ciclosporin inhibitors still remains a major risk factor for the development of PTLD.

Control of Viral Malignancies

The impact of malignancies caused by virus infections can be reduced by:

- public health campaigns on avoidance of infection
  - public health campaigns to reduce infection rates (e.g. HCV and HBV in drug users)
  - early identification of people with asymptomatic HCV infection and using antiviral drugs to eliminate the infection
  - avoidance of breastfeeding in mothers infected with HTLV-1 in high-risk populations to prevent vertical transmission of infection

- use of viral vaccines
  - HBV
  - HPV

- immune restoration in the immunosuppressed so that the native immune system is able to prevent the tumour cell proliferation
  - changing or reducing the doses of immunosuppressive drugs in transplant recipients

Chapter

47

Viral Rashes

Clinical

There are several kinds of skin infections caused by viruses and these are best considered in the following four categories that group together similar symptoms for the purpose of differential diagnosis:

- maculopapular rashes
- vesicular rashes
- wart-like lesions
- haemorrhagic rashes.

Maculopapular Rashes

These skin rashes can be caused by a variety of different viruses. Clinically it is difficult to distinguish between the viral causes of these maculopapular rashes. Studies have shown that only a small percentage of these rashes are clinically diagnosed accurately. Figure 47.1 shows a typical maculopapular rash. Table 47.1 provides information on the laboratory diagnosis of virus infections associated with maculopapular rashes.

Human Parvovirus B19

Infection with human parvovirus B19 can present as a rubella-like rash but the most typical presentation is with a 'slapped cheek' rash, especially in children. It can cause hydrops fetalis in babies when the mother is infected up to 20 weeks' gestation. Pregnant mothers should seek advice from a healthcare professional if they are in contact with a rubella-like illness in the first 20 weeks of pregnancy, especially to check their immunity status and evidence of recent infection. Patients are infectious for 1 week before the onset of rash, but they are not infectious once the rash appears. See Chapter 22 for more information. Figure 47.2 shows a typical slapped cheek rash.

Rubella

Rubella is caused by rubella virus. It produces a mild illness with a maculopapular skin rash. However, it causes severe congenital damage in children born to mothers who acquire infection in the first 12 weeks of pregnancy. Because of this, women should receive rubella virus vaccine before becoming pregnant. They should also seek advice from a healthcare professional if they are in contact with a rubella-like illness in the first 20 weeks of pregnancy, especially to check their immunity status and evidence of recent infection. Patients are infectious for 1 week either side of the onset of rash. See Chapter 28 for more information.

Table 47.1 Laboratory diagnosis of virus infections associated with maculopapular skin rashes

Virus	Diagnosis	Treatment and prevention
Human parvovirus B19	Clotted blood sample tested for parvovirus-specific IgM	No vaccine available. No antiviral treatment available. Always seek medical advice if pregnant.
Rubella virus	Clotted blood sample tested for rubella virus-specific IgM	Prevention by giving MMR vaccine. No antiviral treatment available. Always seek medical advice if pregnant.
Measles virus	Clotted blood or saliva sample tested for measles virus-specific IgM. Throat swab in virus transport medium can be tested by PCR.	Prevention by giving MMR vaccine. No antiviral treatment available. Always seek medical advice to investigate the source of infection and to protect those in contact with a case of measles.
Enteroviruses	Throat swab in virus transport medium or faeces can be tested by PCR. Can test for enterovirus antibody but tests are not very sensitive.	No vaccine available. No antiviral treatment available.
Adenoviruses	Throat swab in virus transport medium can be tested by PCR.	No vaccine available. No antiviral treatment available.
Human herpesviruses 6 and 7	EDTA blood for PCR in severely ill children	No vaccine available. No antiviral treatment available.

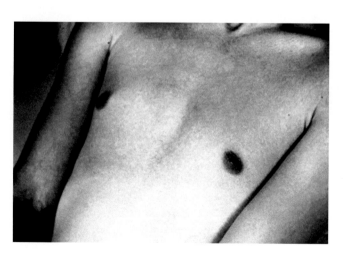

Figure 47.1 Typical maculopapular rash (with permission from CDC; details – Public Health Image Library (PHIL): https://phil.cdc.gov/Details.aspx?pid=22150)

Measles

Measles presents with coryza, conjunctivitis, fever and a blotchy skin rash. Since most people in the UK have either had natural measles infection or have received vaccine, infection is uncommon. However, small outbreaks do occur, especially in the spring and

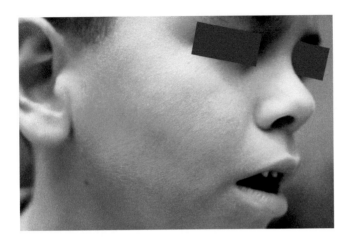

Figure 47.2 A boy with skin rash of erythema infectiosum, or fifth disease, caused by the human parvovirus B19 (courtesy of CDC; details – Public Health Image Library (PHIL): https://phil.cdc.gov/Details.aspx?pid=4509)

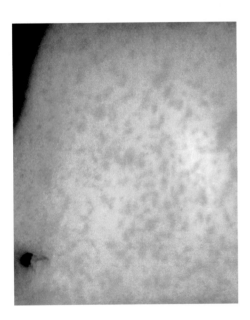

Figure 47.3 Typical measles rash (courtesy of CDC: www.cdc.gov/measles/symptoms/photos.html)

summer, due to the inadequate levels of vaccine-induced immunity in the community. Measles is difficult to diagnose clinically, with accuracy rates as low as 5%. Measles is not a cause of congenital infection. It can be severe and 1 in 1,000 cases may develop encephalitis, which can be fatal. Severe or fatal infection occurs in immunocompromised and severely malnourished people. See Chapter 17 for more information. Figure 47.3 shows a typical measles rash.

Enteroviruses

Enteroviruses can produce a non-specific rash, often with respiratory symptoms. Children are most affected but adults can have more severe symptoms, including meningism and meningitis. See Chapter 4 for more information.

Table 47.2 Laboratory diagnosis, treatment and prevention for virus infections associated with vesicular skin rashes

Virus	Diagnosis	Treatment and prevention
HSV	Lesion swab in virus transport medium or vesicle fluid for PCR (or direct antigen detection tests as immunofluorescence)	No vaccine available. Treatment with aciclovir IV for severe infections in immunosuppressed patients).
VZV	Lesion swab in virus transport medium or vesicle fluid for PCR. Clotted blood sample tested for VZV-specific IgM (may be negative in zoster).	There is a vaccine available. Treatment of chickenpox with aciclovir (IV for severe infections – pneumonia and encephalitis and in immunosuppressed patients). Zoster can be treated with valaciclovir, famciclovir (or IV aciclovir in immunocompromised patients).
Stevens–Johnson syndrome	Investigate infectious cause (e.g. Mycoplasma pneumoniae, CMV, HSV, VZV, Chlamydia psittaci)	
Enteroviruses	Throat swab or faeces tested by PCR for diagnosis. Enteroviruses can be detected in vesicles by PCR.	No vaccine available. No antiviral treatment available.
Pox viruses	Lesion swab, vesicle fluid or scab for PCR or electron microscopy	No vaccine available. No antiviral treatment available.

Adenoviruses

Adenoviruses can produce a non-specific rash, often with respiratory symptoms. Adenovirus infection can mimic measles, especially in immunocompromised persons. See Chapter 1 for more information.

Human Herpesviruses Types 6 and 7

Human herpesviruses types 6 and 7 can give a non-specific rash and fever. They usually produce symptomatic infection in very young children. See Chapter 13 for more information.

Allergic reactions (e.g. to drugs) can give similar symptoms.

Vesicular Rashes

Vesicular skin rashes cause vesicles (small fluid-filled blisters) on the skin and are usually caused by herpes simplex virus and varicella-zoster virus, although Stevens–Johnson syndrome (erythema multiforme) can give similar symptoms and should be considered in the differential diagnosis (see Table 47.2).

Herpes Simplex Virus

Herpes simplex virus (HSV) causes a vesicular skin rash. Primary infection in children often presents as mouth and gum infection. Vesicles usually occur in a small group on the skin (Figure 47.4), mouth or genitals. The virus lies dormant in nerves and can give

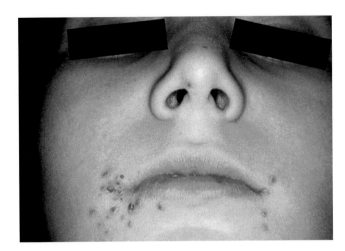

Figure 47.4 Typical HSV skin rash (courtesy of CDC; details – Public Health Image Library (PHIL): https://phil.cdc .gov/Details.aspx?pid=12617)

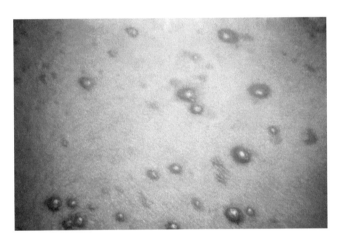

Figure 47.5 Typical chickenpox rash (courtesy of CDC: details – Public Health Image Library (PHIL): https:// phil.cdc.gov/Details.aspx?pid= 5407)

rise to reactivated infection (e.g. cold sores). Rarely, reactivation can lead to encephalitis, but concurrent skin lesions are rare. HSV can cause severe symptoms in immunocompromised patients and those with chronic skin conditions such as eczema. Infection in mothers at the time of childbirth can give rise to severe or fatal infection in neonates (Chapter 39). Antiviral treatment (aciclovir, valaciclovir, foscarnet, etc) is available. See Chapter 10 for more information.

Varicella-Zoster Virus

Primary varicella-zoster virus (VZV) infection gives rise to chickenpox. Chickenpox produces a generalised vesicular rash which starts on the central area of the body and then spreads. Figure 47.5 shows a typical chickenpox rash. After chickenpox infection, the virus lies dormant in the nerve cells and can reactivate later in life to produce zoster (shingles), which produces clusters of vesicles on one side of the body in the distribution of a sensory nerve (see Figure 47.6). In VZV infections, lesions in one cluster are usually at different stages of development (cropping) which can help in distinguishing infection

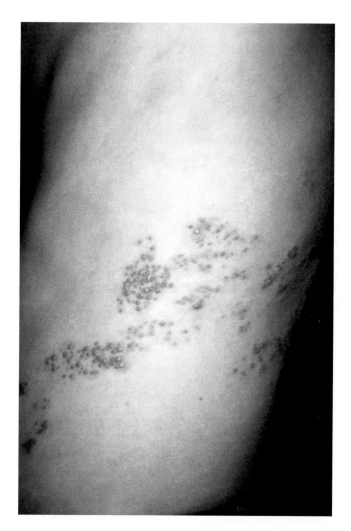

Figure 47.6 Typical zoster rash (courtesy of CDC: details – Public Health Image Library (PHIL): https://phil.cdc.gov/Details.aspx?pid=21506)

from HSV (where all lesions are usually at the same stage of development). However, HSV and VZV skin lesions can be indistinguishable, so caution is required in differential diagnosis based on the appearance of vesicles since the infection control consequences of infections with these two viruses are very different. VZV can cause severe symptoms in immunocompromised patients. Chickenpox in the first 20 weeks of pregnancy can cause severe or fatal damage in the fetus (Chapter 29). Infection in the last 7 days of pregnancy poses a severe risk of neonatal chickenpox in the baby, which can be fatal. Antiviral treatment (aciclovir, valaciclovir, famciclovir, etc) is available.

Stevens–Johnson Syndrome

Stevens–Johnson syndrome can be caused by HSV, *Mycoplasma pneumoniae* and *Chlamydia psittaci* infection. For more information on these organisms, see Chapters 30 and 33. Stevens–Johnson syndrome produces target-like lesions on the skin, especially on the genitals. It can mimic chickenpox, especially in children (but the presence of a cough in children should suggest a respiratory cause).

Enteroviruses

Certain enteroviruses (especially coxsackie A viruses) cause hand, foot and mouth disease. This is common in young children and is usually a mild infection associated with small hard vesicles on the palms of the hand, soles of the feet and in the mouth. Adults (usually parents) can have similar symptoms, sometimes with meningism or meningitis with an intense frontal headache. See Chapter 4 for more information.

Poxviruses

Cowpox should be suspected in patients with single large vesicular lesions, especially if patients have had contact with cats. Cowpox should always be considered in patients who have a single large vesicular lesion which develops a scab, especially in people with no history of contact with farm animals.

Orf is a parapox virus which usually produces a single vesicular lesion on an erythematous base, which soon develops a scab. Orf is common in farmers, acquired from sheep, especially when bottle feeding lambs and acquired from cows (milker's nodule) when milking. The animals also have vesicular skin lesions.

Smallpox has been eradicated from the world and is therefore an extremely unlikely diagnosis. In the last few years, there has been a worldwide outbreak of monkeypox (mpox) infections, especially among men who have sex with men (see Figure 47.7 for typical skin lesions).

See Chapter 23 for more information on pox viruses.

Wart-like Rashes

There are many different papilloma viruses which cause wart-like lesions on the skin (skin warts, genital warts, plantar warts (veruccas)) (see Chapter 20). Infection can be diagnosed by testing the excised skin lesions by electron microscopy or nucleic acid amplification test (PCR). There are effective papilloma virus vaccines against some genital warts (especially those responsible for cervical cancer) but not the others.

Molluscum contagiosum (Figure 47.8) is a pox virus infection which causes clusters of small wart-like lesions on eyelid margins, genitals and lower abdominal skin. It is common in children. See Chapter 23 for more information.

Haemorrhagic Rashes

Haemorrhagic rashes are usually associated with exotic virus infections such as Lassa fever, Marburg disease, Ebola, Crimea-Congo haemorrhagic fever or dengue fever (see Chapter 38). Patients are often severely ill and give a relevant history of recent travel to tropical countries. A careful history of the exact location of recent travel and other factors (e.g. contact with rodents or monkeys) is very important for the correct diagnosis to be made. Lassa fever can be effectively treated with ribavirin if prompt treatment is given. Constant research efforts are ongoing to discover treatments for the other haemorrhagic virus infections. Patients should be isolated in strict isolation facilities until a diagnosis is made. Diagnosis is made in specialist reference laboratories using EDTA blood or throat swabs in virus transport medium.

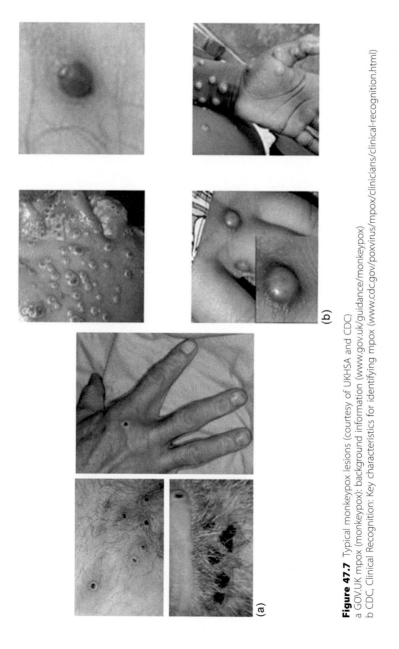

Figure 47.7 Typical monkeypox lesions (courtesy of UKHSA and CDC)
a GOV.UK mpox (monkeypox): background information (www.gov.uk/guidance/monkeypox)
b CDC, Clinical Recognition: Key characteristics for identifying mpox (www.cdc.gov/poxvirus/mpox/clinicians/clinical-recognition.html)

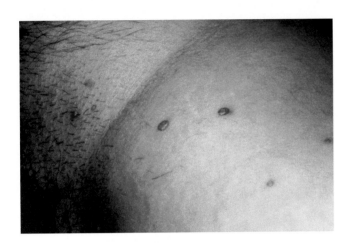

Figure 47.8 Typical molluscum contagiosum skin rash (courtesy of CDC; details – Public Health Library (PHIL): https://phil.cdc.gov/Details.aspx?pid=16687)

Rarely, haemorrhagic chickenpox occurs, almost always in immunosuppressed patients. It is usually a very severe or fatal disease which requires prompt high-dose intravenous aciclovir treatment.

Useful Website

GOV.UK: Guidance on the investigation, diagnosis and management of viral illness (plus syphilis), or exposure to viral rash illness, in pregnancy: https://assets.publishing .service.gov.uk/media/6565bdac1524e6000da101b2/viral-rash-in-pregnancy-guidance-syphilis.pdf

Viral Zoonotic Infections

Zoonoses are diseases spread from animals to humans. Frequently, these viruses cause little or no disease in their natural animal host. Some zoonotic viruses have very limited host range, while others may infect a variety of vertebrate hosts. Spread to humans may be via several routes; some direct (direct contact with animal) and some indirect (via a vector or other humans). Most viral zoonoses require blood-sucking arthropods (mosquitoes, ticks) for their transmission to humans. Arthropod vectors becomes infected when they feed on the viraemic animal and transmit infection to other hosts including humans.

Most zoonotic infections only come to light when humans start to encroach on the enzootic environment. Birds are an important reservoir of zoonotic viruses and bird migration provides an important route of spread and establishment of these zoonoses at long distances and away from their original foci. Many emerging infections (SARS-CoV-2) start as zoonotic infections, that is, have an animal source and first infections occur by close contact with animals, these viruses then adapt to spread human to human. Among emerging infectious diseases, it is suggested that three-quarters may be zoonoses with wildlife being one of the major sources of infection. Some recent examples are Zika virus, SARS-CoV, MERS-CoV and most recently SARS-CoV-2 emergence in 2019.

This chapter is a reminder of important viral zoonotic infections. Most of these have been covered under relevant chapters throughout the book. Some examples of zoonotic infections spread by direct contact and via arthropod vectors are shown in Tables 48.1 and 48.2 respectively.

Disease surveillance in both human and animal hosts with rapid diagnosis of infection is the key to breaking the cycle of transmission. Surveillance requires collaboration between the medical and veterinary fraternity and public health and access to the appropriate laboratory network to identify the emerging infections.

Some examples of strategies that have been employed for control of viral zoonoses are:

- Immunisation of vertebrate hosts (domestic and wild) and humans, e.g. rabies vaccination.
- Elimination of vertebrate hosts – the 1998 Nipah virus outbreak in Malaysia was halted by killing nearly a million pigs. Mass culling of infected herds of cattle in UK to control spread of vCJD and chickens to control avian influenza are other examples. However, such a strategy has financial/commercial consequences and hence is not generally popular with the public. Also, as avian influenza has been introduced into wild birds culling of poultry has limited value since there is the risk of reintroduction to poultry by direct contact with infected wild birds, or indirect contact via carriage of infected material on shoes, etc. to poultry farms.

Table 48.1 Some examples of zoonotic infections spread by direct contact

Virus	Disease caused	Vertebrate host	Mode of spread	Chapter reference
Rabies virus	Rabies	Dogs, cats and other vertebrate animals	Bite, licks on open skin	24
Avian influenza virus	Avian influenza	Birds	Close contact with infected birds	16
Hepatitis E virus, serotype 3 and 4	Hepatitis, jaundice	Pigs, wild boar, deer	Direct contact with animals. Eating undercooked pig and game and processed pork (serotype 3).	9
Cowpox and monkeypox viruses	Pox-like lesions on skin at the contact site	Rodents, cats	Close contact with infected animals	23
Orf virus	Single or multiple skin pustular/scabby lesions generally on fingers/hands/fore arms	Sheep, goats	Direct contact	23
Hantavirus	Hantavirus haemorrhagic fever and hantavirus pulmonary syndrome	Rats and other rodents including wild rodents	Close contact with rodents or contaminated environment	38
Lassa fever virus	Lassa haemorrhagic fever	Rodents (multimammate rats)	Close contact with infected rodents or contaminated environment	38
Ebola virus	Haemorrhagic fever	Non-human primates (monkeys)	Direct contact, subsequent human-human	38
Marburg virus	Haemorrhagic fever	Non-human primates (monkeys), bats	Direct contact, human-human described	38
SARS-CoV	Severe respiratory infection	Civet cats	Direct contact, subsequently human to human	12
MERS-CoV	Severe respiratory infection	Dromedary camels	Direct animal contact, drinking camel milk. Human to human spread may occur	12

Table 48.1 (cont.)

Virus	Disease caused	Vertebrate host	Mode of spread	Chapter reference
SARS-CoV-2	Respiratory infection	Probably bats (?), another intermediary host	Direct contact. Subsequently human-to-human spread.	12
Nipah virus	Fever, pneumonia, encephalitis	Fruit bats and pigs for Nipah virus	Direct contact with infected bats. Also, by eating fruit contaminated by the fruit bats and contaminated date palm sap.	–
Prion	New variant Creutzfeldt-Jakob disease (vCJD)	Cattle (beef)	Eating contaminated meat	32

- Vector (mosquitoes, ticks, etc.) control by use of insecticides to limit the spread of vector-borne zoonotic disease. This may be problematic due to vectors developing resistance to insecticides. Vector control by removing the breeding ground needs public awareness and support.

Human behaviour is a key factor in creating conditions conducive to spread of zoonotic diseases. In Africa, agricultural irrigation projects have created extensive habitats with an increase in mosquito-transmitted diseases. In Senegal dam constructions were followed by an epidemic of Rift Valley fever with multiple cases in humans and ruminant animals. Human encroachment of the natural host environment by converting wild habitat to agricultural land juxtapositions humans and domesticated vertebrate and wild vertebrate with the risk of disease transmission from the wild vertebrate hosts. Many zoonotic diseases therefore only emerge after such behavioural/ecological changes.

Global climate change is bringing ecological changes and population shifts. Increase in rainfall and temperatures provides conditions for introduction and propagation of arthropod vectors and pathogens in regions previously disease free. *Aedes albopictus*, having originated in Southeast Asia, has undergone massive expansion in its worldwide distribution via transportation of used tyres which have acted as carriers. It was first detected in 1979 in a European country (Albania), then found in Italy in 1990. Italy is the most infested country now in Europe. It has since spread to many other European countries. As the mosquito can potentially transmit viruses of dengue fever, yellow fever, Rift Valley fever, Japanese encephalitis and zika there is a risk that these zoonoses may become endemic in areas where they were previously absent. Ticks carrying the tick-borne encephalitis virus have increased in Europe including in the UK. There was a major outbreak of dengue fever in Madeira in 2012/13 after the introduction of *Aedes aegypti* to the island, and sporadic cases still continue to occur.

Table 48.2 Some examples of zoonotic infections spread by indirect contact via an arthropod vector

Virus	Disease caused	Vertebrate host	Mode of spread	Chapter reference
Venezuelan equine virus, Eastern equine virus, Western equine virus, St Louis encephalitis virus, La Crosse virus	Encephalitis	Horses, rodents, birds. Small forest mammals for La Crosse virus.	Mosquito bites	2
Yellow fever virus	Hepatitis, jaundice (yellow fever), haemorrhagic fever and shock	Non-human primates	Mosquito bite	2
Zika virus	Rash, fever, conjunctivitis, muscle and joint pains	Non-human primates, possibly other unidentified vertebrates	Mosquito bite	2
West Nile virus	Acute febrile illness and encephalitis	Birds (birds–mosquito–bird cycle)	Mosquito bite	2
Crimean-Congo haemorrhagic fever virus	Haemorrhagic fever	Livestock. Transmitted via *Hyalomma* ticks.	Tick bite	38
Tick-borne encephalitis	Meningoencephalitis	Rodents, small mammals, livestock	Tick bite, unpasteurised milk products	2
Chikungunya virus	Fever, joint pains, muscle pains	Humans and other vertebrate hosts	Mosquito bite - *Aedes aegypti* and *Aedes albopictus*	2
Rift Valley fever	Rift Valley fever virus	Cattle, goats, sheep	Direct contact, mosquito bite	2

Urbanisation, globalisation and climate change are facilitating vector establishment in previously naïve areas and juxtapositioning human host and domesticated animals with wild potentially disease-carrying hosts, creating a perfect storm for the emergence of zoonotic infections. A concerted global public health effort is required to monitor and eliminate the emergence of new zoonoses.

49

Sending Specimens to the Laboratory

Sending the Correct Specimens

It is important to establish which are the best specimens to send to the laboratory. Check with the laboratory's user manual. Chapters in this book suggest which specimens are suitable for the diagnosis of different virus infections and clinical syndromes. It is important to consider when, in the patient's clinical course, specimens should be sent. There are a few simple rules of thumb:

- When sending specimens for molecular testing, be aware that viral DNA and RNA may only be found in certain body sites in different viral infections.
- Virus antibody is usually not present in serum reliably until about 10 days after the onset of symptoms.
- For those viruses where specific IgM is not tested for, an acute sample taken as soon as possible after the onset of symptoms and a second specimen taken 10 days after the onset of symptoms allows for the detection of a specific IgG rise (paired sera).
- Viruses causing maculopapular rashes (e.g. measles virus) usually produce specific IgM antibody within a few days of the onset of the rash.
- When diagnosing acute hepatitis, HBsAg will be present at the onset of symptoms of HBV infection but HAV IgM is not detectable until at least 5 days after the onset of symptoms.

Filling in the Specimen Request Form Correctly

It is important to fill in the specimen request form with as much detail as possible. The following information should be provided irrespective of whether it is a paper or electronic request:

- Always provide at least three patient identifiers from the list below. Failure to do so (or providing different information on the specimen container and the request form) will result in the specimen being discarded or not being tested:
  - First and last names
  - Date of birth
  - National Health Service number
  - Hospital number
  - Address (including postcode)

- Always provide full details of the healthcare professional to whom the result should be sent. It is useful to provide a telephone number, especially for telephoning urgent or abnormal results.

- Specimen type.
- Tests requested.
- Date and time the specimen was taken.
- Clinical information – this is the most important information because it allows the laboratory doctor to request the most appropriate tests and to interpret the laboratory findings. Failure to provide this hampers the provision of an individualised service.
- Have previous specimens been sent? This is important for paired serological investigations and for monitoring viral load trends.

Packaging Specimens Correctly

Specimens should be placed in the appropriate specimen container, which must be securely fastened and any accidental spillage cleaned immediately, with an appropriate chlorine-containing disinfectant (10,000 ppm available chlorine for blood spillage, 1,000 ppm for surface disinfection). Each specimen should be placed in a clear plastic, double ('marsupial'), self-sealing bag with one compartment containing the request form and the other the specimen, which will allow the request form to be kept separate from the specimen. Any specimens sent by post must comply with infectious substances transport regulations. Transport of Infectious Substances is a guidance note (17/2012) produced by the Department for Transport, the Civil Aviation Authority and the Maritime and Coastguard Agency. It is available to download at https://assets.publishing .service.gov.uk/media/5f60c1c58fa8f51063ce4e83/dangerous-goods-guidance-note-17-document.pdf.

Postal and air freight regulations and those relating to dangerous organisms must be followed at all times, to ensure that the specimens cannot contaminate the outside of the package.

Notifying the Laboratory That Urgent/Important Specimens Are Being Sent

It is useful to telephone the duty virologist or microbiologist if urgent or important specimens are to be sent to the laboratory. This will ensure that specimens are processed correctly and in a timely manner, the required tests are done and the results are telephoned in promptly. Do not rely on automatic electronic transmission of authorised results for urgent and clinically significant results transfer; these may not be read in a timely fashion by the healthcare workers caring for the patient at that time. Tests can often be done urgently if the clinical outcome is likely to be affected by the result.

Chapter

50

Serological Techniques

Very often it is difficult to make a clinical diagnosis of a specific viral infection as many viruses have clinically similar presentation (e.g. hepatitis viruses) and the same virus can have many different clinical presentations (e.g. enteroviruses). It is therefore essential to seek specific laboratory diagnosis to enable correct management of the patient. This may be important from an epidemiological perspective as well.

Serology is the science of measuring antibodies in the serum produced in response to virus infection. The term also includes measurement of viral antigen in the serum. Serological techniques have been adapted to be used on other body fluids as well, for example urine, cerebrospinal fluid and saliva. Measurement of antibody and antigen to diagnose viral infections is an important adjunct to direct detection of viruses by nucleic acid amplification techniques (NAAT) and is widely used as serological techniques are less technically demanding and cheaper and easily automated.

Antibodies are produced as a host response to viral infection. IgA is produced at the local site of infection and provides local immunity, for example in the gut or respiratory tract. The generalised humoral immune response is mounted by B lymphocytes and the first antibody to appear is of the IgM class which can usually be detected as early as a couple of days after an acute infection. Some of the B lymphocyte clones then switch over to producing IgG antibody, which appears from 7 to 15 days after onset of infection. Both classes of antibodies continue to rise in response to the infection, peaking at about 6 weeks post infection. Viral-specific IgM then declines and is normally undetectable about 3 months after infection. IgG antibody persists for life and is responsible for providing lifelong immunity to the particular virus. Figure 50.1 shows the sequence of serological response after viral infection.

Acute or recent infection can therefore be diagnosed by:

- demonstrating the presence of virus-specific IgM (IgG may or may not be present);
- showing a rise in antibody titre between an acute and convalescent specimen; or
- a high antibody titre in a convalescent specimen.

Past infection or immunity is diagnosed by:

- demonstration of virus-specific IgG alone (and absence of IgM).

Principle of Serological Techniques

The antibody class and functionality can be used to measure the immune response after viral infection. Several techniques have been developed, but the fundamental principles are similar for all.

Assays may be *qualitative* (e.g. give only a yes or no answer) or be *quantitative* (e.g. measure the antibody level).

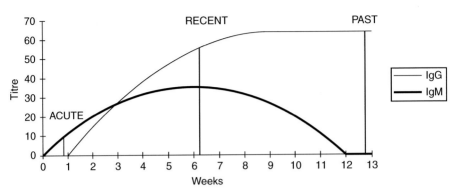

Figure 50.1 Figurative representation of serological response to viral infection

As a rule, assays that utilise the presence of IgM or IgG to make a diagnosis are usually qualitative as presence or absence of these antibodies is sufficient to make a diagnosis.

On the other hand, if diagnosis relies on detection of rising or a high antibody titre, then the assays need to measure the level of antibody response (quantitative). Antibody 'titre' is expressed as the inverse of the highest serum dilution at which the antibody is detected. For example, influenza A antibody titre of 128 means that antibody to influenza A was detected until a 1 in 128 serum dilution but not in higher dilutions.

Many of the quantitative assays have been developed exploiting the functional properties of antibody response (e.g. complement fixation, haemagglutination or neutralisation tests).

Techniques

All serological techniques to detect antibody are based on the principle of adding specific viral antigen(s) to patient serum. If virus-specific antibody is present in the serum then it will bind to the antigen to form an antigen/antibody complex. An indicator system (depending on the technique) is then used to detect whether such a complex has been formed. These techniques can be reversed to detect the presence instead of viral antigen, for example hepatitis B surface antigen in the patient's serum.

Enzyme-Linked Immunosorbent Assays

Enzyme-linked immunosorbent assays (ELISAs, usually now referred to as EIAs) are the most widely used serological assays in routine diagnostic laboratories. There are several variations of the technique, but the essential steps are shown in Figure 50.2a–d.

The colour change in EIAs can be detected by eye or measured in a spectrophotometer and the intensity of the colour can indicate how much antibody is present in the serum. Figure 50.3 shows positive (coloured) and negative (colourless) reactions in the EIA test.

EIAs can be constructed to detect either IgG or IgM depending upon whether the anti-human antibody is directed to IgM or IgG class. Positive and negative controls are added to the assay runs to ensure the quality of the assay system. Most of the EIAs in use have a very high sensitivity and specificity (>95%), some approaching even 100%.

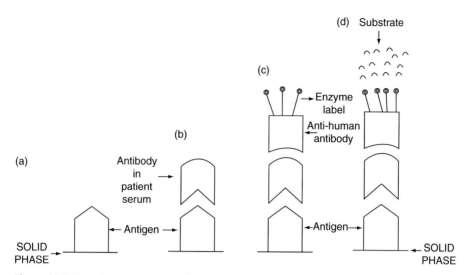

Figure 50.2 Figurative representation of an enzyme-linked immunosorbent assay
a Antigen is attached to the base of a plastic microtitre well (solid phase).
b Patient's serum is added to this microtitre well. If specific antibody is present in the serum it will attach to the antigen on the solid phase. Excess serum is washed off.
c Anti-human antibody coupled to an enzyme is added to bind to this antibody/antigen complex. Excess enzyme is washed off.
d A substrate for the enzyme is added; a colour change indicates a positive reaction due to the action (on the substrate) of the enzyme which has been bound to the antigen/antibody complex.

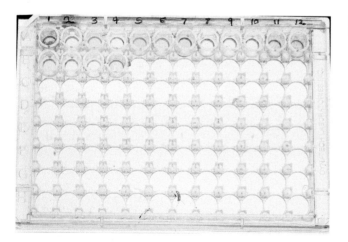

Figure 50.3 Enzyme-linked immunosorbent assay plate

The assay can also be done in reverse to detect viral antigens simply by coating the solid phase with antibody (mono or polyclonal) specific for the antigen to be tested.

Advantages of EIAs are:

- they are rapid – most can be done within 2–3 hours;
- they can be easily automated; and
- they are objective as the reaction can be read by spectrophotometer.

Lateral Flow Tests

These are immune-chromatographic tests working in a similar way to EIAs. These can be used for both antibody detection as for HIV or for antigen detection as for SARS-CoV-2. For Covid-19 testing, a respiratory sample is taken and placed in a small amount of fluid and mixed. A few drops of fluid are then dropped onto the slot in the lateral flow device. The fluid is sucked into the device and rehydrates a conjugate mix and is then drawn, by capillary action, over a strip of immobilised Covid-19 antibody. If the sample is positive for Covid-19 virus, the Covid-19 antigen in the sample will adhere to the immobilised strip containing the enzyme conjugate, which will change colour, giving a positive result line on the device. There is also a control line which must change colour for the test to be valid. The Covid-19 pandemic has accelerated this point of care (POC) test availability, with lateral flow POC tests being widely available for home use as well to facilitate infection control effectiveness.

Immunofluorescence Tests

Immunofluorescence tests (IFs or IFTs) use the same principle as EIAs and, like EIAs, can be constructed to detect either viral antibody or antigen in patient specimen. However, instead of the enzyme/substrate detector system of EIAs, fluorescein-labelled anti-human antibody is used to detect positive reaction which appears as apple green fluorescence under a light microscope. Figure 50.4 shows a positive varicella-zoster virus IF reaction.

To look for viral antigen, cells from the patient's secretions (e.g. nasopharyngeal aspirate) are fixed to a spot on the glass slide and fluorescein- labelled monoclonal antibody against the virus (respiratory syncytial virus (RSV), influenza A, etc.) is added. A mixture of these monoclonal antibodies can be added at the same time to detect a panel of viruses (e.g. respiratory viruses all at one go).

IFs are also rapid serological tests, but the disadvantage is that they require subjective interpretation and are therefore labour intensive and dependent upon operator expertise and have largely been replaced for both antibody and antigen detection by EIAs. See Table 50.1.

Latex Agglutination Test and Gelatin Particle Agglutination Test

Here the antigen or antibody is adsorbed on an inanimate particle (latex or gelatin) and a positive reaction is indicated by agglutination of the particles.

Complement Fixation Test

This test is based on the principle that when an antigen/antibody complex is formed it will 'fix' (bind) complement so free complement is not available to lyse sensitised red cells which are added as indicator.

Complement fixation tests have been extensively used in the past to aid clinical diagnosis; however, because of their complexity and relative insensitiveness they have been replaced by EIAs.

Haemagglutination and Haemagglutination Inhibition Tests

These detect antibodies to viruses (rubella, influenza) that possess a haemagglutinin antigen. They are also relatively insensitive and can give non-specific reactions and have been replaced by more sensitive and specific techniques.

Table 50.1 Diagnostic uses of the serological techniques

Test	Example of use
Complement fixation test	To diagnose recent infection acute and convalescent serum samples are required to show rise in titre. CFT is no longer in routine use in diagnostic laboratories.
Enzyme-linked immunosorbent assays	*IgG/IgM antibody* – rubella, measles, mumps, HIV, hepatitis A, etc. *Antigen* – hepatitis B surface antigen in serum samples, norovirus and rotavirus antigen in faeces.
Immunofluorescence	*Antigen* – RSV, influenza and other respiratory viruses in respiratory secretions. IF techniques for virus detection have limited use in diagnostic laboratories, having been replaced with EIA-based techniques or NAAT.
Latex and gel particle agglutination	*Antibody* – rubella, CMV, toxoplasma *Antigen* – rotavirus, norovirus
Western blot and line assays	Used to confirm HIV and hepatitis C antibody screen positive specimens.
IgG avidity assays	To confirm recent CMV, EBV, HIV, HBV, rubella and toxoplasma infections.

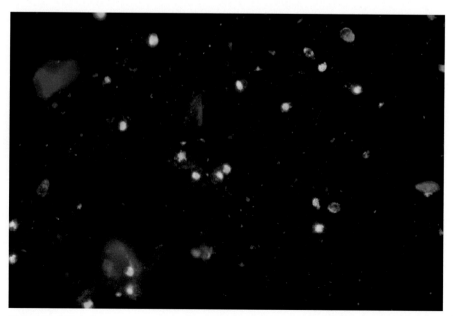

Figure 50.4 Varicella-zoster virus immunofluorescence

Neutralisation Test

Virus-specific neutralising antibodies if present in the serum will neutralise the virus so it is not able to grow in culture. This is a very specific but labour-intensive and technically demanding technique and is generally only used in research settings.

Western Blot or Line Immunoassays

Specific viral proteins are transferred onto blotting paper either from a gel (Western blot) or produced by recombination or peptide synthesis (line immunoassays). Further steps are similar to those of EIAs. The viral antigen band on the blotting paper develops colour if specific antibody to that particular antigen is present in the serum. Assay is able to distinguish antibody directed against specific virus proteins and is therefore very specific and has been used to confirm initial screen positive HIV and hepatitis C antibody results.

Antibody Avidity Assays

The host antibody response matures over several weeks post acute infection. Therefore, antibody detected >3 months after acute infection binds strongly (high avidity) to antigen(s) used in laboratory assays; as a corollary the antibody in the first 3 months has weak binding (low avidity) and can be easily dissociated from the antigen/antibody complexes.

This is used as a principle in tests devised to measure IgG avidity. These tests are helpful in distinguishing primary infections from reinfections or reactivations as in the latter IgG is of high avidity. Antibody avidity assays have been extensively used to distinguish primary infections from reinfections or reactivations for rubella, varicella-zoster virus, cytomegalovirus (CMV), Epstein–Barr virus (EBV) and *Toxoplasma gondii*. They have also been used to time the acquisition of infection, as in that for HIV.

Use of Non-serum Samples for Antibody Tests

EIA antibody tests have been adapted for use on urine (HIV) or salivary samples (HIV, hepatitis B and C, measles, mumps and rubella). This is of great advantage for those who are needle-phobic or difficult to bleed such as intravenous drug users or neonates/small children. A special kit is required to collect the salivary sample for antibody testing.

Automation in Serology

All the steps in the EIA lend themselves to automation and several systems are now available on the market. This has enabled the laboratories to process thousands of specimens very quickly and improve turnaround times for results. The latest genre of automated machines is called 'random access' as the specimens do not have to be batched and an urgent specimen can be put on the machine at any time without disrupting the other specimens already on it. Results can be obtained in under an hour.

Much of this automated serology equipment in use in the virology laboratory is common to clinical chemistry and immunology, therefore the technology is further driving the way that specialist laboratories work. Many hospitals now have blood sciences laboratories where automated machines are linked with specimen tracks which act as assembly lines to load the specimens onto the machines.

Most laboratories will also have interfaces linking their machines to the laboratory computer system. Linking the laboratory computer system to the hospital-based IT system allows the clinician to access these results as soon as they are ready. This also has the advantage that if barcodes are used for specimen recognition, samples are not registered to the wrong patients accidentally.

Future of Serology

- Despite the availability of rapid molecular diagnosis serology remains an important tool for the diagnosis of acute and chronic viral infections.
- Serology is of particular value in assessing the immune status of patients either as a result of natural infection or post-immunisation.
- Serological screening of blood for blood-borne viruses is mandatory in many countries around the world.
- Serology is a very important public health tool for epidemiological studies to provide prevalence of infection data.

Conclusion

The technically demanding serological assays of the past have largely been replaced with rapid diagnostic techniques in serology. Automation of the EIA has further revolutionised the way that the laboratories operate and a test result can be given for patient management to the clinician within hours of the specimen arriving in the laboratory.

Despite the popularity of molecular diagnostic techniques for viral diagnosis, serological techniques will continue to form an important part of the laboratory's armoury for some time to come.

51

Virus Detection – Molecular Techniques

Molecular techniques are those that use the principles of molecular biology to detect viral genomes (RNA or DNA). The use of these techniques has been commonplace in virology for many years and has led to the discovery of new viruses (e.g. hepatitis C virus), the study of antiviral resistance and the designing of new antiviral drugs and vaccines.

Molecular techniques are in use in most, if not all, routine diagnostic laboratories to aid viral diagnosis and are available as point-of-care tests. They are generically known as nucleic acid amplification techniques (NAAT). Those techniques that are in current and common use are detailed next.

Polymerase Chain Reaction

Polymerase chain reaction (PCR) was the first NAAT in routine use. It is a technique by which a single copy of DNA or RNA can be amplified more than a million times. To detect RNA viruses, RNA has to be first transcribed to complementary DNA by means of an enzyme called reverse transcriptase (this type of PCR is referred to as reverse transcription PCR, or RT-PCR). PCR tests use a bacterial enzyme, taq polymerase, to initiate DNA amplification.

The first step in the diagnostic process is the extraction and denaturation of the DNA or RNA in the clinical sample; this extract is then amplified. Amplification involves complex chemical reactions and heating and cooling of the sample mix in a thermo-cycler. Each heating and cooling cycle takes only a few minutes to complete and each cycle doubles the amount of DNA product present in the reaction mix. Greater than a million copies of the DNA sequence can be produced in about 40 cycles, which may typically take 2–3 hours to complete. The amplified DNA product (amplicon) can be detected by use of specific probes labelled with fluorescent or chemiluminescent dyes. Probes need to be carefully selected to identify unique sequences contained in individual viruses' nucleic acid, so that PCR tests are sensitive and specific.

One of the most significant issues in the use of PCR tests for diagnosing viral infections is the accurate interpretation of results. Not only do laboratory personnel who authorise and sign out test results need to analyse carefully the results obtained with the various control samples in each assay to ensure the test run is valid and complies with the quality control rules, but they also need to look carefully at the shape of the reaction curve and the cycle threshold value to make a judgement of the likelihood of the result being a true positive.

Several variations of the PCR technique are in use:

- *Nested PCR* – this type of PCR uses two separate amplification steps, so in theory can generate twice the amount of amplicons as compared to traditional PCR.

- *Multiplex PCR* – this can detect several different viral genomes in a single reaction mixture. This allows detection of several different viruses at the same time, in a single test (e.g. respiratory viruses). It is also useful for syndromic testing, examining specimens from patients in whom a suspected infection may be caused by different unrelated viruses, bacteria or parasites (e.g. gastroenteritis).
- *Real-time PCR* – in this test, the amplification and detection steps of PCR occur simultaneously (rather than sequentially). Therefore, the time taken to get a result is much shorter.
- *Quantitative PCR* – this test provides a comparison of the amount of RNA or DNA present in the patient sample compared with a set of standard control samples with known amounts of viral RNA or DNA which results in the viral load for the patients' sample being elucidated.

Loop-Mediated Isothermal Amplification Test

The loop-mediated isothermal amplification (LAMP) test is a one-step process used to multiply specific nucleic acid sequences. The patient's sample is mixed with primers, reverse transcriptase and DNA polymerase and incubated at a single temperature, so does not need thermal cyclers. LAMP uses six primers (rather than two for PCR), allowing the use of multiple genome sequence regions as specificity targets. The increased number of starting points for DNA synthesis can deliver improved specificity and sensitivity compared to most PCR-based detection assays. Reverse transcription loop-mediated isothermal amplification (RT-LAMP) combines LAMP with a reverse transcription step to allow the detection of RNA. LAMP is so called because as synthesis begins, pairs of primers form loops to facilitate each round of amplification. It is quicker and cheaper than PCR.

Transcription-Mediated Amplification

Transcription-mediated amplification (TMA) is an isothermal single-tube nucleic acid amplification system using RNA polymerase and reverse transcriptase. It does not need a thermal cycler and is quicker than PCR, producing 100–1,000 copies per cycle. TMA involves RNA transcription (via RNA polymerase) and DNA synthesis (via reverse transcriptase) to produce an RNA amplicon and can be used to target both RNA and DNA. One of its uses is in testing for SARS-CoV-2.

Microarrays

DNA microarrays can be used to detect DNA or RNA (usually as cDNA after reverse transcription). A DNA microarray is a collection of microscopic DNA spots (probes) attached to a solid surface used to measure the presence of a large number of molecular targets simultaneously. The probes are usually short sections of viral DNA that are used to hybridise a cDNA or cRNA sample (target) under high-stringency conditions. Probe-target hybridisation is usually detected and quantified by detection of fluorophore-, silver-, or chemiluminescence-labelled targets to determine relative amounts of nucleic acid sequences in the patient's sample. These tests are most useful for syndromic screening tests (e.g. testing simultaneously in one assay for a range of viral, bacterial, fungal and parasite respiratory pathogens on samples from patients with respiratory

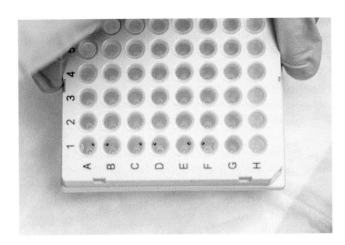

Figure 51.1 Magnetic DNA-binding beads pelleted together inside a plate, using a strong magnet used in whole-genome sequencing to determine the DNA fingerprint of a specific virus (courtesy of CDC; details – Public Health Image Library (PHIL): https://phil.cdc.gov/Details.aspx?pid=26142)

symptoms). These tests have rather fallen out of favour in recent years, with the rapid advancement of faster and cheaper adaptations of rapid next-generation sequencing.

Nucleic Acid Sequencing

Sanger sequencing was developed in the 1970s for sequencing nucleic acid; however, it was slow and expensive to perform, limiting its usefulness. In the early 1990s, high-throughput capillary sequencing was developed, which, as time has gone by, has become cheaper and quicker to perform, making it suitable for routine virus diagnosis and epidemiology analysis. Complete virus genome sequencing allows typing and comparison of virus isolates for epidemiological purposes (e.g. typing measles virus isolates to identify clusters of measles cases) and to identify the infection transmission chain (e.g. in hepatitis B virus needlestick transmission inquiries). Another important clinical application is for antiviral resistance testing to identify if any infecting virus may have any mutation that may confer resistance to the antiviral drugs that are being proposed to be used (e.g. HIV). This technique is most important for RNA viruses because of their increased tendency to mutate.

Next-Generation Sequencing

Next-generation sequencing relies on PCR clustering on flow cells (Illumina) and is similar to that of the Sanger sequencing method, using array-based sequencing to process millions of reactions in parallel. After the amplification process, sequencing is performed; several different sequencing techniques can now be used. After sequencing, the sequence readouts that are obtained are aligned to reference genomes to identify the likely cause(s) of infection. The main disadvantage of next-generation sequencing is that it requires computer capacity and storage and staff to analyse and interpret the sequencing data. Figure 51.1 shows magnetic beads inside a plate during whole-genome sequencing tests.

Molecular Point of Care Tests

In recent years, there has been a rapid increase in the number and variety of molecular point of care tests available for diagnosing viral infections (e.g. Cepheid, Biofire), which has been further accelerated with the tests introduced to diagnose SARS-CoV-2 infections. These PCR-based multiplex tests are available for syndromic screening for respiratory, gastrointestinal and central nervous system infections caused by viruses, bacteria, fungi and parasites and are used in laboratories and clinical settings including Accident and Emergency Departments and clinics to facilitate clinical diagnosis and infection control practice. The test panels can either test for a single virus (e.g. the Cepheid enterovirus meningitis test) or syndromic testing for a small group of viruses (e.g. the Cepheid SARS-CoV-2, influenza A and B viruses and respiratory syncytial virus test) or for over 20 possible infectious viruses, bacteria, fungi and parasites, with results available in 45–60 minutes (e.g. the Biofire syndromic assays).

Chapter

52

Virus Detection – Non-molecular Techniques

Detection of viruses in the patient secretions or tissue provides direct evidence of current or ongoing infection. This can be by:

- virus culture (also referred to as cell or tissue culture)
- electron microscopy – visualisation of whole virus particles
- detection of viral antigens
- detection of viral genome (RNA or DNA) by molecular techniques.

Detection of viral genome by molecular techniques is collectively known as nucleic acid amplification techniques (NAAT) and detection of viral antigens by enzyme-linked immunosorbent assay (ELISA or EIA) has replaced both cell culture and electron microscopy for viral diagnosis in routine diagnostic laboratories; however, as they still have an important role in research setting and are basic tools of virus detection they are described here.

Virus Cell Culture

Viruses, like bacteria, can be cultured in the laboratory. However, viruses are fastidious intracellular organisms and therefore living cells are required to grow viruses in the laboratory. Many cell lines have been developed to support the growth of different viruses. A single type of cell line is not adequate as viruses need receptors on the cell surface to which they attach to gain entry into the cell and to initiate replication. The presence of specific cell receptors on the cell surface determines which viruses will be able to infect them and this is called viral cell tropism. For this reason, many cell lines have to be maintained in a diagnostic laboratory. Another problem in the laboratory is to maintain these living cells in culture long enough to allow sufficient virus growth.

A suspension of cells in growth medium (consists of buffer + calf serum to provide protein and amino acids and antibiotics to prevent bacterial overgrowth) is put in glass or plastic tubes/flasks; the cells attach to the side of the container and grow until they become confluent. The patient's specimen is then added and cells incubated at 37°C to allow the virus to grow (33°C for respiratory viruses). The tubes are examined daily to look for evidence of virus growth, which may take from a day to weeks. If virus is present, then it kills off the cells, depending upon the cell line and the virus growing in it. This gives a typical appearance in the cell sheet and is referred to as the cytopathic effect (CPE). An experienced virologist can make a provisional diagnosis on the basis of CPE, but confirmation is required and this can be by electron microscopy, immunofluorescence, neutralization, etc. of the growth medium to see if the suspected virus is present in it.

Figure 52.1a Uninfected Graham 293 cells

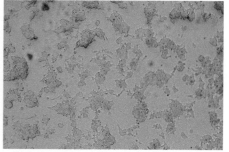

Figure 52.1b Graham 293 cells showing adenovirus cytopathic effect

Cell lines can be from human or non-human sources and can be broadly divided into:

- *Continuous* – these are immortalised cell lines derived mostly from tumour cells or cells that have been transformed in the laboratory. They can be maintained in indefinite growth cycles in the laboratory. Examples are HeLa (human cervical cancer cell line), hep2 and Graham 293 cells (transformed human epithelial cell line). Figure 52.1a shows the uninfected Graham 293 cells and 52.1b shows the adenovirus CPE.

- *Primary or semi-continuous* – as the name implies they can be maintained for only one or a limited number of growth cycles. They are more sensitive to infection by viruses and fastidious viruses like varicella-zoster virus, cytomegalovirus and the influenza virus will only grow in them. Examples are MRC5 (human lung fibroblast cell line) and PMK (primary monkey kidney cell line).

Cell culture, although a very sensitive and specific technique, is labour intensive and requires considerable technical expertise. Results may take up to a few weeks and the specimens need to be transported quickly and under correct conditions to the laboratory to maintain the viability of the infecting virus. Many viruses, such as the hepatitis viruses, papillomaviruses, parvovirus B19, rotavirus and norovirus cannot be grown in cell culture and others like the Epstein–Barr virus and HIV need special cells, therefore are not suitable for culture in routine diagnostic laboratories.

Electron Microscopy

Viruses are below the resolution of light microscopy and therefore require electron microscope (EM) for visualisation. A limiting factor of EM is that the viruses belonging to the same family (e.g. herpes group) cannot be distinguished from each other as they will have the same morphology (size, shape and surface characteristics – see Figure 52.2a). Therefore, EM cannot be used to make the differential diagnosis of a herpes simplex or chickenpox lesion as both will contain a 'herpes' virus with exactly the same morphology (Figure 52.2a). On the other hand, it is a useful tool in making differential diagnosis of viral gastroenteritis as rotavirus, norovirus and enteric adenoviruses all belong to different families and can be distinguished from each other on the basis of their morphology (see Chapter 43). It is a 'catch all' technique and many viruses (rotavirus, norovirus) were discovered by EM.

EM was first used in the 1950s to distinguish the vesicular rashes of smallpox from chickenpox which are caused by morphologically distinct viruses. Figures 52.2a and 52.2b

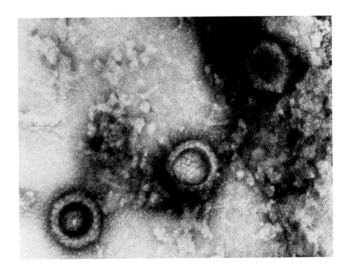

Figure 52.2a Electron micrograph of herpes viruses (courtesy of CDC; details – Public Health Image Library (PHIL): https://phil.cdc.gov/Details.aspx?pid=6493)

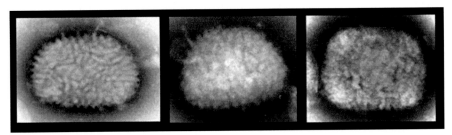

Figure 52.2b Electron micrographs of poxviruses (courtesy of CDC; details – Public Health Image Library (PHIL): https://phil.cdc.gov/Details.aspx?pid=2143)

show EMs of varicella-zoster virus (a herpes group) and poxviruses respectively. During the 1980s and 1990s it was the only tool to diagnose the viral gastroenteritis viruses (rotavirus, norovirus, calicivirus, enteric adenoviruses 40/41). However, due to the availability of rapid sensitive and specific antigen detection and molecular tests for these viruses, EM has largely become redundant for diagnosis of viral gastroenteritis.

EM is expensive, technically demanding, requires specialist training and is relatively insensitive (requires a minimum of one million viral particle/ml) and has therefore largely been limited to research institutions.

Antigen Detection

Detection of viral antigen in patient specimen is sufficient to provide evidence of viral presence. Various techniques such as:

- enzyme-linked immunosorbent assay (ELISA or EIA)
- immunofluorescence tests
- latex agglutination tests
- lateral flow tests

are in wide use and have already been described in Chapter 50.

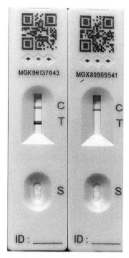

Figure 52.3 SARS-CoV-2 test results. The left- hand result is positive, with both the test (T) and control (C) lines visible. The right-hand result is negative, with just the control line visible (image courtesy of Dr Tim Wreghitt)

Point of Care Tests

Point of care tests (POCTs) are tests for virus detection that are performed at or near patient side. Currently they are mainly in use for detection of respiratory viruses (e.g. influenza viruses, respiratory syncytial virus and SARS-CoV-2). These can be EIA or immunofluorescence based. However, the more recent tests are NAAT based and have very good sensitivity and specificity (see Chapter 51). The NAAT-based POCTs require portable instrumentation for implementation. As POCTs are generally deployed in clinical areas and away from laboratory they require clear testing policy and algorithms and staff training and quality assurance.

Figure 52.3 shows a positive SARS-CoV-2 test result.

53

Quality Control and Laboratory Accreditation

In any well-run clinical virology laboratory, it is vital to pay careful attention to quality control, effective laboratory management and compliance with laboratory accreditation criteria.

Quality Control

Quality control relates to the overall quality of a laboratory's output. It is part of quality management that is focused on satisfying all quality requirements and centres around inspections and the operations needed to fulfil quality requirements. It is a strategy that systematically identifies the processes and procedures used to ensure that the laboratory service meets its stated quality goals. Maintaining service standards is an essential aspect of meeting user needs and stakeholder expectations. Quality control measures should include equipment, environment and quality assessment (internal and external).

Quality Assurance

Quality assurance is another aspect of quality management that focuses on providing a level of confidence to meet all quality requirements. Quality assurance is defined as planned activities within the laboratory diagnostic process that help to ensure the overall quality and safety of the laboratory results. Quality assurance aims to prevent problems by adhering to rules, regulations and standard operating procedures (SOPs). If the laboratory follows the rules of quality assurance correctly, it should always deliver a safe and efficient laboratory diagnostic service. Quality assurance is more preventive and proactive, as the strategy aims to reduce errors by assessing the process rather than the output.

A major part of the quality assurance process is auditing, which is the process of monitoring current conditions to ensure that they conform to regulatory requirements. There are several kinds of audit that good laboratories perform regularly:

- *Vertical audit* – these audits are conducted by choosing a laboratory report at random and checking to see if all the procedures in the relevant SOPs have been followed correctly (a good example is to choose the last confirmed HBsAg positive result – this will lead to examination of all the procedures used to test for hepatitis B virus (HBV) markers as well, including molecular tests). Auditing molecular testing is important, especially the interpretation of results.
- *Horizontal audit* – these audits are conducted by looking at one process across the laboratory (e.g. this could be looking at documentation control).
- *Witnessing audit* – these audits are conducted by sitting next to a healthcare scientist and observing if, when carrying out a laboratory procedure, they are correctly following the SOP for that procedure.

- *Clinical audit* – these audits are conducted by choosing a service carried out in the laboratory (e.g. confirmation of hepatitis C virus (HCV) antibody–reactive results). You need to decide on the appropriate audit standard (e.g. all HCV antibody screening test reactive samples should be tested in a second HCV antibody/antigen test or HCV PCR test) and then audit compliance against that audit standard. These audit standards can be local or national. Clinical audits can also be conducted in collaboration with clinical colleagues (e.g. compliance with HBV and HCV testing in a dialysis unit).
- Audits that focus on confidence around the area of reporting and interpretation, particularly around cut-off levels or clinically critical result values are important in assuring the effectiveness of clinical reporting.

If non-compliances are found in these audits, it is important to take corrective action and then re-audit to make sure that these changes have been effective.

Root cause analytical investigation of errors is an important tool to steer corrective and preventive actions.

Sources of Errors in Laboratory Results

Even in the best-run laboratory, with good policies and procedures in place, erroneous results can be sent out, almost always because of human errors. Possible reasons for these incorrect results include, but are not limited to:

- Errors in completing the laboratory request form for a specimen. This could include incorrect or incomplete clinical summary, incorrect age or incorrect or absent sample category. It could also include a test request which is inappropriate and not the one most likely to produce the ideal result.
- Errors in registering the request on the laboratory computer. Requests are almost always generated by the sender, so this should not be common now.
- Errors in allocating laboratory tests for the specimen. This can be very serious and can have severe or fatal consequences (e.g. allocating anti-HBc rather than HCV antibody tests for an organ donor specimen).
- Errors in performing assays. Careful attention needs to be paid to the inclusion of and validity of internal and external control specimens when deciding if test runs are valid and able to be reported.
- Errors in transferring laboratory results from the laboratory testing machines or manual assays to the laboratory test reporting computer. In the majority of cases these days, test results are transmitted automatically, but where this is not the case, careful checking of the correct results transfer must be done by two different people, to check for transposition errors.
- Errors in authorising and validating results and issuing them to clinicians and other virologists and microbiologists.
- Errors in transmitting the results across an interface (e.g. from laboratory computers to the requesting clinician's computers) and adequate accessibility of consultant virologists' interpretative comments on the transmitted reports.

It is important that when a laboratory error is discovered, which could have an adverse impact on a patient's health or well-being, that the error and the correct result are transmitted as soon as possible to the requesting clinician, microbiologist or primary care physician and that the patient is informed as soon as possible.

The Technical Competence of a Laboratory

The technical competence of a laboratory depends on a number of factors, including:

- good quality assurance procedures (quality control and quality assessment);
- suitable testing facilities;
- appropriate qualifications, training and experience of staff;
- appropriate testing procedures;
- the right equipment – properly calibrated and maintained;
- appropriately selected and quality assured test methods;
- traceability of measurements to relevant national and international standards; and
- accurate recording and reporting procedures.

Laboratory Accreditation

The United Kingdom Accreditation Service (UKAS) is the national accreditation body for the United Kingdom. It is appointed by the Government, to assess the testing procedures in organisations that provide laboratory diagnostic services. UKAS accredits laboratory testing procedures against the current version of the international quality standard ISO 15189. If UKAS successfully assesses a laboratory, it provides assurance to users that the laboratory's test procedures meet the relevant requirements, including the operation of its quality management system, and the ability to demonstrate that specific activities are performed within the criteria set out in the relevant standard.

UKAS carries out assessments on an annual basis with a full reassessment of the laboratory organisation every fourth year.

UKAS introduced the new international standard (ISO 15189:2022) in November 2022. This new standard contains the minimum requirements for quality and competence in clinical virology laboratories (and other relevant medical testing laboratories), but it should be noted that in order to provide the best possible clinical diagnostic service, continuous improvement should always be sought. The new international standard will be used as criteria to award accreditation. The requirements of the previous standard are largely unchanged; most (if not all) of the existing quality management systems implemented in laboratories remain valid. The new standard is risk-based and patient-focused and encourages continuous improvement within medical laboratories. There are requirements that are there to ensure that the risk to patients is central to the ethos of the laboratory's quality management system. The new standard is much less prescriptive; there is more flexibility as to how to meet and evidence the requirements set out in the revised standard. This added flexibility will allow for clinically justifiable variations in the ISO 15189:2022 standard. This will require laboratories to have an understanding of what is appropriate for their local service and, if something is considered not to be appropriate, they need to justify why this requirement is not met. Point of care testing is now included in this standard; therefore, the related ISO 22870:2016 standard will be withdrawn.

All medical laboratories will need to review their local quality management system against the requirements of the new standard. This analysis must involve input from the wide range of laboratory staff, including staff in clinical advisory and interpretation roles, due to the importance of clinical decision-making in many of the clauses.

There is a transition period for accredited organisations, which requires the transition to the new standard to be completed within 3 years of publication (2025). By the end of this period, all organisations accredited to ISO 15189:2012, and those also accredited to ISO 22870:2016, will need to have been assessed and be accredited to the updated version of ISO 15189.

Chapter

54

Antiviral Drugs

The most successful antiviral agent to date, aciclovir, was a serendipitous discovery. It was manufactured as an anti-cancer drug but was found to have good in-vitro activity against herpes simplex virus (HSV) and after clinical trials was licensed for use in the 1980s. Subsequently the antivirals have been designed and manufactured with specific viral targets in mind that will inhibit viral replication (see Table 54.1).

One disadvantage of the antivirals that act by DNA polymerase inhibition is that they affect the cellular DNA replication at the same time and therefore can cause cytotoxic side effects such as nausea, vomiting and bone marrow suppression. For this reason, they are not licensed to be used in pregnancy (except life-threatening situations or in HIV where the risk to the fetus is outweighed by the benefit of treatment) because of risk of fetal teratogenesis. These side effects are limited in certain drugs like aciclovir because the drug is preferentially activated in virus-infected cells and has little or no side effects on normal uninfected cells.

New therapeutic agents to treat viral infections are constantly being discovered or manufactured and others discarded as more effective and less toxic drugs become available. The aim of this chapter, therefore, is to describe in brief the mechanism of action of some of the antiviral drugs and their uses based on the knowledge at the time of publication.

Herpes Viruses

Aciclovir

Mechanism of Action

Aciclovir (acicloguanosine) is an acyclic analogue of the purine nucleoside guanine and is inert until phosphorylated to aciclovir triphosphate. Fortunately, as the first step in phosphorylation to aciclovir, monophosphate is initiated specifically by a viral enzyme called thymidine kinase (TK). The drug only gets activated in viral-infected cells (further phosphorylation to its triphosphate form is aided by cellular enzymes) and therefore there are very few side effects as relatively little active drug is formed in the uninfected cells. Furthermore, the drug reaches a higher concentration in infected as compared to uninfected cells. This specific action of the drug gives it its safety profile and narrow spectrum for treatment (HSV and varicella-zoster virus (VZV)) as these are the only two herpes viruses that possess the TK enzyme required to change the drug to its active form.

Aciclovir triphosphate inhibits viral replication in two ways:

- Aciclovir triphosphate competes with guanosine triphosphate to be incorporated in the DNA chain. Incorporation leads to DNA 'chain termination' as further nucleosides cannot be attached to allow the DNA chain to complete.

Table 54.1 Examples of antiviral drugs targeted to different replication steps in the viral life cycle

Stage	Drug	Target	Agent
Viral attachment/ adsorption	Maraviroc	Blocks CCR5 receptor	HIV1
Viral uncoating/ penetration	Amantadine	Matrix protein	Influenza A
Viral nucleic acid	Zidovudine	Reverse transcriptase	HIV
Synthesis	Aciclovir/penciclovir	Viral DNA polymerase	HSV and VZV
	Ganciclovir	Viral DNA polymerase	CMV
	Adefovir	Viral DNA polymerase	HBV
	Ribavirin	mRNA	RSV/HCV
Virus release/budding	Indinavir	Protease inhibitor	HIV
	Oseltamivir/ zanamivir/ peramivir	Neuraminadase (NA)	Influenza A/B
Miscellaneous	Interferon alpha	Immune modulator	HBV/HCV
	Rituximab	CD20 molecule B cell	EBV
	Palivizumab	monoclonal antibody	RSV

- It directly inhibits the viral DNA polymerase enzyme which is responsible for initiation of viral DNA synthesis. It is able to inhibit cellular DNA polymerase as well but to a much lesser degree hence has little effect on cellular DNA synthesis.

Resistance

Clinical resistance is uncommon and may be due to a variety of viral factors:

- Viral TK mutants
  - The loss of viral TK enzyme (TK-mutants) will result in the inability of the virus to activate aciclovir to its active form and hence treatment failure. Fortunately, such strains are generally not virulent and therefore do not cause clinically significant infection.
  - Altered viral TK gene so that the viral TK enzyme is not able to effectively start the phosphorylation step.
- Mutations in the viral DNA polymerase (DNA pol mutants) so that it does not preferentially take up aciclovir triphosphate for incorporation in the DNA chain. Such HSV mutants are a clinical problem, especially in severely immunocompromised patients (e.g. with AIDS) where recurrent or persistent infection may occur.

Valaciclovir

Valaciclovir is a prodrug of aciclovir – it is aciclovir with an attached valine ester. This results in greater absorption through the gut and about 70% of the drug is absorbed when taken orally as compared to 20% of aciclovir. In the body, valaciclovir is hydrolysed (the valine ester is removed) to aciclovir and therefore has exactly the same mechanism of action and resistance profile as aciclovir. The advantage is that oral valaciclovir does not have to be given as frequently as aciclovir.

Penciclovir and Famciclovir

Famciclovir is the prodrug of and is converted to penciclovir in the body. Penciclovir is very similar to aciclovir in structure and mechanism of action and is active against HSV and VZV once it is phosphorylated to its triphosphate form.

Ganciclovir and Valganciclovir

Mechanism of Action

Ganciclovir is an anti-cytomegalovirus (CMV) drug and is a nucleoside analogue derived from aciclovir. It does not need the viral TK enzyme for activation to its triphosphate form. Instead, it is activated by a virally encoded enzyme (encoded by the UL97 gene of CMV). Ganciclovir triphosphate inhibits the CMV viral DNA polymerase.

Unfortunately, as cellular enzymes can activate it equally, it does have serious cytotoxic side effects. Its use is therefore limited to treatment of life- and sight-threatening CMV infections.

Ganciclovir is poorly absorbed when given orally (<10%), however valganciclovir (the valyl ester of ganciclovir) is used orally as it is much better absorbed (40%); once absorbed it is converted to ganciclovir in the body by removal of the valine moiety.

Resistance

Resistance develops rarely (usually after prolonged use in immunocompromised persons) and is due to mutations in the UL97 gene of CMV so the drug cannot be activated. Resistance may also occur due to mutations in the DNA polymerase enzyme to make it resistant to the drug action.

Cidofovir

Cidofovir is a nucleotide analogue. It is activated by cellular enzymes. However, the drug preferentially acts upon the viral rather than cellular DNA polymerase. Like aciclovir, it inhibits the DNA synthesis by acting as a 'chain terminator'. As the drug is activated in uninfected cells it has cytotoxic side effects; it is also nephrotoxic and should be administered with probenecid to prevent renal damage.

Cidofovir is active against CMV and some other DNA viruses such as adenovirus, BK virus and smallpox virus.

Brincidofovir

Brincidofovir is a lipid conjugated prodrug of cidofovir with good oral bioavailability and is active against a broad range of double-stranded DNA viruses including pox viruses (smallpox and monkeypox) and adenoviruses. It has a lower rate of nephrotoxicity and myelotoxicity as compared to cidofovir.

Foscarnet

Foscarnet inhibits viral DNA synthesis but is a different class of drug. It is a pyrophosphate analogue so does not need phosphorylation to an active form. It is active against all herpes viruses including CMV.

Rituximab

Rituximab is a monoclonal antibody directed against CD20 B-cells. As the Epstein–Barr virus (EBV) infects the B-cells, rituximab has been used in treatment of post-transplant lymphoproliferative disease caused by EBV (Chapter 45).

Respiratory Viruses

Ribavirin

Ribavarin is a nucleoside analogue of guanosine and is phosphorylated intracellularly to its active form. Its active triphosphate form interferes with protein synthesis by acting upon mRNA and therefore it is active against a range of RNA and DNA viruses. However, in clinical use, its role is limited to treatment of respiratory syncytial virus (RSV) infections although it has also been used to treat other RNA viruses like parainfluenza, measles and Lassa fever viruses.

Amantadine

Amantadine was the first anti-influenza agent to be licensed for use. It acts specifically to inhibit the matrix protein M2 of influenza A virus, a key protein involved in the uncoating of the virus in the cell cytoplasm as the first step in the influenza virus replication cycle. It is not effective against influenza B virus since it does not possess the M2 protein. Resistance develops readily and, as amantadine has dopaminergic side effects such as restlessness, agitation, insomnia, confusion, etc., it has not found wide acceptance either among clinicians or patients as an anti-influenza agent.

Oseltamivir, Zanamivir, Peramivir

These are 'designer' anti-influenza drugs. They inhibit the neuraminidase (NA) enzyme of influenza viruses. After replication, the virus particles bud out of the cell and NA breaks the sialic acid bond between the virus and the cell surface to allow the release of the virus particles from the cell surface to initiate further infection cycles. Inhibition of NA results in infectious viral particles not being released.

These drugs act against both influenza A and B viruses and have relatively few side effects. Resistance develops due to point mutations in the NA enzyme of the virus so it becomes resistant to the action of the drug. Resistance to oseltamivir associated with a specific mutation causing a histidine to tyrosine substitution (H274Y) in neuraminidase was reported among seasonal influenza A (H1N1) virus strains in many countries at the time of the 2009 H1N1 influenza A pandemic. These oseltamivir-resistant H274Y virus infections have been susceptible to zanamivir.

Baloxavir Marboxil

This is an endonuclease inhibitor anti-influenza drug so it has a different mechanism of action from the previous three drugs listed.

Paxlovid

A combination of two protease inhibitor drugs, nirmatrelvir and ritonavir, paxlovid is available for treatment of SARS-CoV-2 infections in outpatient settings to reduce the risk of Covid-19–associated hospitalisation and death.

Remdesivir and Molnupiravir

Remdesivir is an RNA polymerase inhibitor that disrupts the production of viral RNA, preventing multiplication of SARS-CoV-2. Molnupiravir (a prodrug) is a ribonucleoside analogue that increases the number of mutations in viral RNA thus preventing multiplication of the virus.

Palivizumab

Palivizumab is a humanised monoclonal antibody against RSV. It is used in prophylaxis of RSV infection in children at risk of severe life-threatening RSV infection.

Cidofovir and Brincidofovir

These are used to treat adenovirus infection (pneumonitis and other systemic infection) in immunosuppressed patients. See the earlier section on these two drugs for more information.

Hepatitis B Virus

Interferon Alpha and Peginterferon Alpha

Interferon alpha was the first drug to be used for treatment of chronic hepatitis B and C infections. It is an immune modulator and acts through various immune mediated pathways; the initial expectation that it will therefore be effective against a large range of virus infections has not been borne out in clinical terms although it has been used for treating hepatitis B (HBV) and hepatitis C (HCV) infections. Pegylated or peginterferon alpha is produced by attaching the polyethylene glycol molecule to interferon alpha and has a longer half-life.

Lamivudine

Lamivudine is a nucleoside analogue reverse transcriptase (RT) inhibitor and was first manufactured as anti-HIV agent (see Table 54.2). As HBV also has a reverse transcriptase step in its replication it is now used as a first-line anti-HBV agent. However, resistance develops very rapidly due to point mutations in the viral RT and adding or switching over to second-line agents may be required.

Adefovir, Entecavir, Telbivudine and Tenofovir

These are nucleoside (NA) analogue agents used to treat HBV infection. Adefovir dipivoxil (ADF) acts on the reverse transcriptase enzyme. Tenofovir is available as two

Table 54.2 Antiviral drugs for use with herpes, respiratory and hepatitis viruses

Herpes group viruses	Drug	Preparations	Indication for use	Toxicity
Herpes simplex virus (HSV) type 1 and 2 and varicella-zoster virus (VZV) (chickenpox and shingles)	Aciclovir	Topical Oral Intravenous	Treatment and prophylaxis of HSV and VZV infections. Intravenous preparation should be used to treat HSV encephalitis and HSV and VZV infections in the immunosuppressed. Topical preparations are available over the counter and should be used for treatment of localised HSV skin lesions only in immunocompetent patients.	Very little. Good safety profile (see mechanism of action section). Some renal toxicity as drug is excreted through kidneys. Dose may need adjustment in renal failure.
	Valaciclovir and famciclovir	Oral	Indications are same as for aciclovir except where intravenous aciclovir is indicated.	Same as aciclovir
Cytomegalo-virus (CMV)	Ganciclovir	Intravenous, given as infusion	Life- or sight-threatening CMV infection in the immunocompromised	Leucopenia especially neutropenia is the most serious side effects, white blood count should be monitored whilst on treatment.
	Valganciclovir	Oral	Prophylaxis and maintenance therapy for CMV infection in the immunocompromised	As ganciclovir
	Cidofovir and brincidofovir	Intravenous, given as infusion	Ganciclovir-resistant CMV infection, BK virus and adenovirus infections in the immunocompromised	Renal toxicity, bone marrow suppression. Less renal toxicity with brincidofovir.
	Foscarnet	Intravenous, given as infusion	Ganciclovir-resistant CMV infection	Renal toxicity

Table 54.2 (cont.)

	Drug	Preparations	Indication for use	Toxicity
Herpes group viruses				
Epstein–Barr virus (EBV)	Rituximab	Intravenous, given as infusion	PTLD due to EBV	Infusion-related side effects
Respiratory viruses				
Respiratory syncytial virus (RSV)	Ribavirin	Particle aerosol for RSV infection. Oral for HCV (see below)	Severe RSV infection in neonates and immunocompromised adults	Anaemia
	Palivizumab	Intramuscular	Prophylaxis of RSV in children at risk of severe RSV infection	
Influenza A virus	Amantadine	Oral	No longer recommended for treatment and prophylaxis for influenza A	Restlessness, agitation, confusion
Influenza A and B viruses	Oseltamivir	Oral	Treatment and post-exposure prophylaxis (of high-risk individuals) for influenza A and B	GI symptoms
	Zanamivir	Inhalation of powder	As above	Bronchospasm and respiratory impairment may occur rarely
SARS-CoV-2	Paxlovid	Oral	Treatment of Covid-19 in outpatient setting	Nausea, vomiting, diarrhoea, altered taste
Hepatitis viruses				
Hepatitis B virus (HBV)	Interferon alpha	Intramuscular	Treatment of chronic HBV infection	Chills, rigors, fever, fatigue, flu-like symptoms
	Lamivudine	Oral	Chronic HBV infection	Bone marrow suppression
	Adefovir	Oral	Chronic HBV infection, alone or in combination with lamivudine	GI symptoms, rash

Table 54.2 (cont.)

Herpes group viruses	Drug	Preparations	Indication for use	Toxicity
	Tenofovir (TDF and TAF)	Oral	HBV and HIV co-infected patients	Renal toxicity with TDF
	Entecavir	Oral	Chronic HBV infection	GI symptoms, raised serum amylase and lipase
Hepatitis C virus (HCV)	Sofosbuvir, dasabuvir pibrentasvir, ombitasvir, elbasvir, velapatasvir, ledispasvir, glecaprevir, paritaprevir, voxilaprevir, grazoprevir.	Oral	HCV infection	See drug data sheets
Miscellaneous				
Adenovirus	Cidofovir	Intravenous, given as infusion	Clinical adenovirus disease in immunocompromised patients	As above
BK virus	Cidofovir	Intravenous, given as infusion	Clinical BK virus disease in immunocompromised patients	As above

compounds: tenofovir alafenamide (TAF) and tenofovir disoproxil fumarate (TDF). TAF is less nephrotoxic than TDF therefore is preferred in patients with renal compromise. Tenofovir is also effective against HIV and therefore it is the drug of choice for treating patients who are co-infected. Entecavir and telbivudine are the newest nucleoside analogue drugs. Lamivudine, adefovir and telbivudine have a low barrier against HBV resistance and entecavir, TDF and TAF have a high barrier to it.

Hepatitis C Virus

The initial peginterferon alpha and ribavirin combination regimes have been replaced by combinations of direct acting antivirals (DAAs).

The DAAs can be classified into those that:

- act on RNA-dependent RNA polymerase non-structural protein NS5B protein (examples are sofosbuvir and dasabuvir);
- act on non-structural protein NS5A (examples are pibfentasvir, ombitasvir, elbasvir, velapatasvir and ledispasvir); and
- are non-structural protein 3/4A protease inhibitors (examples are glecaprevir, paritaprevir, voxilaprevir and grazoprevir).

The HCV protease inhibitors block the activity of the viral encoded protease that is essential in the post-translational modification of the viral polypeptide that is cleaved into a series of structural and non-structural (enzyme) regions required for virus replication.

Antiretrovirals

Zidovudine or AZT was the first drug to be used in the treatment for HIV. Since then, several drugs have become available targeting different replication steps in the viral cycle and are shown in Table 54.3. None of the drugs eradicate the virus and the aim of the therapy is to keep viral replication suppressed. Drug resistance is a major issue because of mutations in the viral gene under drug selective pressure therefore the drugs are used in combination which is popularly referred to as highly active antiretroviral therapy.

Triple therapy using at least two different class of drugs (see Table 54.3) is the norm with two NRTIs forming the backbone of treatment combined with one NNRTI or PI. Increasingly, integrase inhibitors are replacing NNRTIs and PIs as the drugs of choice. The route of administration is oral for all the antiretroviral drugs and, to reduce the pill burden, zidovudine and lamivudine have been combined (combivir) to give the backbone of two NRTIs. Indication for treatment and follow-up are given in Chapter 11.

Useful Websites

Further details of drug routes and dosage are available from the British National Drug Formulary at www.bnf.org or the Electronic Medicines Compendium at www.emc.medicines.org.uk or refer to the manufacturer's data sheet.

Table 54.3 Antiretroviral drugs in common use

Drug class	Mechanism of action	Drugs in the class	Drug resistance	Drug side effects
Nucleoside reverse transcriptase inhibitors (NRTIs) or nucleoside analogues (NAs) *This class of drugs inhibits (thereby stopping viral replication) the HIV reverse transcriptase (RT) enzyme which facilitates the transcription of HIV RNA to DNA as the first step in viral replication cycle.*	Phosphorylated first to their triphosphate compounds by cellular enzymes. Inhibit HIV RT by binding to the substrate binding site. Also acts as DNA chain terminator.	Abacavir Didanosine (DDI) Lamivudine (3TC) Stavudine (D4T) Zalcitabine (DDC) Zidovudine (AZT)	Several point mutations in RT gene are required to confer resistance. Resistance to one drug does not necessarily mean resistance to all drugs within the class.	Lactic acidosis and mitochondrial toxicity
Non-nucleoside reverse transcriptase inhibitors (NNRTIs) – not effective against HIV-2. *Inhibit the RT of HIV-1 (see above).*	Inhibits the RT (HIV-1 only) but by acting on a site different than NRTIs above	Efavirenz Nevirapine	Point mutations in RT gene confer resistance. Cross-resistance between the drugs in the class is very high, e.g. resistance to one will confer resistance to others in the class.	Rashes, abnormal LFTs. Affect cytochrome p450 function.
Protease inhibitors (PIs). *Are active at very low concentration, work in synergy with NRTIs.*	Act on HIV protease enzyme and prevent production of functional viral protein so that the virus particle is not able to mature	Indinavir Nelfinavir Saquinavir Ritonavir Amprenavir	Single-point mutations in the protease gene confer resistance to more than one PI (cross-resistance)	Abnormality of fat and sugar metabolism leading to lipodystrophy and diabetes. Affect cytochrome p450 function.

Table 54.3 (cont.)

Drug class	Mechanism of action	Drugs in the class	Drug resistance	Drug side effects
Integrase strand transfer inhibitors /integrase inhibitors	First-generation raltegravir, elvitegravir, and second-generation dolutegravir and bictegravir	Act on HIV-1 integrase enzyme to block viral DNA integration into the host chromosome, an essential step in replication	See drug data sheet	See drug data sheet
Fusion inhibitors. *Prevent the fusion of virus to the receptors on cell surface and hence prevent viral entry into the cell and cell infection.*	Blocks attachment of viral gp41 to CD4 molecule cell receptor therefore preventing viral entry into the cell	Enfuvirtide		
	Blocks the CCR5 co-receptor and hence viral entry into the cells.	Maraviroc	Those viruses that do not require the CCR5 co-receptor to gain cell entry will be resistant.	

Viral Vaccines

The first vaccination known to humankind was against a viral infection, when Edward Jenner, in 1796, injected material from a lesion of cowpox into an 8-year-old boy, to protect him from smallpox. The culmination of this first step was in 1980, with the declaration that smallpox was the first human infection to be eradicated from the world.

Subsequently, many viral vaccines have been developed and there have been successful public health campaigns to reduce the burden of infections. The World Health Organization has an ongoing vaccination programme for the elimination of polio and measles. Polio is now considered to be non-endemic apart from in Pakistan and Afghanistan.

Vaccines against hepatitis B and papillomaviruses can arguably be considered as the first vaccines that protect against cancers (hepatocellular carcinoma and cervical cancer respectively).

In recent years, there have been huge advances in the development of and use of viral vaccines (e.g. Covid-19 vaccines).

There are several types of viral vaccines.

Vaccine Types

Live Attenuated Virus Vaccines

Attenuation of viruses implies the loss of pathogenicity, but for successful vaccination, the immunogenicity has to be maintained. The first viral vaccine was to protect against smallpox; it was made from a related less-pathogenic virus, the cowpox virus.

Attenuation can be achieved by selective pressure on the virus during repeated passages in cell culture. The whole process has to be carefully controlled, so that there are no extraneous pathogenic viruses or 'wild type' pathogenic viruses in the attenuated vaccine product.

The main advantage of attenuated vaccines is that the vaccine virus replicates in vaccinees and causes a subclinical infection and therefore produces a good immune response. On the other hand, there are always concerns about the possibility of the vaccine virus strains reverting to wild type virus, causing symptomatic infection. This concern is certainly present with live polio vaccines; the polio type 3 vaccine strain is particularly liable to revert to the wild type and cause clinical disease. Some live viral vaccines may cause a mild infection mimicking the natural infection, although usually with much less severe symptoms (e.g. some people who receive varicella-zoster virus vaccine develop fever and a localised vesicular rash around the inoculation site).

Live vaccines are generally contraindicated in the immunosuppressed, since the vaccines are more likely to cause serious symptoms in them. Some live vaccines are also contraindicated in pregnancy, despite there being no evidence of fetal damage but because a theoretical risk may exist that the vaccine virus could infect and damage the baby (e.g. rubella vaccine). Expert guidance should be obtained when considering the use of live virus vaccines in these two groups.

Killed or Inactivated Virus Vaccines

Viruses can be killed with chemicals such as formalin or B-propriolactone. These killed virus vaccines can then be injected into humans, to produce an immune response with the advantage that they are incapable of causing disease. The major disadvantage of killed vaccines is that they are usually more expensive to produce than live virus vaccines, because much higher titred virus preparations need to be grown. Inactivated vaccines can be either whole virus vaccines (e.g. polio) or subunit vaccines (e.g. only use particular viral proteins) to induce an antibody response capable of neutralising an infecting virus (e.g. Covid-19, influenza or hepatitis B and zoster vaccines).

Even for killed virus vaccines, the viruses have to be first grown in cell cultures or embryonated hens' eggs.

Recombinant and Subunit Vaccines

Part of the viral genome is transfected into yeast or bacterial cells, so that when they multiply, they also produce the viral protein encoded by the transfected viral gene. Hepatitis B vaccine (comprising HBsAg) is made in this way.

The human papillomavirus (HPV) vaccines comprise virus-like particles assembled from recombinant HPV coat proteins. The natural virus capsid is composed of two proteins, L1 and L2, but vaccines only contain L1, synthesised in the yeast *Saccharomyces cerevisiae*.

mRNA Vaccines

mRNA vaccines use a copy of a messenger RNA (mRNA) to produce an immune response. The mRNA is delivered by a mixture of the RNA encapsulated in lipid nanoparticles that protect the RNA strands and help their absorption into the cells. The vaccine delivers molecules of antigen-encoding mRNA into host cells, which use the designed mRNA as a blueprint to build protein that would normally be produced by a pathogen (e.g. a virus) or by a cancer cell. These protein molecules stimulate the host's immune response to identify and destroy the corresponding pathogen or cancer cells.

DNA Vaccines

Pure viral DNA, when injected into cells, can use cellular protein translating systems to produce viral proteins that are capable of producing an effective neutralising antibody response. Therefore, in effect, viral DNA acts as an attenuated viral vaccine but is incapable of causing disease by itself.

Adenovirus Vector Vaccines

Viral vector vaccines enable antigen expression within cells and induce a robust cytotoxic T-cell response, unlike subunit vaccines which only produce a humoral immunity. In order to transfer a nucleic acid coding for a specific viral protein to a cell, the vaccines employ a variant of a virus containing the desired viral nucleic acid sequence as its vector. This process helps to create immunity against the disease, which helps to protect people from contracting the infection. Viral vector vaccines do not cause infection with either the virus used as the vector or the source of the antigen and the genetic material it delivers does not integrate into the recipient's DNA.

For example, the AstraZeneca Covid-19 vaccine is a viral vector vaccine containing a modified, replication-deficient chimpanzee adenovirus ChAdOx1, containing the full-length coding sequence for the SARS-CoV-2 spike protein along with a tissue plasminogen activator leader sequence. The adenovirus is called replication-deficient because some of its essential genes required for replication were deleted and replaced by a gene coding for the spike protein.

Viral Vaccines in Use in the UK

Table 55.1 shows a list of virus vaccines in current use in the UK.

Table 55.1 Viral vaccines currently in use in the UK

Virus	Vaccine type	Route of administration	Vaccine usage
SARS-CoV-2 virus	mRNA Adenovirus vector Recombinant	im*	See the Green Book website link at the end of this chapter for details
Hepatitis A virus	Killed	im	Protection for travellers, occupational risk groups and for prophylaxis
Hepatitis B virus	Recombinant	im	Protection for risk groups, travellers and for prophylaxis
Influenza A and B virus quadrivalent (2 influenza A and 2 influenza B strains)	Recombinant Killed Live attenuated	im im intranasal	All are quadrivalent and either egg-grown, cell-based or recombinant (refer to the Green Book for details) Recommended for young children (refer to the Green Book for details)
Japanese encephalitis virus	Killed	im	Recommended for travellers to high-risk countries and for laboratory workers handling live virus
Measles virus	Live attenuated	im	Childhood vaccination and prophylaxis
Mumps virus	Live attenuated	im	Childhood vaccination and prophylaxis
Papilloma virus	Subunit	im	Childhood vaccination (teenagers)

Table 55.1 (cont.)

Virus	Vaccine type	Route of administration	Vaccine usage
Polio virus	Live attenuated	oral	For those countries where polioviruses are still circulating
	Killed	im	For those countries where polioviruses have been eliminated
Rabies virus	Killed	im	For travellers to countries where rabies is endemic, veterinary quarantine workers and for prophylaxis
Rotavirus	Live attenuated	oral	Childhood vaccination
Rubella virus	Live attenuated	im	Childhood vaccination and prophylaxis
Smallpox and monkeypox viruses	Live attenuated	Deep subcutaneous	For pre-exposure in risk groups and for prophylaxis
Varicella	Live attenuated	im	For pre-exposure
Zoster virus	Live attenuated	im	For prevention of zoster
	Recombinant subunit	im	
Yellow fever virus	Live attenuated	im	For pre-exposure in travellers

Note: * intramuscular.

Vaccination Strategy

Vaccines are a powerful armament in the prevention of viral infections and vaccine strategy can be broadly divided into childhood vaccinations and vaccinations for pre- and post-exposure prophylaxis.

Childhood Vaccinations

Universal childhood vaccination programmes are aimed at eradicating the endemic infections and this can only be done by breaking the chain of transmission. For infections that are spread by the respiratory route (e.g. measles, rubella) a herd immunity of >90% is required and therefore high vaccination rates need to be achieved.

Vaccinations for Pre- and Post-exposure Prophylaxis

There are many reasons why individuals may remain unprotected, even against common infections. In such cases, pre- or post-exposure immunisation can be offered. Such vaccinations may not be recommended for all but may only involve specific groups who are at risk (e.g. travellers to endemic countries, healthcare workers, etc.).

Table 55.2 shows details of viral vaccines recommended for pre- and post-exposure prophylaxis in the UK. For up-to-date information readers should always refer to the Green Book to check the current guidelines for immunisation against infectious disease (www.gov.uk).

Useful Website

GOV.UK: Immunisation against infectious disease: www.gov.uk/government/collections/immunisation-against-infectious-disease-the-green-book

Table 55.2 Vaccines recommended for pre- and post-exposure prophylaxis in the UK

Patient category	Vaccine	Vaccination schedule	Comment
Childhood vaccinations	Measles/ mumps/ rubella (MMR)	First dose at 12 months with a second dose before school entry (3 years 4 months)	Single vaccines are no longer available in the UK
	Inactivated polio (IPV)	2, 3, 4 months at the same time as diphtheria/pertussis, Hib, Hep B and tetanus vaccines. Fourth dose at 3 years 4 months.	All vaccination is with IPV; live oral vaccine is no longer in routine use in the UK
	Rotavirus	2 and 3 months	
	Hepatitis B virus	2, 3 and 4 months.	
	Live attenuated intranasal influenza vaccine (LAIV)	Should be offered each season for children from 2 to 17 years	Local country guidelines may vary
	Papillomavirus	One dose at 12–13 years	Girls and boys
Vaccination for those at occupational risk			
Sewage workers, food handlers	Hepatitis A	HAV and HAV + typhoid vaccine – 2 doses 6–12 months apart	Protects long term, probably for life
Healthcare workers and those who are likely to be exposed to blood or blood-contaminated material during the course of their work	Hepatitis B	Three doses, at least 1 month apart. Combined hepatitis B and hepatitis A vaccine is available.	

Table 55.2 *(cont.)*

Patient category	Vaccine	Vaccination schedule	Comment
Susceptible healthcare workers	MMR	Two doses at least 1 month apart	Ideally, immune status should be checked before offering vaccine
Healthcare and those that work in emergency services	Influenza A and B	Annually	
Susceptible healthcare workers	Varicella zoster	Two doses 1–2 months apart	
Vets and others in contact with animals in quarantine facilities, laboratory workers working with rabies virus	Rabies	Three doses – 0, 7 and 21–28 days	
Travel vaccines			
Those without evidence of past infection and travelling to endemic countries	Hepatitis A	Two doses 6–12 months apart	Protects long term, probably for life. Single vaccine containing both hepatitis A and B virus is available and can be given as a three-dose schedule, as for hepatitis B.
Travel to endemic countries and likely to engage in at risk behaviour	Hepatitis B	3 doses, at least 1 month apart. Combined hepatitis B and hepatitis A vaccine is available.	Accelerated schedule of 0, 1, 2 months can be used if required
Travelling to endemic countries only if in remote areas where immediate healthcare not available	Rabies	Three doses – 0, 7 and 21–28 days	
Travel to endemic countries	Japanese encephalitis (JE)	Two doses at 0 and 28 days	
Travel to endemic countries	Yellow fever	One dose	Vaccination is mandatory for entry into and exit out of endemic countries

Table 55.2 (cont.)

Patient category	Vaccine	Vaccination schedule	Comment
Vaccinations for at-risk groups			
Susceptible contacts of patients with acute hepatitis A, IDUs and men who have sex with men (MSM), those with chronic hepatitis B and C infection.	Hepatitis A	Two doses 12 months apart	Protects long term, probably for life. Single vaccine containing both hepatitis A and B virus is available and can be given as a three-dose schedule as for hepatitis B
Susceptible contacts of patients with hepatitis B, those whose lifestyle puts them at risk of infection, chronic hepatitis C infection	Hepatitis B	One dose of HBV vaccine or accelerated course. See guideline link.*	
>65 years of age, immunocompromised, those with chronic debilitating illnesses, those with high BMI or underlying heart and respiratory diseases	Influenza A and B	Annually	
>65 years of age	Zoster	One dose	To reduce the risk of developing zoster
Susceptible women of reproductive age group	Rubella	MMR immediately after delivery for rubellavirus antibody–negative women	
Those likely to come in contact with monkeypox or smallpox either socially (e.g. MSM) or professionally	Smallpox	Two doses at least 28 days apart	
Non-immune susceptible contacts of chickenpox or zoster	VZV	Not indicated	Aciclovir or specific varicella-zoster immunoglobulin given as an intramuscular injection
Contacts of rabies	Rabies	2–5 doses of vaccine, depending on risk factors and patient category. See Green Book link.**	Always seek expert advice. Rabies immunoglobulin may also be advised, depending on risk factors.

Table 55.2 (cont.)

Patient category	Vaccine	Vaccination schedule	Comment
Non-immune contacts of measles	Measles	MMR given within 3 days of contact. See weblink for detailed recommendations.***	Intravenous normal immunoglobulin may also be given. See weblink for detailed recommendations. ***

Notes: * HBV prophylaxis guidance following exposure can be found at: Interim guidance on the public health management and control of acute hepatitis B, October 2019: https://assets.publishing.service.gov.uk/government/uploads/system/uploads/attachment_data/file/843970/Interim_guidance_on_the_public_health_management_control_of_acute_hepatitis_B.pdf.

** Management of rabies contacts can be found at: Rabies, *The Green Book on Immunisation*, chapter 27 (Public Health England): www.gov.uk/government/publications/rabies-the-green-book-chapter-27.

*** Advice on the post-exposure use of measles vaccine and normal immunoglobulin can be found at: National measles guidelines, February 2024: https://assets.publishing.service.gov.uk/media/65bb924dcc6fd600145dbe4d/20240123_national-measles-guidelines-February-2024.pdf.

Chapter 56

Infection Control

Infection control is a significant part of a clinical virologist's work. It is an important public health tool in the preventative measures to stop the spread of viral infections. To do this, we must first understand how viruses spread and gain entry to infect susceptible hosts. Viruses may gain entry through mucous membranes or directly through blood. Skin, although a good barrier to infection, may also allow viral entry, especially if there are breaks in the skin surface. Infections may then be localised to the site of entry or spread via the blood stream (*viraemia*) to distant sites and cause systemic infection. The route by which viruses enter the host to establish infection is dictated very much by viral cell tropism.

Viruses and Their Route of Entry and Spread

Respiratory Route

There are a large number of viruses apart from the respiratory viruses that enter the host via the respiratory route. Primary infection is established in the respiratory tract epithelium and virus is also shed from the respiratory tract. Infection may remain localised to the respiratory tract or spread to other sites through viraemia and cause systemic infection (e.g. chickenpox, smallpox, measles, mumps, rubella and parvovirus B19 infections).

The infection is spread by small droplets which are released into the environment while sneezing and coughing. These droplets containing the infectious virus may either be inhaled or be inoculated into the respiratory mucous membranes via contaminated hands or fomites such as handkerchiefs.

Gastrointestinal or Faecal-Oral Route

Viruses that replicate in the gut are shed in the faeces and enter the host via ingestion of contaminated food or water. Faecal or vomit contamination of the environment aids the spread of viruses such as noroviruses.

Blood-Borne

Blood is an important source of infection for viruses that have a viraemic phase. This may be chronic as in the blood-borne viruses or transitory during the acute viraemic phase of infection with other viruses. This is the most significant route of spread for the blood-borne viruses. Virus is spread via blood and blood-contaminated secretions either by direct entry to the bloodstream or via entry into the bloodstream via exposure to mucous membranes and abraded skin.

Genital Tract

Direct exposure of genital tract mucosa or abraded skin to infected secretions is required to allow the virus to gain entry and establish infection.

Vertical Route of Infection

Infection is spread from the mother to the baby, either in utero or at the time of delivery (perinatal) or in the neonatal (postnatal) period. Virus may gain entry either directly through the bloodstream or through exposure of the mucous membranes.

Vector-Borne

Mosquitoes, ticks and animals are important vectors of transmission of infection for alpha, flavi and arenaviruses, arbo and other bunya viruses and rabies virus. This may be through bites of infected insects, ticks or mammals or exposure to contaminated secretions, such as urine from infected rodents.

Control of Infection

In the Community

Viruses in the community are ubiquitous in nature; it is therefore difficult to impose control of infection measures, except in extreme cases (e.g. Covid-19). Efforts in the community for controlling viral infections should be directed at:

- Public education – for the avoidance of infection, including vector control and measures to prevent bites (e.g. from mosquitoes and ticks etc) for vector-borne infections such as arboviruses.
- Screening programmes – for identifying infected patients with a view to treating or isolating them, to limit the spread of infection.
- Vaccination.

In Hospitals

The aim of infection control in hospitals is to avoid infection spread while under medical care (nosocomial infection). Certain groups of patients, such as the immunosuppressed, pregnant, neonates and elderly, are more vulnerable than others and may require special attention.

Universal Precautions

Most patients are admitted to hospital for reasons other than infection, but may have an incidental infection. Many viral infections are very mild or asymptomatic, so it is not possible to identify everyone who is suffering from an infection. Universal precautions assume that all patients are potentially infected and therefore work on the principle of applying certain basic rules of hygiene and infection prevention for all healthcare-related tasks:

- Handwashing or use of alcohol gel before and after examining patients.
- Wearing gloves and other protection, such as plastic aprons and eye protection (if indicated) when dealing with blood or other body secretions.

Respiratory Precautions

- Patients should be isolated in single rooms (ideally in negative pressure room) wherever practicable.
- Gloves and other appropriate protection (e.g. eye protection) should be worn during respiratory procedures (e.g. taking nasopharyngeal aspirates). Face masks should be worn in addition if a virus which spreads readily by the respiratory route (e.g. SARS CoV-2) is suspected.

Enteric Precautions

- Strict handwashing.
- Patients with infective diarrhoea and/or vomiting should be isolated in single rooms wherever practicable or cohort nursed in isolated bays or wards.

Precautions for Highly Dangerous Pathogens

Patients suspected of being infected with viral haemorrhagic fevers, smallpox, rabies, avian influenza or SARS require special isolation facilities. Patients with viral haemorrhagic fever should be admitted only to designated centres as a specially adapted room with Trexler isolators and other specialised equipment is required to isolate these patients. High-consequence respiratory viruses (e.g. avian influenza) should be managed as other respiratory pathogens, but FFP3 masks should be worn in addition.

Use of Post-exposure Prophylaxis

Post-exposure prophylaxis is an important part of controlling the spread of infection in hospitals. This can be in the form of:

- antiviral drugs (e.g. for influenza and HIV)
- vaccine (e.g. for measles)
- immunoglobulin (e.g. for varicella-zoster virus infection).

Details of post-exposure prophylaxis are given under the individual virus or clinical syndrome chapters.

Outbreaks

Outbreaks of infection occur in both community and hospital settings. An outbreak is defined as the occurrence of two or more cases of the same infection associated in time and space. Outbreaks may occur from a common source (point source outbreak) or be due to person-to-person spread. Point source outbreaks, by their nature, tend to be explosive (several persons are infected together and display symptoms at the same time) and are usually food- or water-borne infections. Certain outbreaks that spread from person to person may also spread rapidly because of high infectivity (e.g. norovirus).

Outbreak Investigation

This requires the establishment of a link between cases, preferably by molecular epidemiology to demonstrate either a common source or person-to-person spread. Careful questioning of infected patients will often point to the potential source and mode of spread of infection. Once these facts are established, then measures can be put in place to control the outbreak.

Control of Outbreaks

Measures that are put in place will depend on the infecting agent, its source and suspected route of transmission. These consist of:

- isolation of infected cases;
- prophylaxis by vaccination, immunoglobulins or antiviral drugs, as indicated; and
- surveillances and isolation of new cases by:
  - o careful follow-up of those who may have been exposed and may be incubating the disease, for clinical signs; and
  - o laboratory screening tests on those exposed to identify those who may have developed asymptomatic infection.

Outbreak Committee

Management of outbreak control requires good team working between the laboratory clinician and public health specialists. An outbreak committee should be instituted as soon as possible to investigate and manage the outbreak and should include:

- a control of infection doctor (usually a virologist or microbiologist);
- a control of infection nurse;
- a public health specialist (doctor or nurse) – in the UK, this is usually a consultant in communicable disease control (CCDC) or their representative;
- a clinician looking after the cases; and
- others, such as nurse managers, laboratory staff and appropriate experts, who should be co-opted onto the committee as required.

Notifiable Infections

In the UK, it is mandatory to report cases of the following viral infections to the CCDC, who is the designated 'proper officer' in public health:

- acute infectious hepatitis (hepatitis A, B, C, D and E)
- acute poliomyelitis
- Covid-19
- measles
- monkeypox
- mumps
- rabies
- rubella
- SARS
- smallpox
- viral haemorrhagic fevers
- yellow fever

Occupational Health

57

There are several health-related aspects of being employed as a healthcare professional which affect the health and well-being of staff, carers and patients. All health provider organisations should have an Occupational Health department or have arrangements with another provider to provide this function. There are two important occupational aspects of virus infections:

- protection of staff from infection; and
- protection of patients from acquiring infection from staff.

Many aspects of these two issues are interrelated as protection of staff from infection prevents staff inadvertently passing on the infection to other patients. Next we list some aspects of the service which should be provided in relation to virus infections for the two issues. The recommendations in this chapter are based on the UK guidelines, although the general principles would apply broadly. Always refer to the latest local and national guidelines as these change over time.

Pre-employment Health Check

All employees should have a pre-employment health check before their employment contract is confirmed. A good clinical history should be taken. This should include any health problems in the healthcare worker (HCW) as these may impact on their vulnerability to infection (e.g. if immunosuppressed) or ability to pass on infection to patients (e.g. if they have chronic hepatitis B virus infection). Laboratory tests should include checks for immunity for vaccine-preventable virus infections as well as evidence of chronic infection with blood-borne viruses (e.g. HIV, hepatitis B and C) as these can be passed on from the HCW to patients in the clinical setting.

Vaccination for Vaccine-Preventable Virus Infections

There are vaccines which can be given to health professionals to protect them against the risk of occupationally acquired virus infections. There should be good practice guidelines to offer vaccination for vaccine-preventable infections to all HCWs, especially those who are in direct patient contact and those who work in the laboratory and who may handle material containing the viruses. These guidelines may vary for different countries depending upon risk assessment and vaccine licensure for HCWs. The following is based on the UK guidelines:

- *Hepatitis B virus (HBV) vaccination* – All healthcare staff in contact with patients or specimens are recommended to be vaccinated, followed by a check for immunity (blood sample to test for antibody to hepatitis B virus surface antigen). HBV vaccination should be offered as soon as a medical or nursing or allied health professional career is embarked upon (e.g. to medical, nursing, physiotherapy students).

- *Varicella-zoster virus (VZV) vaccination* – All VZV non-immune HCWs should be vaccinated if they are not immune, to protect against chickenpox.
- *Influenza* – All healthcare staff are recommended to have annual influenza vaccination. This is to prevent staff from acquiring infection from patients or in the community, but most importantly to reduce the risk of staff transmitting influenza to patients, many of whom will be particularly susceptible to severe infection.
- *Covid-19* – As for the influenza virus, all healthcare staff should be vaccinated against SARS-CoV-2 and offered booster vaccination as appropriate.
- *Measles* – All healthcare staff are recommended to have MMR vaccination. Measles is very infectious and is a serious infection which can be fatal in immunocompromised patients.
- *Mumps* – All healthcare staff are recommended to have MMR vaccination.
- *Rubella* – All healthcare staff are recommended to have MMR vaccination. This is particularly important for those staff caring for pregnant women.
- *Poliomyelitis* – All healthcare staff are recommended to be vaccinated.

There are other bacteriological vaccine-preventable diseases for which vaccines and health checks are advised. They include:

- TB
- diphtheria
- meningococci
- tetanus.

It is important that staff who are immunocompromised or pregnant, or who are actively trying to become pregnant should advise occupational health staff of this; many of these vaccines contain live attenuated viruses and may be contraindicated as they could theoretically pose a risk to the HCW or their unborn fetus.

Needlestick and Sharps Injuries

Needlestick and other sharps injuries as well as contamination of mucosa with blood or blood-stained body fluids are an occupational hazard for healthcare staff. The greatest concern about the risk of infection from these incidents centres around the three blood-borne viruses (BBVs) HBV, hepatitis C virus (HCV) and HIV. Since there is a vaccine for HBV, prophylactic antiviral regimes for HIV and antiviral regimes for treatment of acute HCV infection, prompt and active management of these incidents is essential in order to provide maximum protection for staff.

If a member of staff has a needlestick or other sharps injury or mucosal contamination with blood or blood-stained body fluids, they should seek urgent medical attention, preferably through the relevant Occupational Health department. If that department is closed, the advice of a local medical member of staff should be sought. The most important aspects to be considered urgently are:

- Patient risk factors – Does the patient whose blood or blood-stained body fluids contaminated the member of staff have any risk factors for BBVs (e.g. intravenous drug use, men who have sex with men, born in a country with high prevalence of these infections, etc.)?

- What was the nature of the incident – was it a deep intramuscular injection with an open bore needle with a risk of microinjection of blood or a slight scratch from a probe? Did the splash involve mucous membrane or was it on intact skin?
If secretions were involved, were they bloodstained? In case of a bite, it is important to establish if blood was drawn or saliva was bloodstained.
- Has the staff member been vaccinated against HBV?
- When and in what circumstances did the incident happen?

If there is judged to be a possible risk of infection with a BBV to the member of staff, permission should be sought, from the index source patient, to test a 10 ml clotted blood sample for HBsAg, HIV antibody/antigen and HCV antibody (HCV RNA if the index case is immunosuppressed or if HCV antibody positive). If the patient is not competent to give consent, urgent discussions should be held with the patient's clinician in charge and testing agreed if it is in the best interest of the patient. If the index case is a child, consent from the parent or legal guardian of the child, and consent or assent from the child, depending on their age, should be sought. If the source is unknown or it is not possible to test the source patient, then a proper risk assessment should be done as to the risk of transmission of BBVs.

There should be procedures in place to test the patient's blood sample urgently and the result should be telephoned promptly to the relevant person agreed in the incident management. These test results should be available within hours of arriving in the testing laboratory. A baseline blood sample should be taken from the HCW at the same time and stored for future testing. In the vast majority of cases, the patient tests negative and no action is required.

HBV: In case of a significant exposure from an HBsAg positive source, if the member of staff has not received HBV vaccine and is not already infected, an accelerated HBV vaccination schedule (0, 7 and 21 days with HBV booster at 12 months) is recommended as well as hepatitis B immunoglobulin (HBIG).

In the vaccine non-responders (those who did not achieve >10 mIU/ml of anti-HBs), a booster dose of HBV vaccine should be given along with HBIG, with a second dose of HBIG given 1 month later.

If the staff member has been vaccinated but has not received the full course, or had a primary vaccination course but no booster previously, one dose of HBV vaccine should be given immediately and the course completed in those with an incomplete course.

Even if the exposure is low risk or the source is HBsAg negative, HBV vaccination status of the HCW should always be reviewed and the opportunity taken to vaccinate or to give a booster dose, depending upon the vaccination history. This is especially important in those who are at continued risk due to the nature of their work.

HIV: In case of high-risk injury, that is, where the source patient is HIV positive and is not on antiretroviral therapy (ART) for >6 months with a suppressed viral load, post-exposure prophylaxis (PEP) should be initiated as soon as possible (within hours of exposure), but definitely within 24 hours; it should not be denied up to 72 hours post exposure, after which time it is not recommended. If there is a risk of HIV infection from the incident and a delay in getting the patient's blood sample tested, the staff member should be offered PEP without waiting for results; PEP can be reviewed once the results are known.

PEP is generally not recommended in other case scenarios, that is, where the index case is known to be positive for HIV but on ART for >6 months with suppressed viral load, or where the source of exposure is unknown, but each incident needs to reviewed on a case-by-case basis to assess the risk of transmission and for the decision to offer PEP.

Local policies should ensure that there is 24-hour access to advice from Occupational Health and if required from an experienced HIV clinician, particularly for complex cases. The PEP regimen generally consists of three drugs, with a backbone of two nucleoside/nucleotide reverse transcriptase inhibitors and an integrase inhibitor (see Chapter 54) and should be given for 28 days. For the PEP to be effective complete adherence to the PEP regimen is required.

HCV: There are no vaccines or prophylactic antiviral regimes for protecting staff against HCV infection.

Post-exposure Follow-up

A baseline blood should be taken from exposed staff and stored for future testing for BBVs to establish seroconversion in case the HCW tests positive on follow-up testing.

- *HBV* – Follow-up samples at 12 weeks for HBsAg and anti-HBs; further samples may be tested if indicated.
- *HIV* – Test for HIV antibody/antigen at 6 weeks and 12 weeks. In those who receive PEP a sample should be tested, but not before 45 days after stopping PEP.
- *HCV* – If the source patient is HCV RNA positive, test the HCW's clotted blood at week 6 post exposure (for HCV RNA) or at 12 weeks (HCV RNA and antibody). Any positive test result must be confirmed by testing a second blood sample. If the HCW has confirmed HCV infection (HCV RNA positive), prompt treatment with ribavirin and pegylated interferon alpha has a success rate of above 95% in curing the infection.

Additional samples for testing should be considered on clinical grounds (e.g. if evidence of seroconversion illness) or if longer-term follow-up is required.

Management of Healthcare Workers Infected with Blood-Borne Viruses

Health professionals who are infected with BBVs are at risk of transmitting the infection to patients if they are performing exposure-prone procedures (EPPs). However, with successful antiviral treatment regimens for HIV, HBV and HCV infections, these infections can either be cured (e.g. HCV) or long-term viral suppression achieved as in the case of HIV and HBV infection, so that there is no longer a risk of transmission from the HCW to the patient.

EPPs are those invasive procedures where there is a risk that injury to the HCW may result in the exposure of the patient's open tissues to the blood of the HCW. These include procedures where the HCW's gloved hands may be in contact with sharp instruments, needle tips or sharp tissues (e.g. spicules of bone and teeth) inside a patient's open body cavity, wound or confined anatomical space where the hands or fingertips may not be completely visible at all times.

UK guidelines state that HBsAg positive HCWs should not perform EPPs or undertake clinical duties in renal units if they have an HBV DNA level at or above 200 IU/mL regardless of their treatment status.

HCWs who have antibodies to the HCV and are HCV RNA negative should be allowed to continue performing EPPs. HCWs who have active, or current, infection (those who are HCV RNA positive) should be restricted from performing EPPs.

HCWs living with HIV with a plasma viral load above 200 copies/mL should be restricted from performing EPPs.

For further detailed guidance readers are referred to 'Integrated guidance on health clearance of HCWs and the management of HCWs living with bloodborne viruses (hepatitis B, hepatitis C and HIV)', by the UK Advisory Panel for Healthcare Workers Living with Bloodborne Viruses (UKAP), the website address for which is given at the end of the chapter.

Infection and Outbreak Control in Healthcare Settings

HCWs are frequently in contact with patients with infectious diseases. Airborne and faecal-orally transmitted infections can transmit readily to them. Some of these pose particular risks to HCWs themselves and other patients, especially if they are immuno-suppressed. Here are some problem infections and their management:

- *VZV* – Chickenpox can be fatal in immunocompromised patients and can cause congenital abnormalities in babies if the mother is infected in the first 20 weeks of pregnancy. Any HCW with chickenpox or zoster on an exposed area should be excluded from work and especially must not work with immunocompromised or pregnant patients. If an HCW is in contact with chickenpox or zoster in the healthcare setting and they are unsure if they have had chickenpox before or they are unaware of their VZV antibody status, their blood should be tested for VZV IgG to establish their immune status to VZV. Infection control procedures differ in different healthcare facilities, but in most, an HCW looking after immunocompromised or pregnant patients would be removed from patient contact from days 8–21 from the date of contact (remember that by the time a person develops chickenpox, they have been infectious for 2 days). Zoster-immune globulin is available in the UK for providing prophylaxis against severe VZV infection for non-immune immunocompromised and pregnant persons (both staff and patients) in contact with VZV. Aciclovir can also provide prophylaxis and may be recommended in some circumstances.

- *Hepatitis A* – This is transmitted by the faecal-oral route. There is good evidence that post-exposure vaccination given within a week of exposure is effective in preventing or attenuating infection in exposed individuals and effective in interrupting outbreaks. Hepatitis A immunoglobulin is recommended, in addition, for those less able to respond to the vaccine, for example the immunosuppressed.

- *SARS-CoV-2* – HCWs who have symptomatic or asymptomatic confirmed SARS-CoV-2 infection should be excluded from work for an appropriate length of time (depending upon local and/or national guidelines).

- *Influenza* – HCWs should receive annual vaccination for influenza. For those not vaccinated, if they are in contact with a case of influenza, prophylactic oseltamivir (75 mg once a day for 7 days) should be offered along with influenza vaccination.

- *Measles* – This is one of the most infectious viral diseases and can cause severe or fatal infection in immunocompromised patients. Any HCW who is suspected of having measles should be removed from patient contact immediately. Prophylactic human normal immunoglobulin is recommended for non-immune immunocompromised patients in contact with a case of measles. Healthcare staff in contact with measles should have their immune status established. Susceptible HCWs should be offered MMR vaccine and those who work with at-risk patients should be excluded from work during the incubation period if exposed to measles. All infected HCWs should be excluded from work during the infectious period.

Useful Websites

British HIV Association: UK Guideline for the use of HIV post-exposure prophylaxis 2021: www.bhiva.org/PEP-guidelines

GOV.UK: BBVs in healthcare workers: health clearance and management: www.gov .uk/government/collections/bloodborne-viruses-bbvs-in-healthcare-workers

GOV.UK: Immunisation against infectious disease: www.gov.uk/government/ collections/immunisation-against-infectious-disease-the-green-book

UKHSA: Integrated guidance on health clearance of healthcare workers and the management of healthcare workers living with bloodborne viruses (hepatitis B, hepatitis C and HIV): https://assets.publishing.service.gov.uk/media/65423f21d36c91 000d935b8f/integrated-guidance-for-management-of-bbv-in-hcw-november-2023.pdf

58 Public Health and Pandemic Preparedness

In recent years, there has been a focus on pandemic preparedness because of the Covid-19 outbreak. Pandemics have circled the globe for many centuries and have occurred at infrequent and unpredictable intervals in the past. Many of these infections are zoonotic (including the 2009 influenza pandemic, HIV and Covid-19), with the initial human infection acquired from animals. As the human population of the world increases, man is brought into closer contact with animals, increasing the risk of zoonotic infection causing another pandemic.

In recent years, the UK Government has regarded pandemic influenza as one of the greatest risks to human health. It published 'The UK Influenza Preparedness Strategy' in 2011, which provided a UK-wide strategic approach to planning for and responding to the demands of an influenza pandemic. However, not all pandemic viruses have similar outbreak characteristics to pandemic influenza, which was demonstrated when the Covid-19 pandemic arrived.

Pandemic Preparedness

Pandemic preparedness plans usually involve some or all of the following aspects:

- Advance risk assessment of the likelihood of there being a pandemic in the future caused by a virus and the likely type of virus. Making preparations for dealing with a future pandemic, including provision of molecular diagnostic services, contract tracing capability and coordination, epidemiological modelling capability and stockpiling of protective equipment and antiviral drugs.
- When a new pandemic virus is identified:
  - Surveillance and modelling – to detect and assess the impact of any new virus which poses a potential risk, by identifying the molecular composition, symptoms and transmission characteristics of the novel virus and identifying and quantifying the groups of people most at risk of severe illness, hospitalisation and death.
  - Reducing the risk of transmission – through adopting effective infection prevention and control practices and provision of relevant personal protective equipment for front-line health and social care staff, to be acquired and held in stockpiles.
  - Minimising serious illness and deaths – by holding stockpiles of relevant antivirals to treat patients and for prophylactic use.
  - Vaccination – when appropriate to develop potential vaccines to protect the public (or the groups most likely to be most vulnerable) and determining evidence-based vaccination schedules.

- Surge plans – to plan for increased demand on health and care services in hospitals and community settings.
- Modifying prescribing regulations – so that antivirals, vaccines and antibiotics can be made more available to those dealing with the pandemic.

Responding to a New Pandemic

Strategies for responding to a new likely pandemic may have several phases:

- *Detection* – This phase starts when a pandemic is declared by the World Health Organization, or earlier on the basis of reliable evidence from viral surveillance studies. Early recognition of the molecular structure of the new virus is of paramount importance, so that molecular screening methods can be developed rapidly and employed for screening potential new cases. As in the case of Covid-19, this phase often depends on the recognition of the cluster of symptoms associated with the novel virus and the likely countries, where cases may have travelled from recently.
- *Assessment* – This phase starts when the first patient with the pandemic strain is identified in the UK. Enhanced surveillance is instituted, which should include regional virology laboratories being equipped with screening PCR tests for the novel virus.
- *Treatment* – Where it has not been possible to contain the spread of the pandemic strain upon arrival, the focus is on identifying, isolating and treating cases and responding to the increasing number of patients as well as providing prophylaxis if appropriate. Advice should be issued by the Government to citizens on how to respond to this enhanced threat.
- *Escalation* – Pressures on services and wider society may be extreme. The focus of the response at this stage of a pandemic is on adjustments to service delivery arrangements to meet increasing demand. All contingency measures should be implemented.
- *Recovery* – Following the peak of the pandemic, services will be scaled back as the number of new cases declines and/or the virus becomes less virulent. After this, the recovery phase is entered, where the focus is on returning services to normal, restoration of business, and planning for preventing and responding to a possible resurgence of the pandemic (a second 'wave'), which usually occurs.

These plans should be regularly reviewed to reflect the latest expert advice. One way of ensuring plans are fit for purpose is through exercises, which are run both locally and nationally across various parts of the health system to stress-test policies.

Preparing Virology Laboratory Services for the Next Pandemic

The UK has a history of preparing for potential pandemics. As a response to the fear of bacteriological warfare in the Second World War, the Emergency Public Health Laboratory Service was established in 1939 under the direction of the Medical Research Council and was consolidated as the Public Health Laboratory Service (PHLS) as part of the National Health Service in 1946. There was a central laboratory at Colindale in North London and a network of regional and local laboratories, in most places, located within hospital laboratories which had a diagnostic focus and a university affiliation (e.g. Cambridge, Manchester and Bristol). The laboratory network was expanded and by

1955 there were about 1,000 staff. These laboratories were primarily preventive with an epidemiological focus. Around 1970, regional and trainee epidemiologists were appointed and the Communicable Disease Surveillance Centre (CDSC) was created at the Colindale site. In 1991, there were 52 diagnostic laboratories throughout England and Wales (10 regional laboratories and 42 area laboratories) as well as the Central Public Health Laboratory at Colindale with the associated CDSC. By 1998, funding had been reduced and the area and regional PHLS laboratories had been reorganised into nine regions, each with a regional laboratory and a total of 39 local laboratories.

The PHLS was replaced by the Health Protection Agency in 2003, which was morphed into Public Health England (PHE) in 2013 as an executive agency of the Department of Health, as part of the wider NHS reorganisation. PHE became the UK Health Security Agency (UKHSA) in 2021.

One of the problems identified in the response to the Covid-19 outbreak in the UK was the lack of laboratory preparedness and the inability to scale up molecular testing rapidly in the early stages of the pandemic. When the pandemic was declared, there was insufficient planned molecular diagnostic capacity and insufficient trained staff to ensure a safe, accurate and clinically relevant diagnostic service. Despite government pledges to provide 100,000 tests per day by May 2020 as part of the UK test and trace scheme, demand quickly outstripped capacity to set up testing safely in new laboratories, conduct quality assurance of the tests, and process samples. Surge capacity was already required by the time the first tests were available. Availability of laboratory facilities and resources, from basic reagents to IT support, was a substantial challenge, but the biggest bottleneck was finding trained staff to carry out the tests. Maintaining surplus laboratory capacity for emergencies is expensive, and therefore politically and economically unpalatable. Nevertheless, Covid-19 has shown that effective surge capacity is a vital part of pandemic preparedness. As well as being a problem during the Covid-19 pandemic, staffing was identified as a key weakness in laboratory preparedness after the 2009 influenza pandemic.

Additional capacity can be generated by keeping trained reserve staff permanently available, ready to function independently when required rather than relying on voluntary action or competing with other health sector needs. The initial German response to Covid-19, which saw faster expansion of testing capacity than in the UK, called on existing trained staff.

Since retaining a permanent reserve of diagnostic staff would be very expensive and politically unpalatable in economically strained times, a hybrid retained reservists and voluntary reserve model would best meet the UK's requirements for diagnostic surge capacity across the different phases of a pandemic. Typical models of voluntary reserves and retained reserves could cover a spectrum of skill levels, training and time commitments. Highly skilled staff such as clinical and biomedical scientists, who require substantial training and regular practice to develop and maintain their skills, are required in smaller numbers, typically in the earliest stages of an emergency response. This small, select group could be assembled and paid on retainer. For example, people from academia and industry and those who recently retired with appropriate skillsets could be employed as retained reservists to help in the initial phases of an emergency. Many more staff members with less specialised skillsets are needed, including a large number of technicians to provide local testing in an outbreak, epidemic or pandemic scenario. Such staff could be given training relatively quickly with only periodic training refreshers. These staff are essential and should be recruited to a large volunteer reserve that can be accessed quickly during an emergency in a way that is relatively low cost and does not generate parallel infrastructure with its potential problems of poor quality control, as seen during the Covid-19 pandemic response.

It is vital, before the next pandemic appears, that there is a national plan to have a coordinated diagnostic virology service which involves the UKHSA laboratories (regional and central) and NHS, university and research laboratories in a coordinated way with adequate quality assurance and governance oversight.

Index

Page numbers in **bold** = tables, while those in *italics* = figures.

Printed in the United States
by Baker & Taylor Publisher Services